Clinical Cases in
Orthodontics

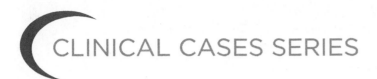

CLINICAL CASES SERIES

Clinical Cases in
Orthodontics

Martyn T. Cobourne
BDS (Hons), FDSRCS (Eng), FDSRCS (Edin), MSc, MOrthRCS (Eng), FDSOrthRCS, PhD, FHEA
Professor of Orthodontics, King's College London
Honorary Consultant in Orthodontics, Guy's and St Thomas' NHS Foundation Trust
King's Health Partners

Padhraig S. Fleming
BDentSc (Hons), MSc, MFDSRCS (Eng), MOrthRCS (Eng), FDSOrthRCS
Consultant Orthodontist, Royal London Dental Institute and East Kent Hospitals University
Foundation NHS Trust, Canterbury

Andrew T. DiBiase
BDS (Hons), FDSRCS (Eng), MSc, MOrthRCS (Eng), FDSOrthRCS
Consultant Orthodontist, East Kent Hospitals University Foundation NHS Trust, Canterbury

Sofia Ahmad
BSc, BDS (Hons), FDSRCS (Eng), MSc, MOrthRCS (Eng), FDSOrthRCS, FHEA
Consultant Orthodontist, Queen Victoria Hospital NHS Foundation Trust and Guy's and
St Thomas' NHS Foundation Trust
Honorary Specialist Clinical Teacher in Orthodontics, King's College London

WILEY-BLACKWELL
A John Wiley & Sons, Ltd., Publication

This edition first published 2012
© 2012 by Martyn T. Cobourne, Padhraig S. Fleming, Andrew T. DiBiase and Sofia Ahmad

Wiley-Blackwell is an imprint of John Wiley & Sons, formed by the merger of Wiley's global Scientific, Technical and Medical business with Blackwell Publishing.

Registered office: John Wiley & Sons, Ltd, The Atrium, Southern Gate, Chichester, West Sussex, PO19 8SQ, UK

Editorial offices: 9600 Garsington Road, Oxford, OX4 2DQ, UK
                  The Atrium, Southern Gate, Chichester, West Sussex, PO19 8SQ, UK
                  2121 State Avenue, Ames, Iowa 50014-8300, USA

For details of our global editorial offices, for customer services and for information about how to apply for permission to reuse the copyright material in this book please see our website at www.wiley.com/wiley-blackwell.

Library of Congress Cataloging-in-Publication Data
Clinical cases in orthodontics / Martyn T. Cobourne ... [et al.].
    p. ; cm. – (Clinical cases uncovered)
Includes bibliographical references and index.
    ISBN 978-1-4051-9779-3 (pbk. : alk. paper)
    I. Cobourne, Martyn T.   II. Series: Clinical cases uncovered.
    [DNLM: 1. Orthodontics, Corrective–methods–Case Reports.   2. Orthodontics, Corrective–methods–Problems and Exercises.   3. Malocclusion–therapy–Case Reports.   4. Malocclusion–therapy–Problems and Exercises.   5. Orthognathic Surgical Procedures–methods–Case Reports.   6. Orthognathic Surgical Procedures–methods–Problems and Exercises. WU 18.2]
    617.6′43–dc23
                                                                2011048153

A catalogue record for this book is available from the British Library.

Wiley also publishes its books in a variety of electronic formats. Some content that appears in print may not be available in electronic books.

Cover images supplied by the authors
Cover design by Meaden Creative

Set in 10/13 pt Univers Light by Toppan Best-set Premedia Limited, Hong Kong
Printed and bound by CPI Group (UK) Ltd, Croydon, CR0 4YY

C9781405197793_271023

CONTENTS

Acknowledgements

We are indebted to our many colleagues who have also been involved in the treatment of cases presented within this book. In particular, we are grateful to the maxillofacial surgeons who carried out the orthognathic surgery for the combined cases that are shown and the technicians who performed the model surgery and wafer construction. At King's College Hospital, Christoph Huppa operated on cases 10.3, 10.7, 10.11 and 10.12 and Shaun Matthews on cases 6.18 and 10.8. At East Kent Hospitals, Jeremy McKenzie operated on cases 10.1, 10.6 and 10.9 and Nicholas Goodger on cases 10.2 and 10.10. At Bart's and the Royal London Hospital, Michael Millwaters operated on case 10.5. At the Queen Victoria Hospital, East Grinstead, Ken Sneddon operated on case 10.4 and Darryl Coombes on case 6.14. MTC is also grateful to Natalie Short and Cristina Nacher for model surgery and wafer construction and both Jerry Kwok and Chris Sproat at Guy's Hospital, who expertly carried out the necessary oral surgery on a number of cases illustrated here. In addition, the orthodontic treatment for several of the cases was carried out by specialist registrars. At East Kent Hospitals, Omar Yaqoob treated cases 4.5, 5.2 and 5.3 and Saba Qureshi treated case 5.4 under the supervision of ATD. At Guy's Hospital, Cleopatra Darwish treated case 10.3 and Poh Then treated case 6.18 under the supervision of MTC. Some of the cases shown were treated by SA at the Queen Victoria Hospital, East Grinstead in conjunction with Lindsay Winchester.

SA would also like to acknowledge Nadia Alwash for her contribution to the completion of case 6.7, and Aneel Jaisinghani for his contribution to the treatment of case 7.11. Philip Ellisdon kindly provided Figure 8.8 and Archie Cobourne was good enough to allow his uncle to take numerous photographs of his developing dentition (he knows where he is!). We are also grateful to the *Journal of Orthodontics* and Maney Publications for permitting the re-use of images in cases 4.1 and 7.3 (Fleming PS. BOS MOrth cases prize 2008. *Journal of Orthodontics* 2010; 37:188–201.http://jorthod.maneyjournals. org).

MTC would like to acknowledge Jackie, Miles and Max; PSF would like to acknowledge Oliver, Sophie, John, Anne and particularly Caroline Fleming; and ATD would like to acknowledge Sarah, Wilf, Arthur and Stanley. Without their collective unwavering help, encouragement and support, this book would not have been possible. SA would also like to acknowledge the Department of Medical Photography at the Queen Victoria Hospital, East Grinstead and her secretary Beverley Cressey for their support. Finally, we would like to thank all of the patients, who generously consented to the use of their clinical photographs within the pages of this book. Without them we would have been unable to illustrate the clinical aspects of orthodontic treatment.

Preface

We think that orthodontics is one of the most interesting and challenging of the dental specialties. Although we might be biased in this assumption, there are some persuasive reasons for believing that it is true. The treatment of malocclusion represents a combination of science and artistic flair, and is often, although not exclusively, carried out on a young and vibrant population. The results of orthodontic treatment and the positive impact that it can have on the patient can also be intensely rewarding for the clinician. Moreover, developments in diagnostic tools, appliance systems and orthodontic materials continue at some considerable pace within the profession, which provides considerable stimulus to the contemporary clinician.

We have written this textbook primarily to be used as a tool for dental professionals who wish to broaden their experience and understanding of clinical orthodontics. The intention has been to show a wide variety of individual cases and clinical scenarios that illustrate many of the problems commonly seen during development of the craniofacial region, with emphasis on the jaws, dentition and occlusion. All of these cases have been treated or directly supervised by the authors, primarily in secondary care, following referral from general practitioners and specialists. We have attempted to illustrate a wide variety of problems that present in the orthodontic clinic, both common and rare, and demonstrate different approaches to their management. Relevant discussion around the etiology, diagnosis and planning of these cases is included in each presentation. We hope that this book will be of particular benefit to postgraduate orthodontic students preparing for their MSc, MClinDent, DDS and Membership examinations in orthodontics. Indeed, a number of the cases included have been successfully used in recent sittings of these examinations. However, the clinical focus underlying this text should mean that it will also be of benefit to other dental professionals involved in management of the developing occlusion, including therapists and undergraduate dental students – who indeed, represent the orthodontists of the future.

It was not our intention to write a definitive textbook on orthodontics, but rather to illustrate contemporary practice using clinical cases and individual examples. Therefore, the introduction to each chapter gives a general overview of the subject area, which is then followed by a series of cases with appropriate questions and answers. We have included the answers to these questions within the cases to avoid the need for constant reference to other parts of the book. Hopefully, this will make it relatively straightforward for the reader to follow the treatment strategies that have been used. In some of the clinical scenarios, more emphasis has been given to clinical examination and diagnosis; whilst in others, questions focus on the treatment that has been carried out. Indeed, many of these cases have been chosen to illustrate specific aspects of etiology, diagnosis, treatment planning or use of mechanics in the management of malocclusion. This problem-based approach of discussing aspects of malocclusion should allow practising clinicians to develop their skills in the management and care of orthodontic patients, from initial assessment, through to the completion of treatment. However, whilst we strive to achieve clinical excellence for the cases that we treat, we did want to illustrate those that had been treated 'in the real world' and therefore have not excluded examples where difficulties have been experienced. In addition, some cases have the cephalometric values provided in the diagnostic information, whilst some do not. We believe that cephalometrics should be used to supplement the clinical diagnosis and felt that the reader would benefit from having them provided in some, but not all, of the case records included.

In setting out this book, we have attempted to arrange the chapters into a series that progresses logically, although there can be considerable flexibility in the precise order in which they can be read, particularly those chapters dealing with specific malocclusions. Chapter 1 provides an introduction to clinical examination and diagnosis of the orthodontic patient, including the use of radiographic and cephalometric analysis in treatment planning. This chapter also covers aspects of the patient medical history that can be of relevance to orthodontic treatment. Chapter 2 is concerned with postnatal development of the dentition and has been designed to include individual examples of anomalies that can occur during establishment of the dentition (both common and rare), the use of interceptive treatment and major aspects of tooth agenesis. Chapters 3–6 are organized according to the conventional classification of malocclusion and include the management of class I, class II division 1, class II division 2 and class III cases. Chapter 7 covers problems associated with tooth impaction in the permanent dentition and Chapter 8 focuses on fixed orthodontic appliances, using individual examples to demonstrate issues

relating to their use and the application of treatment mechanics. Chapter 9 covers the subject of post-treatment stability and the management of retention, whilst Chapter 10 explores diagnosis and treatment of cases requiring a combined orthodontic and surgical approach to correct significant skeletal discrepancies. Finally, Chapter 11 is concerned with the etiology and management of developmental conditions that can affect the craniofacial region.

Inevitably, amongst all of the cases that have been used, there is some repetition of problems that can occur in relation to malocclusion; however, we hope that this adds rather than subtracts from the quality of the text. Indeed, many different philosophies and approaches exist regarding the management of malocclusion and we hope that many of these have been suitably illustrated. This book does not represent a comprehensive text, but hopefully does cover most aspects of contemporary clinical orthodontics through the documentation of treated cases. We hope that the style and content of the book is stimulating and that you as the reader are broadly in agreement with the treatment decisions that have been made and satisfied with the final results that have been achieved.

Martyn T. Cobourne
Padhraig S. Fleming
Andrew T. DiBiase
Sofia Ahmad

1

Clinical and Cephalometric Analysis

Introduction

Orthodontics is the area of dentistry concerned with the management of deviations from normal occlusion or malocclusion and involves treatment of children, adolescents and, increasingly, adults. Malocclusion is a variation on normal occlusion and is not a disease entity. Consequently, orthodontic planning and management does not involve binary decisions, but rather evaluation of a range of possibilities to decipher the most appropriate option for each individual.

An ideal static occlusion is characterized by class I molar and incisor relationships, with well-aligned teeth. An acceptable occlusion, however, develops naturally in only 30–40% of the population in Western societies. The occurrence of an acceptable occlusion is multi-factorial, although important factors include the size of the jaws; the relationship of the jaws to each other; the size, number and morphology of the teeth; and the morphology and behaviour of the lips, tongue and peri-oral musculature.

Given that malocclusion does not represent a pathological process but rather a variation from an accepted norm, there is little agreement, even among orthodontists, as to when orthodontic treatment becomes necessary (Richmond et al., 1984). As a consequence, a variety of orthodontic indices have been developed to ration treatment where care is provided as part of a public health service, such as in the UK and Scandinavia (Brook and Shaw, 1989), based primarily on aesthetic and dental health impairment.

The demand for orthodontic treatment has increased universally, particularly over the past two decades. A desire to enhance dental appearance is the underlying motivation for most patients who seek orthodontic treatment (Shaw et al., 1991). Furthermore, the lay public has developed an increasing awareness of the importance of the dentition to overall attractiveness. Carefully planned and well-executed orthodontics can also enhance facial appearance, which in turn has been linked to improved social skills, greater desirability, higher intellectual ability and enhanced occupational prospects (Shaw et al., 1979).

Deviation from occlusal norms may leave children susceptible to harassment, teasing and bullying, with obvious psychosocial implications (Shaw et al., 1980; Seehra et al., 2011). Consequently, orthodontic treatment may have significant psychosocial benefits (Shaw et al., 1980; O'Brien et al., 2003) and can often lead to improved oral health-related quality of life. Similarly, combined orthodontic–surgical treatment has been linked to notable enhancement of both self-esteem and quality of life (Arndt et al., 1986).

The undoubted benefits of orthondontics are, however, reliant on careful diagnosis, planning and management. Clinical assessment and radiographic analysis are central to the formulation of appropriate treatment decisions leading to the best aesthetic and functional outcome from treatment.

As in any other area of medicine or dentistry, to reach a diagnosis in orthodontics requires a thorough history, examination and special tests. A comprehensive history should be undertaken to clarify the motivation for treatment, the dental and orthodontic history, and any relevant medical history that might impact on the provision of orthodontic treatment (Patel *et al.*, 2009).

Dental History

A history of dental attendance is relevant in relation to caries experience and the presence of restorations. Caries experience is the best predictor of future caries. Poor oral hygiene predisposes to two risks of treatment: gingivitis and demineralization. Premature loss of primary teeth due to caries may also have consequence for the developing dentition. In particular, early loss of primary teeth may hasten or retard eruption of permanent teeth and lead to space loss, which can result in centre line discrepancies or potential tooth impaction.

What has led to crowding of the second premolars in Figure 1.1?

Early loss of the second primary molars has allowed the first permanent molars to drift forward in the dental arch. The second premolars are most vulnerable to space loss in this region.

Restorations

Heavily-restored teeth may pose problems in relation to bonding, necessitating alteration of the bonding protocol, with sandblasting of amalgam and precious metal restorations proven to enhance bond strength (Zachrisson *et al.*, 1995; Büyükyilmaz *et al.*, 1995).

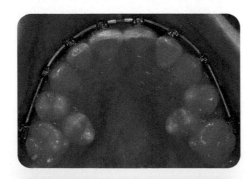

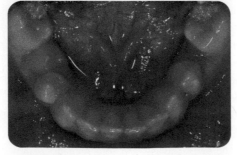

Figure 1.1

There is conflicting evidence in relation to the susceptibility of root canal-treated teeth to root resorption during treatment. Nevertheless, the health of root-treated teeth should be monitored throughout treatment.

Trauma

A history of trauma to the dentition should be investigated. Previously traumatized teeth risk loss of vitality irrespective of orthodontic treatment. This potential eventuality should be discussed at the outset as part of the informed consent process. In addition, traumatized teeth may also be at risk of undergoing more apical root resorption during treatment. The nature and timing of the traumatic injury has a bearing on further treatment (Kindelan *et al.*, 2008) (Table 1.1).

Previous orthodontics

Increasingly, potential orthodontic patients, particularly adults, may have undergone previous treatment. Details of the original malocclusion may help to decipher the aetiology of both the presenting and residual malocclusion. Potential consequences of incomplete treatment include residual malalignment and spacing, traumatic overbite, residual overjet, crossbite and relapse. Previous failure to complete a course of orthodontic treatment may raise questions with respect to compliance (Murray, 1989). Where compliance is questionable, it may be inadvisable to embark on an ambitious course of orthodontic treatment.

Furthermore, contemporaneous records are important to reveal deleterious effects of the primary phase. Rarely, significant root resorption may limit the feasibility for retreatment.

Table 1.1 Timing of further treatment for traumatic injury

Type of injury	Recommended observation period before orthodontic treatment
Fracture without pulpal involvement	3 months
Subluxation	3 months
Extrusive luxation	3 months
Minor lateral luxation	3 months
Moderate/severe lateral luxation	1 year
Intrusion	1 year
Avulsion	1 year

CASE 1.1

This 17-year-old female presented with a class III malocclusion on a moderate skeletal class III pattern with an average lower facial height. She has had previous orthodontic treatment to align her maxillary teeth, involving extraction of maxillary first premolars. She remains concerned in relation to her facial appearance and occlusion.

What do you notice with respect to the radiographic appearance of the maxillary incisors (Figure 1.2)?

The maxillary incisors, particularly the UR1, UL1 and UR2, have experienced extensive root resorption during the first phase of treatment.

How will this finding influence further management?

The patient is keen to undergo combined orthodontic–surgical treatment to address her malocclusion comprehensively. Prior to instituting such treatment, the patient will be counselled in relation to the likelihood of further resorption. If the patient opts

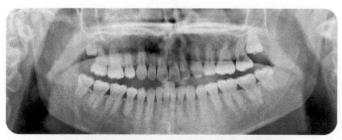

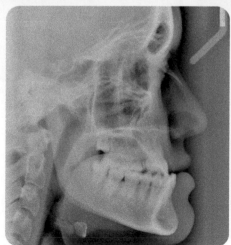

Figure 1.2

to undergo combined treatment, attempts will be made to avoid an upper fixed appliance. If an appliance is to be placed, light forces will be applied, there will be a premium on excellent oral hygiene and the duration of treatment will be necessarily short with realistic objectives.

Family History

The contribution of genetic factors to malocclusion has been established in family and twin studies. Concordance of occlusal patterns in monozygotic twins provides support for the influence of genetics on malocclusion, while discordance between monozygotic twins suggests occlusal relationships may be under greater environmental influences. A family history of severe class III malocclusion; abnormalities of tooth number and form; and ectopic dental development should be considered when planning treatment for relatives.

Cranio-facial morphology in class II and class III groups tends to have strong heritability, although the association is less clear in class I subjects. In particular, familial cephalometric studies have shown that mandibular length may be reduced, with a smaller mandibular body and retruded mandible in class II patients (Harris, 1975).

Furthermore, mandibular prognathism in monozygotic twins is six times higher than among dizygotic twins (Litton *et al.*, 1970). A Japanese study showed that 70% of patients undergoing orthognathic surgery for class III malocclusion have a first-degree relative with mandibular prognathism (Watanabe *et al.*, 2005). Therefore, a history of orthognathic intervention in a family member should be considered when planning early treatment and anticipating future growth in class III malocclusion.

There is also a familial link in relation to supernumerary teeth. Inheritance does not follow a simple Mendelian pattern, being variously described as an autosomal dominant trait with incomplete penetrance, a sex-linked trait and an autosomal recessive trait with lesser penetrance in females (Fleming *et al.*, 2010). Hypodontia has also been linked to specific mutations related to *MSX1* and *PAX9* genes, and tends to co-exist with microdontia (Brook, 1984). Genetic factors are also implicated in palatal impaction of maxillary canines; dental transpositions; infra-occlusion of primary molars; and impaction of first permanent molars.

Genetic susceptibility to severe root resorption during orthodontic treatment has also been attributed to mutations of genes encoding interleukin-1 beta (IL-1β). Consequently, the potential for extensive resorption should be anticipated in family members. Treatment objectives may be modified accordingly.

Medical History

A comprehensive medical history should be taken for each patient. Whilst there are few medical conditions that contraindicate orthodontic treatment in a compliant dentally fit individual, several can impact on the delivery of care.

Heart defects with risk of infective endocarditis

Infective endocarditis is a rare cardiac condition with mortality rates of up to 40%. Previously, antibiotic prophylaxis was recommended for patients with structural heart defects predisposing to formation of valvular vegetations, which may culminate in infective endocarditis. High-risk conditions include previous infective endocarditis, prosthetic heart valves and acquired valvular disease with stenosis or regurgitation. However, under new National Institute of Health and Clinical Excellence (NICE) guidelines in the UK, the use of prophylactic antibiotics is no longer recommended for dental procedures (NICE, 2008).

Is antibiotic cover required prior to any orthodontic procedure?

Historically, antibiotic cover has been recommended for dental procedures involving gingival manipulation on patients with structural defects of the heart. The rationale for use of antibiotics was to counteract transient bacteraemia that may lead to infective endocarditis. Susceptible orthodontic procedures included placement of separators and bands, and removal of appliances. However, NICE now advises that use of prophylactic antibiotics is not indicated (NICE, 2008). The cost-efficacy of prophylaxis is unproven. The use of antibiotics has a reported attendant morbidity with fatal anaphylaxis of up to 12–25 cases per million (Ahlstedt, 1984). This risk is thought to outweigh the benefits of their use. Therefore, in current practice, antibiotic cover is not routinely recommended for patients with a structural heart defect undergoing orthodontic treatment.

Bleeding disorders

Conditions such as haemophilia do not preclude orthodontic treatment; however, treatment should involve haematological input. These patients are also at higher risk of carrying blood-borne viral infections, including HIV or hepatitis.

CASE 1.2
This 15-year-old male presented with haemophilia A. He has mild crowding of both arches and is anxious to have orthodontic treatment (Figure 1.3).

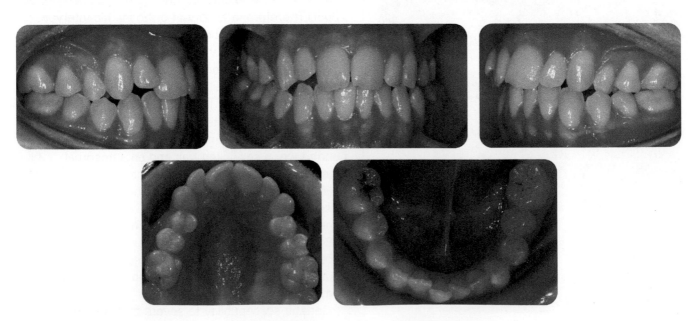

Figure 1.3

How will his history of haemophilia A affect his management?

Oral hygiene
Prior to instituting treatment, the importance of excellent oral hygiene should be emphasized. This may necessitate sessions with a dental hygienist or oral hygiene educators. A plaque score below 10% should be achieved before committing to treatment.

Treatment planning
If possible treatment should be undertaken on a non-extraction basis, obviating the risks of extractions and complex haematological management of extractions. Space creation may therefore be achieved by arch lengthening involving transverse or anteroposterior arch expansion or by inter-proximal reduction.

Management of extractions
Where extractions are necessary, these should be managed with input from physicians. Factor VIII production may be increased with 1-desamino-8-D-arginine vasopressin (DDAVP). Cryoprecipitate, Factor VIII in isolation or fresh frozen plasma may be used to replace missing Factor VIII. An anti-fibrinolytic, tranexamic acid, is also useful to stabilize clot formation.

Gingival trauma and soft tissue irritation
Efforts should be made to make the appliance as safe and unobtrusive as possible. In particular, wire ligatures should be avoided and use of self-ligating brackets can be considered. Soft tissue trauma from sharp and long wire ends should be avoided.

Allergies
The most important allergies in relation to orthodontic treatment are those associated with exposure to latex and nickel. Hypersensitivity reactions occurring with either allergen may be immediate (Type I) or delayed (Type IV); however, those related to nickel are typically Type IV reactions. Type I sensitivity is antibody mediated and may present as a localized urticaria or as anaphylaxis. Type IV hypersensitivity typically results in localized allergic contact dermatitis.

Latex allergy: Allergy to natural rubber latex is becoming increasingly prevalent with powdered gloves harbouring latex allergens. Individuals susceptible to allergic reactions include atopic individuals with allergic rhinitis, asthma and eczema; and patients with spina bifida.

How should potential orthodontic patients with suspected latex allergy be managed?
- **Definitive diagnosis:** Latex allergy can be diagnosed with either patch testing or pin prick testing, although the latter is more reliable.
- **Staff training and communication:** Staff should be aware of emergency protocols for dealing with anaphylactic reactions and auxiliary staff should be aware of the diagnosis.
- **Appointment and surgery management:** Appointments should be scheduled for the early morning with use of a latex-screened area to segregate latex-free products to avoid contamination.
- **Appliance design and handling:** The use of latex products should be avoided. Latex-containing gloves should be replaced with alternatives, including nitrile or vinyl. The use of elastomeric ties could be avoided with use of self-ligating brackets. Space closure should be undertaken with nickel–titanium coils. Where inter-maxillary elastics are required, latex-free elastics can be used, although they are subject to greater force degradation.

Nickel allergy: Nickel allergy is relatively common, affecting over 10% of females (Nielsen and Menne, 1993). Typically, Type IV hypersensitivity reactions present on the skin as contact dermatitis; however, intra-oral manifestations are less common. There appears to be a higher threshold nickel concentration required intra-orally to induce a reaction. Nickel–titanium archwires and auxiliaries, and stainless steel products, including archwires, brackets and headgear, all contain nickel. Hence, vigilance should be exercised when using these materials in at-risk patients.

What is the recommended protocol in a 25-year-old female patient with a suspected nickel allergy?
- **Definitive diagnosis:** Patch testing may be performed by a dermatologist to confirm the diagnosis.
- **Treatment:** Consideration could be given to use of nickel-free brackets, e.g. ceramic, gold, titanium or polycarbonate brackets. The use of nickel–titanium archwires should be avoided where intra-oral signs of a reaction are noted. These wires may be replaced by fibre-reinforced composite wires,

stainless steel wires with reduced nickel content, titanium molybdenum alloy or titanium niobium wires. Rarely, in severe cases, consideration could be given to the use of clear plastic aligners.

Diabetes

Poorly controlled diabetics are more susceptible to periodontal breakdown. Excellent oral hygiene therefore needs to be maintained during orthodontic treatment.

Immunosuppression

Certain immunosuppressive drugs such as cyclosporin can cause gingival hyperplasia or drug-induced gingival overgrowth in the presence of good oral hygiene (Figure 1.4). Again, excellent oral hygiene is imperative for these patients throughout treatment, as gingival swelling may become more marked with poor plaque control (Figure 1.5).

Epilepsy

Epilepsy is a common neurological condition, occurring in 2–5% of individuals. It is considered active if a patient is taking medication or has had a seizure within the last 2 years. If treatment is to be considered, the

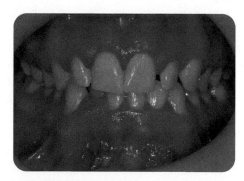

Figure 1.4

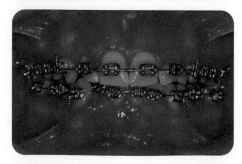

Figure 1.5

condition should be well-controlled. Removable appliances are best avoided in epileptics as displacement of the appliance during a seizure risks airway compromise. Consequently, fixed functional appliances or class II correctors are preferred to removable alternatives. Anti-convulsants, including phenytoin, may result in gingival hyperplasia, with 50% of individuals affected within 3 months of commencing the medication. Second-line medications, including carbamazepine, may result in glossitis, xerostomia or oral ulceration.

Childhood malignancy

Childhood malignancy and its treatment may have significant implications for orthodontic treatment. The most common malignancy is leukaemia, with acute lymphoblastic leukaemia accounting for 25% of childhood tumours. Treatment of acute leukaemia may involve bone marrow transplantation or chemotherapy. Immunosuppressants and total body irradiation are used following bone marrow replacement to prevent graft-versus-host disease.

Treatment of malignant disease in childhood with either radiotherapy or chemotherapy can result in either tooth agenesis or root shortening. Other tumours of the head and neck requiring early radiotherapy may include retinoblastoma and sarcomas.

What side effects of head and neck radiotherapy are of relevance to orthodontics?

- Root shortening and arrested tooth development
- Reduced growth hormone production and impaired bone growth: This may result in reduced craniofacial dimension
- Reduced bone density
- Mucositis
- Arrested root development
- Premature apical closure
- Microdontia
- Hypodontia
- Delayed dental development
- Enamel defects

(Sheller and Williams, 1996)

What are the orthodontic implications of childhood malignancy and its treatment?

- Premium on excellent oral hygiene
- Use of light forces
- Early termination of treatment

- Consideration of compromised treatment
- Relevant medications

Bisphosphonates

Bisphosphonates inhibit the resorption of trabecular bone by impairing osteoclastic activity to maintain bone density. They have found particular application in the management of osteoporosis, and may be prescribed to reduce hypercalcaemia following bone metastasis. Potential side effects of bisphosphonates relevant to orthodontics include osteonecrosis of the jaws, delayed eruption and retarded tooth movement. Cessation of the medication is likely to be of little benefit due to the protracted half-life of some bisphosphonates, with alendronate having a half-life of 10 years.

While osteonecrosis is a serious potential consequence, it is rare, being more likely with IV administration and prolonged use. Nevertheless, care should be taken to reduce its likelihood.

CASE 1.3

A 45-year-old female presented with osteoporosis. She has been taking oral alendronate. She has a crowded class I malocclusion.

How will her medical history affect her management?

Bisphosphonates pose two major risks to her treatment. There is a very small but serious risk of developing osteonecrosis of the jaws and tooth movement is likely to be difficult. Consequently, informed consent is important prior to embarking on treatment; it is also wise to discuss treatment with the patient's physician. As alendronate has a long half-life, temporary discontinuation is ineffective.

It is wise to avoid invasive procedures, including extractions or temporary anchorage devices. If required, space may be created by transverse or anteroposterior arch expansion or inter-proximal reduction. Alternatively, the goals of treatment can be modified to accept a compromised outcome, obviating the need for extractions and reducing the overall treatment time. In addition, great care should be taken to ensure appliances are smooth and well-fitting, limiting the risk of ulceration and soft tissue trauma.

Occasionally, orthodontics is best avoided with a restorative approach being an alternative.

Non-steroidal anti-inflammatory drugs (NSAIDs)

NSAIDs may be used on a long-term basis for chronic illness, including rheumatoid arthritis. They are also recommended for analgesia following manipulation of orthodontic appliances. They act by inhibiting cyclo-oxygenase activity, inhibiting production of prostaglandins. Animal studies have suggested that use of NSAIDs, including aspirin and ibuprofen, for pain control may retard tooth movement (Arias and Marquez-Orozco, 2006). Nevertheless, as their analgesic properties are proven, they continue to have application in orthodontic pain control.

Clinical Examination

Orthodontic treatment planning decisions are governed by both facial and occlusal goals with the aims of optimizing facial harmony and dental aesthetics, and creating a healthy and stable occlusion both in centric relationship and in function. More specifically, treatment planning decisions, including extraction and anchorage requirements, also need to take account of intra-arch features, including degree of crowding, spacing, canine angulation and occlusal curves in relation to the tooth movements planned to achieve the treatment aims. In addition, the influence of inter-arch features in all three spatial planes has a significant bearing on treatment decisions. These features may then be amalgamated in formal space planning to make robust and consistent treatment plans.

Extra-oral examination

The face should be examined both at rest and in animation from the front and in profile. Although absolute measurements can be made and compared to anthropometric means, of more importance are the proportions of component parts relative to each other. Any areas of disproportion should be noted.

What is natural head posture and why is it important?

Natural head posture is the physiological position in which the head is held during normal function. During clinical and cephalometric examination, the orthodontist tries to replicate this using natural head position. This can be reproduced by asking the patient to look straight ahead into the distance,

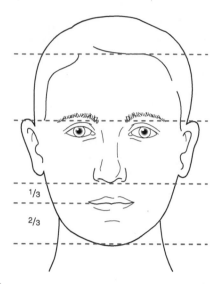

Figure 1.6

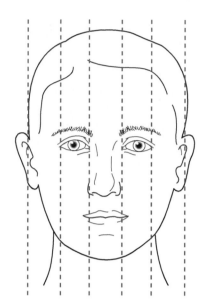

Figure 1.7

or look at themself in a mirror placed in front of them at eye level. Natural head position has been shown to be remarkably reproducible, allowing the orthodontist to compare the soft and hard tissues to an extra-cranial true vertical reference line. This avoids reliance on intra-cranial planes for reference, which are not only subject to significant biological variability but also the same distortion as the facial skeleton in the presence of anomalies of skeletal growth.

Frontal view:
- **Vertically:** The face can be divided into thirds. The lower face can be divided further into thirds with the lower lip making up two-thirds and the upper lip one-third of the total (Figure 1.6).
- **Transversely:** The face can be divided into fifths, with each fifth being approximately the width of the eye (Figure 1.7). Any asymmetry should be noted.

 The patient's lips are described as:
- Competent when they meet at rest
- Incompetent when they are apart at rest.

Lip incompetence occurs due to either anteroposterior skeletal discrepancy or increased vertical skeletal proportions. The amount of maxillary incisor display at rest should be approximately 3–4 mm in males and 4–5 mm in females in late adolescence and early adulthood. Incisor show decreases with age, although over 90% of upper lip length is established in females by the age of 7 years (Nanda *et al.*, 1990). Lip competence tends to increase with maturation of the soft tissues and increasing social awareness in adolescence.

What factors contribute to an attractive smile?

Smiling is an integral part of human communication and one of the principal aims of orthodontics is to create a pleasing smile. The patient should therefore be examined in animation during smiling (Sarver, 2001). The three areas that need to be assessed are:
- **Vertical incisor position:** On smiling, most of the upper incisor should be displayed but without excessive gingival display. However, the amount of tooth and gingival display decreases with maturation; this should be borne in mind when examining a younger patient. The gingival contour of the maxillary anterior teeth should also be assessed, the gingival margins of the central incisors and canines ideally being slightly higher than the lateral incisors.
- **Smile width:** The width of the maxillary arch in relation to the lips should be assessed. If the arch is too narrow or set back, the space between the buccal dentition and angle of the mouth, known as the buccal corridor, can be excessive, making the arch look narrow. However, some space to frame the smile is important; otherwise the smile can look artificial. Arch expansion, appropriate torque in the buccal segments, as well as the anteroposterior position of the maxilla relative to the lip drape influence the size of the buccal corridors (Isiksal *et al.*, 2006).
- **Smile arc:** On smiling the incisal edges of the upper anterior teeth should lie on the arc of the lower lip. This is called a consonant smile and is considered

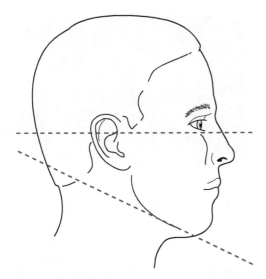

Figure 1.8

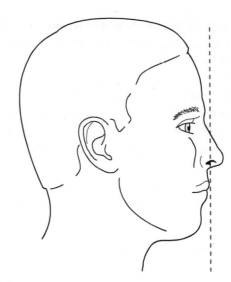

Figure 1.9

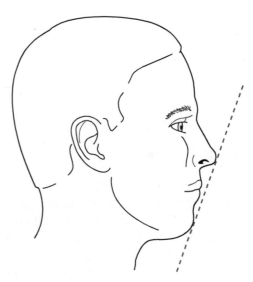

Figure 1.10

the most pleasing (Frush and Fisher, 1958). If the upper anterior teeth follow a straight line, the smile can also look artificial.

Profile view
- **Vertically:** The face can also be divided into equal thirds. The angle between the lower border of the mandible and the Frankfort horizontal plane can be measured with imaginary lines intersecting at the occiput in the presence of a normal vertical relationship (Figure 1.8).
- **Anteroposterior:** The relative position of the dental bases should be described in relation to the cranial base and to each other. These can be visualized by direct palpation or by dropping a vertical line from the forehead through the intersection of the upper lip and base of nose (subnasale) (Figure 1.9). The upper lip should rest on or slightly in front of this line, whilst the chin point should be just behind it. The maxillary dental base should lie approximately 4 mm in front of the mandibular dental base.

The soft tissues of the lower third of the face are described in relation to the relative protrusion of the lips and the angle of the upper lip to the base of the nose, the naso-labial angle. The lips are described as protrusive if they rest in front of a line from the tip of the nose to the chin (Rickett's E-line) (Figure 1.10). With age the lips become less protrusive relative to this line. The naso-labial angle should be between 90 and 110 degrees, although this depends on the shape

of the nose. More practically, the upper lip drape should be parallel to the true vertical previously described (Arnett and Bergman, 1993). Similarly, the labial face of the upper incisors should also be parallel to this line for optimal dental aesthetics.

Temporo-mandibular joints
Both joints should be examined for:
- Clicking
- Crepitus
- Pain
- Locking or limited opening.

What is the relationship between malocclusion and temporo-mandibular joint dysfunction?

Temporo-mandibular joint dysfunction (TMD) is a very common condition in Western societies and its aetiology is considered to be multi-factorial. Certain traits of a malocclusion have been shown in large cross-sectional epidemiological studies to have a weak association with TMD, including anterior open bites, increased overbites, large overjets and posterior crossbites with displacement (Egermark-Eriksson *et al.*, 1983; Mohlin *et al.*, 2007). However, there is no simple relationship. As such, there is no evidence that orthodontic treatment is effective at treating TMD (Luther *et al.*, 2010) and importantly, there is again no evidence that orthodontic treatment induces or exacerbates TMD, including treatment involving extractions (Egermark *et al.*, 2005; Hirsch 2009).

Intra-oral examination

Initial intra-oral examination involves an assessment of dental health. Evidence of active dental disease should be recorded as well as the level of oral hygiene. A plaque index provides an objective score. Each dental arch is then described in isolation and in relation to the opposing arch, both in static and functional occlusion. Key intra- and inter-arch features that should be recorded are outlined below.

Crowding: Dento-alveolar disproportion usually involves a relative excess of tooth tissue, culminating in dental crowding. Crowding has been defined as primary, secondary or tertiary (van der Linden, 1974). Primary crowding refers to an underlying discrepancy of tooth dimension and jaw size. Secondary crowding is caused by environmental factors, including local space conditions in the dental arches and the position and function of the tongue, lips and buccal musculature. Tertiary crowding refers to the propensity for an increase in crowding with dental maturation; imbrication of the lower anteriors in late adolescence and in the third decade is typical.

Crowding can be defined as mild (<4 mm), moderate (4–8 mm) or severe (>8 mm) (Figure 1.11). Crowding is one of a variety of occlusal traits that has implications for orthodontic space requirements and treatment planning. To relieve crowding, treatment protocols that could be considered include dental extractions, typically of premolars; transverse expansion; antero-posterior arch lengthening, either by distal movement

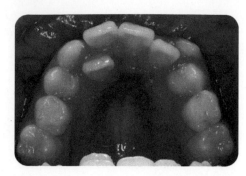

Figure 1.11

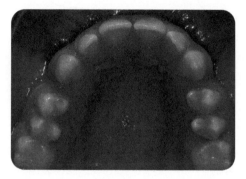

Figure 1.12

of the posterior teeth or advancement of the anteriors; or inter-proximal reduction.

Severe crowding usually warrants extractions as part of the orthodontic treatment plan, relieving crowding while facilitating placement of the dentition in a stable soft tissue environment. Extractions are also considered with moderate degrees of crowding, while mild crowding is usually dealt with without extractions if possible, depending on the proposed final position of the labial segments.

Spacing: Spacing is less common than crowding. It may be generalized (Figure 1.12) or local. Physiological spacing tends to occur between the maxillary central incisors during development; a maxillary median diastema and tends to close upon eruption of the maxillary canines. In approximately 8% of individuals, this persists into the permanent dentition (Keene, 1963). It may be closed with fixed appliances, although there is a premium on prolonged fixed retention to retain this correction.

Generalized spacing may be a manifestation of relatively large dental bases, with normal tooth size and shape being more common in Afro-Caribbeans (Richardson *et al.*, 1973; Mugonzibwa *et al.*, 2008).

Occasionally, spacing may reflect reduced tooth number, size and width. Missing and diminutive maxillary lateral incisors are a common finding. Relocation of space following treatment may be necessary to facilitate build-up of these teeth, improving dental aesthetics and long-term stability (Figure 1.13).

Rotations, contact point displacements and labio-lingual displacements: Rotations and displacements of teeth should be recorded. Correction of rotations in the buccal segments will generate space as rotated premolars and molars occupy more space than aligned teeth; the reverse is true in the anterior dentition.

Canine position and angulation: Particular note should be made of the position of the maxillary canines, even if unerupted. Maxillary canines should be palpable buccally from 8 to 10 years. If this is not the case, it may indicate canine ectopia warranting further investigation.

The angulation of erupted canines has implications for anchorage management. The canines have long and broad roots; significant change in the position of their roots is therefore anchorage demanding. The desired final canine position involves slight mesial positioning of the crown relative to the root (mesial angulation); therefore, correction of distal canine crown angulation necessitates a significant bodily root movement. This should be considered when planning extractions and requirements for anchorage support.

How would you classify the crowding in the maxillary arch in the intra-oral records shown in Figure 1.14?

The maxillary arch is moderately crowded; there is approximately 7 mm of crowding.

What do you notice about the maxillary canines? What is the clinical relevance of this?

Both maxillary canines are distally angulated. The anchorage requirement in the maxillary arch is

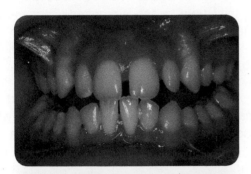

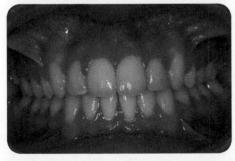

Figure 1.13

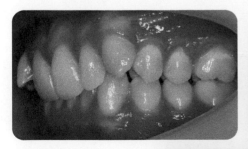
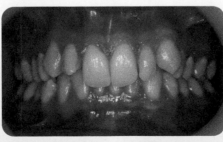
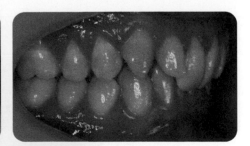

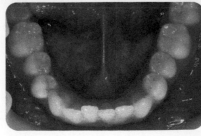
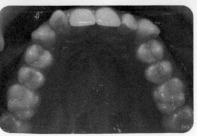

Figure 1.14

increased as there are likely to be significant reciprocal forces during attempted distal root movement of both canines.

What do you think of the mesio-distal width of the maxillary lateral incisors? What is the clinical relevance of this finding?

The mesio-distal width of both maxillary lateral incisors is reduced. Both teeth will require build-up to restore ideal dental aesthetics and occlusal harmony. If a decision is made to avoid build-up of these teeth, either a reduced overjet and overbite will result or inter-proximal reduction of the lower anteriors could be performed to eliminate the inter-arch tooth-size discrepancy.

Incisor inclination: Labial segment inclination is the inclination of the maxillary and mandibular incisors relative to the dental bases. Incisors may be upright, proclined or retroclined. The inclination of the anterior teeth represents the influence of soft tissue relationships on the dentition. The teeth are held in soft tissue equilibrium by the lips and cheeks externally and the tongue on the inside. Mismatch in the soft tissue forces acting on the teeth may result in changes in incisor inclination. In Figure 1.14, the maxillary central incisors have been retroclined, almost certainly by a high lower lip line. In Figure 1.15, incisor proclination has occurred as a result of a lip trap. Furthermore, incisor inclination may compensate for a skeletal discrepancy. Typically, retroclination of the maxillary incisors tends to occur in the presence of a milder skeletal class II pattern (Figure 1.14), whilst

proclination is more common with a more severe class II discrepancy (Figure 1.15). In contrast, mandibular incisor retroclination is often seen in association with a skeletal class III discrepancy; this also occurs under soft tissue influence (Figure 1.16).

Curve of Spee: The curve of Spee is an imaginary line formed in the sagittal plane between the cusp tips of the mandibular first molars and incisors. An increased curve represents a deeper curve with relative inferior positioning of the mandibular premolars; this is associated with increased overbite. To reduce the depth of this curve, space is required (Germane *et al.*, 1992). Rarely a reversed curve of Spee may be seen; this is associated with reduced overbite or anterior open bite.

Occlusion (inter-arch features): The static and functional occlusion should both be described, with the static occlusion recorded in three spatial planes. Sagittal relationships, including molar, canine and

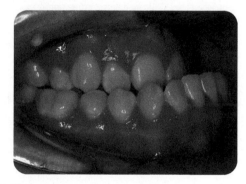

Figure 1.16

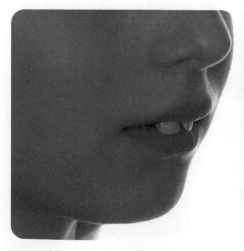

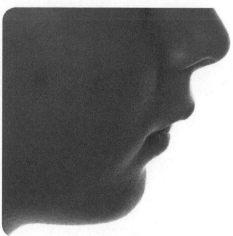

Figure 1.15

incisor relationships, and overjet should be recorded. These terms are defined as follows:

- **Molar relationship** (Angle's classification):
  - **Class I:** The relative position of the dental arches is normal, with first molars in normal occlusion; the mesio-buccal cusp of the upper first permanent molar occludes in the mid-buccal groove between the mesial and distal buccal cusps of the lower.
  - **Class II:** The relationship of the dental arches is abnormal; the mandibular teeth occlude distal to normal. Angle recognized two subdivisions under class II:
    Class II division 1 is characterized by protruding upper incisors
    Class II division 2 is characterized by lingually inclined upper incisors.
  - **Class III:** The relationship of the dental arches is also abnormal, with mandibular first molars occluding mesial to the Class I position.
- **Incisor relationship.** This is described using the British Standards Institute Glossary of Dental Terms:
  - **Class I:** The mandibular incisor tip occludes or lies on or below the cingulum plateau of the maxillary incisors.
  - **Class II:** The mandibular incisor tip occludes or lies posterior to the cingulum plateau of the maxillary incisors. This classification is further subdivided into:
    Class II division 1: The overjet is increased with upright or proclined maxillary incisors
    Class II division 2: The maxillary incisors are retroclined, with a normal or occasionally increased overjet.
  - **Class III:** the mandibular incisor tip occludes with or lies anterior to the cingulum plateau of the maxillary incisors.

Overjet is measured from the labial surface of the most prominent maxillary incisor to the labial surface of the mandibular incisors. If there is an anterior crossbite the overjet is given a negative value.

The aim of comprehensive orthodontic treatment invariably involves creating a class I incisor relationship with an overjet of 2–4 mm. With an intact dentition and correct inclination of the anterior dentition, this also necessitates class I molar and canine relationships. However, in certain malocclusions, class II or III molar relationships may be accepted with removal of maxillary premolars or mandibular premolars, respectively, camouflaging the incisor relationship and

also achieving class I canine relationships bilaterally. Therefore, if the molar relationships deviate from class I, the treatment plan will revolve around the decision to either correct the molar relationships to class I or to accept the molar relationship but camouflage the malocclusion with single-arch extractions.

Class II molar relationships may be corrected by distal movement of the maxillary molars, mesial movement of the mandibular molars or more often a combination of these approaches. Methods to correct class II molar relationships include headgear, functional appliances, temporary anchorage devices (TADs) and class II correctors, e.g. Forsus springs. Differential extractions with removal of maxillary first premolars and mandibular second premolars also promote molar correction and overjet reduction in class II malocclusion. In a non-growing patient with severe mandibular retrognathia, a mandibular advancement osteotomy may be required to correct the incisor and molar relationships.

Class III molar relationships may be addressed in growing patients using protraction headgear or class III functional appliances. Differential extractions, typically loss of maxillary second premolars and mandibular first premolars, and inter-arch class III elastic may be used to correct class III molar relationships, promoting establishment of a positive overjet and overbite. In non-growing patients in the presence of a severe skeletal class III base relationship, orthognathic surgery may be required.

In class II malocclusions, extraction of maxillary premolar units can be carried out in isolation, accepting the class II molar relationship (Figure 1.17). This

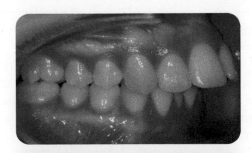

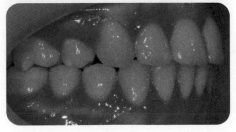

Figure 1.17

approach facilitates correction of the canine relationship; limited controlled advancement of the mandibular incisors may also be planned, reducing the anchorage requirement to reduce the overjet. Conversely, in class III malocclusion, a decision may be made to remove mandibular premolars only to retract the mandibular incisors, maintaining the antero-posterior position of the maxillary incisors. While the aim is to correct both incisor and canine relationships to class I, class III molars would be accepted.

Transverse relationships: Transverse discrepancy should be noted using the following descriptions:
- Buccal crossbite: Buccal cusps of the maxillary dentition occlude palatally to the buccal cusps of the mandibular dentition
- Lingual crossbite: Palatal cusps of the maxillary dentition occlude buccally to the buccal cusps of the mandibular dentition (this can also be referred to as a scissors bite)
- Unilateral crossbite: Affects one side of the dental arch
- Bilateral crossbite: Affects both sides of the dental arch.

Teeth in crossbite should be recorded along with any associated displacement that may exist on the mandibular arc of closure from retruded contact position (RCP) to inter-cuspal position (ICP). If there is a displacement, its location and magnitude should be recorded.

Correct transverse arch co-ordination facilitates occlusal inter-digitation, function and aesthetics. Occlusal displacements, which are often related to crossbites, may be associated with occlusal and gingival trauma and have been weakly linked to temporo-mandibular dysfunction. While correction of crossbites without associated displacement is not essential, this will usually be an aim of comprehensive orthodontics. Crossbite correction may require either maxillary arch expansion, with fixed or removable appliances; mandibular arch constriction, often with extractions; or a combination of both approaches. Arch constriction is thought to be more stable than expansion and may also be encouraged by addition of lingual crown torque to the lower dentition. Conversely, lingual crossbite (scissors bite) correction may be reliant on maxillary arch constriction and broadening of the mandibular arch.

Vertical relationships: Overbite is the vertical overlap of the lower incisors by the maxillary incisors with the teeth in occlusion. Normal overjet is characterized by vertical overlap of one-third to one-half of the mandibular incisors.

Overbite may be:
- **Increased** if the maxillary incisors overlap the mandibular incisor crowns vertically by more than one-half of the lower incisor crown height
- **Decreased** if the maxillary incisors overlap the mandibular incisors by less than one-third of the lower incisor crown height
- **Complete** if there is contact between the mandibular incisor edges (or maxillary if there is a class III incisor relationship) and the opposing dentition or mucosa
- **Incomplete** if there is no contact between the mandibular incisor edges (or maxillary if there is a class III incisor relationship) and the opposing dentition or mucosa
- **Traumatic** if there is evidence of trauma to either the palatal mucosa or to the gingivae of the lower labial segment.

Traumatic overbite is most common in class II division 2 malocclusion and may be compounded by poor oral hygiene resulting in gingival inflammation and attachment loss (Figure 1.18). Overbite reduction may be achieved by intrusion and proclination of the incisors, extrusion of the posterior teeth or by both mechanisms. While overbite reduction carries a space

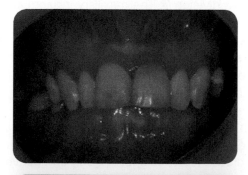

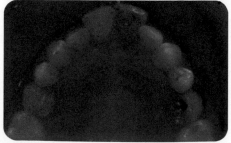

Figure 1.18

requirement to level an increased curve of Spee, lower arch extractions are often best avoided as these may complicate overbite reduction.

Anterior open bite is a vertical gap between the maxillary and mandibular incisors with the teeth in the ICP. The distance between the incisal edges and the posterior extent of the open bite should be recorded. Overbite may be increased using auxiliaries such as occipital pull headgear, intrusion splints and temporary anchorage devices, as well as specific mechanics, e.g. Kim mechanics. Extractions may also be beneficial with resultant space facilitating retraction, extrusion and uprighting of the anterior dentition. In addition, mesial movement of the buccal segments may allow increase in the overbite (Sarver and Weissman, 1995).

What are Andrews's six keys of normal occlusion?

Lawrence Andrews, based in San Diego, noted that many treated cases, despite having an Angle class I molar relationship, did not have an ideal buccal segment inter-digitation. Andrews (1972) came to this conclusion following assessment of 120 dental study casts of individuals who had not undergone orthodontic treatment and who had normal occlusions. From these he described six keys of normal occlusion:

1. **Molar relationship:** The distal surface of the disto-buccal cusp of the upper first permanent molar makes contact and occludes with the mesial surface of the mesio-buccal cusp of the lower second molar. The mesio-buccal cusp of the upper first permanent molar lies in the groove between the mesial and middle cusps of the lower first permanent molar.
2. **Crown angulation or mesio-distal tip:** The gingival portion of the long axis of each crown is distal to the incisal portion.
3. **Crown inclination:** Labio-lingual or bucco-lingual inclination. The upper and lower anterior crown inclination is sufficient to resist over-eruption of the anterior teeth and to allow proper distal positioning of the contact points of the upper teeth in relation to the lower teeth, permitting proper occlusion of the posterior crowns. A lingual crown inclination exists in the upper posterior crowns, is constant and similar from canines through to the second premolars, and slightly more pronounced in the molars. For the lower posterior teeth, the lingual crown inclination progressively increases from canines through to second molars.

4. **Rotations:** There are no rotations.
5. **Spaces:** There are no spaces, contact points are tight.
6. **Occlusal plane:** The plane of occlusion is either flat or there is a slight curve of Spee.

Space planning

Formal space planning involves assimilation of both intra-arch features and inter-arch relationships to produce an overall space requirement to justify treatment and extraction decisions. Furthermore, space planning may help to determine anchorage requirements and treatment mechanics. The Royal London Space Plan involves integration of these features, assigning specific space requirements to each aspect of the malocclusion (Kirschen et al., 2000a,b), including change in the sagittal position of the incisors; crowding or spacing; changes in arch width; occlusal curves; and torque and angulation changes.

What factors contribute to the space requirement in Figure 1.14?

Maxillary arch
- Crowding (7 mm)
- Torque requirement: 10 degrees of torque is required to the maxillary incisors; 2 mm of space is needed to achieve this
- Requirement for build-up of the UR2 and UL2. Both lateral incisors are 4 mm in width; 1.5 mm would be required per tooth if space opening is chosen

Mandibular arch
- Crowding (2 mm)
- Arch levelling: the curve of Spee is 3 mm deep; 1 mm of space will be required to reduce this

What treatment plan would you suggest based on this space analysis?

The space requirement in the maxillary arch is 12 mm if build-up of the lateral incisors is planned. However, just 3 mm of space is required to achieve the treatment goals in the mandibular arch. Hence, consideration could be given to removal of both maxillary first premolars, treating the mandibular arch on a non-extraction basis. If maxillary first premolars alone are extracted, only 1 mm of mesial maxillary molar movement is permissible bilaterally, and consideration should be given to anchorage support in the upper arch.

Functional occlusion

Based on the concepts of a mutual protective functional occlusion, the following features should be recorded:

- Canine guidance or group function in lateral excursion
- Presence of non-working side interferences
- Large discrepancies between the RCP and ICP, particularly in the presence of crossbite.

Diagnostic summary

At the end of the clinical examination a short diagnostic summary should be produced containing the salient points ascertained from the interview and examination (Box 1.1).

BOX 1.1 KEY DIAGNOSTIC FEATURES

Name
Age and sex
Medical history
Referral source
Patients concerns and motivation

Extra-oral

Skeletal relationship:
  Antero-posterior
  Vertical   FMPA
                    Lower face height
  Transverse   Facial symmetry
Soft tissues   Lip competence
                    Lip lengths
                    Naso-labial angle
Upper incisor show   At rest
                    Smiling
Temporo-mandibular joint

Intra-oral

Teeth present
Dental health
(restorations, caries)
Oral hygiene – periodontal
Lower arch   Crowding
                    Incisor inclination
                    Curve of Spee
Upper arch   Crowding
                    Incisor inclination
Occlusion   Incisor relationship
                    Overjet
                    Overbite
                    Molar relationship
                    Canine relationship
                    Centre lines
                    Functional occlusion
                    Other features

Radiographic Analysis

Following clinical assessment, radiographic analysis is usually warranted. A panoramic view is indicated prior to instituting orthodontic treatment to assess the presence and position of unerupted teeth, and root length and morphology.

What are the potential shortcomings associated with a panoramic view?

- **Lack of sharpness:** Due to various factors including ghost imaging, summation images, static distortion and processing errors.
- **Horizontal distortion:** This tends to be non-linear.
- **Vertical distortion:** Believed to be twice as severe as horizontal distortion.
- **Superimposition of the cervical spine.**
- **Limited focal trough:** Lingually-positioned roots falling outside the focal trough are usually magnified. Similarly, excessively inclined teeth not contained within the boundaries of the focal trough may appear narrow or foreshortened on the resultant image. Consequently, the anterior region of the orthopantomogram may be unrepresentative; reliability may be complicated further by inaccurate patient positioning within the machine.

Therefore, panoramic radiography can be supplemented with intra-oral views to provide greater detail, particularly in the maxillary anterior region. Furthermore, intra-oral views, including peri-apical radiographs and occlusal views (Witcher et al., 2010), may highlight the position of unerupted teeth using the parallax technique.

Cephalometric analysis

A cephalometric radiograph is taken in a standardized and reproducible manner using a cephalostat, which orientates the subject at a fixed distance from the X-ray tube and film during the exposure. This means that image magnification is constant for each individual machine, which allows the direct comparison of cephalometric views taken of one individual at different time points or between individuals. The most common view used in orthodontics is the cephalometric lateral skull radiograph, although occasionally postero-anterior views of the skull are taken to aid in the diagnosis of facial asymmetries or the localization of impacted teeth.

This section describes a simple and easily applied analysis for a cephalometric lateral skull radiograph that can be used to supplement the clinical examination.

A simple cephalometric analysis and mean Caucasian values

SNA	[81]
SNB	[78]
ANB	[3]
SN Mx	[8-11]
Wits Appraisal	[0-1]
FMA	[27]
MMPA	[27]
UI Mx	[109]
LI Md	[93]
Interincisor Angle	[135]
LI to APo	[2]
Upper lip E-plane	[-4]
Lower Lip E-Plane	[-2]
Nasolabial Angle	[108]
TAFH	[119]
UAFH	[54]
I AFH	[65]
% LAFH	[55]

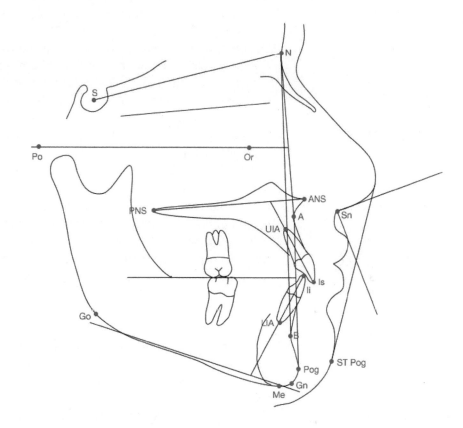

Figure 1.19

The analysis provides useful numerical information on the skeletal base relationship, position of the dentition within the face and the soft tissue profile. This aids in understanding the aetiology of a malocclusion and therefore is a valuable component of diagnosis and treatment planning. In addition, cephalometrics can be used as a definitive measurable baseline record to monitor treatment progress and growth by superimposition of serial radiographs.

When should a cephalometric radiograph be taken?

A cephalometric lateral skull radiograph should not be taken routinely on all patients. The decision can be justified in a number of circumstances, but this view is normally recommended if treatment of the malocclusion will involve:

- Significant anterior or posterior incisor movement
- Correction of a skeletal discrepancy with growth modification or orthognathic surgery

- Monitoring, or possible early interventional treatment in a young patient for a marked skeletal discrepancy.

A simple cephalometric analysis is described for routine orthodontic cases (Figure 1.19). The component cephalometric points, constructed lines and both angular and linear measurements are described. Mean Caucasian values are also provided.

Cephalometric landmarks

A number of hard and soft tissue cephalometric points need to be identified on the cephalometric lateral skull radiograph prior to applying an analysis (Box 1.2). These form the basis of construction for the relevant lines and planes, and allow the appropriate linear and angular measurements for the chosen analysis to be made.

The following points provide the basis for a simple analysis:

BOX 1.2 CEPHALOMETRIC HARD AND SOFT TISSUE LANDMARKS

Sella (S)	Midpoint of sella turcica (= posterior limit of the anterior cranial base)
Nasion (N)	Most anterior point on the fronto-nasal suture (= anterior limit of the anterior cranial base)
A point	Deepest point on the curved profile of the maxilla between the anterior nasal spine and alveolar crest (= anterior limit of the maxillary skeletal base and forms the superior landmark for construction of the A–Po line)
B point	Deepest point on the curved profile of the mandible between the chin and alveolar crest (= anterior limit of the mandibular skeletal base)
Porion (Po)	Uppermost and outermost point on the external auditory meatus (= posterior landmark for the Frankfort plane)
Orbitale (Or)	Most inferior and anterior point on the orbital margin (= anterior landmark for the Frankfort plane)
Gnathion (Gn)	Most anterior and inferior point on the chin
Menton (Me)	Most inferior point of the mandibular symphysis in the midline (= anterior landmark for the mandibular plane)
Pogonion (Pog)	Most anterior point on the chin (= inferior landmark for the A–Po line)
Gonion (Go)	Most posterior and inferior point on the angle of the mandible (= posterior landmark for the mandibular plane)
Posterior nasal spine (PNS)	Tip of the bony posterior nasal spine in the midline (= posterior landmark of the maxillary plane)
Anterior nasal spine (ANS)	Tip of the midline bony anterior nasal spine (= anterior landmark for the maxillary plane)
Incisor superius (Is)	Tip of the crown of the most anterior maxillary central incisor (= lower landmark for maxillary central incisor long axis)
Upper incisor apex (UIA)	Apex of the most anterior maxillary central incisor root (= upper landmark for the maxillary central incisor long axis)
Incisor inferius (Ii)	Tip of the crown of the most anterior mandibular central incisor (upper landmark for mandibular central incisor long axis)
Lower incisor apex (LIA)	Apex of the most anterior mandibular central incisor root (= lower landmark for mandibular central incisor long axis)

The soft tissue profile should also be traced and the following points identified:

Subnasale (Sn)	The point of intersection between the nasal septum and upper lip along the mid-sagittal plane
Soft tissue pogonion	Most anterior point on the soft tissue chin

Skeletal base relationships

The antero-posterior and vertical skeletal relationship can be measured on a cephalometric lateral skull radiograph (Box 1.3).

Antero-posterior skeletal base relationship: The antero-posterior relationships of the maxilla and mandible are assessed in relation to the anterior cranial base by measuring the SNA and SNB angles. A significant increase in these values when compared to population norms can indicate maxillary or mandibular protrusion (prognathia) relative to the anterior cranial base; whilst a reduction is indicative of retrusion (retrognathia).

The subtracted difference between the SNA and SNB angle (the angle ANB) will give an indication of the antero-posterior relationship between maxilla and mandible:

- ANB = 2–4 degrees: Skeletal class I
- ANB >4 degrees: Skeletal class II
- ANB <2 degrees: Skeletal class III.

BOX 1.3 WHAT DIAGNOSTIC INFORMATION CAN BE OBTAINED FROM A CEPHALOMETRIC ANALYSIS?

SNA   Position of the maxilla in relation to the anterior cranial base

SNB   Position of the mandible in relation to the anterior cranial base

ANB   Relative position of maxilla and mandible in relation to the anterior cranial base:
- Values <4 degrees indicate a class II relationship
- Values >2 degrees indicate a class III relationship

This therefore confirms the skeletal discrepancy

MMPA   Vertical relationship of the maxilla and mandible:
- Increased MMPA value (high angle) cases are associated with posterior growth rotation, which results in a tendency towards a reduced overbite or anterior open bite. In a growing individual this suggests that the overbite may reduce with further growth. There is often more rapid space loss in high angle cases and it is sensible to avoid extrusive mechanics during treatment as these may reduce the overbite further.
- Reduced MMPA value (low angle) cases are associated with anterior growth rotations. These are more associated with increased overbite, which may worsen with future growth. In these cases there may be difficulty with space closure during treatment, which can indicate treatment on a non-extraction basis.

UI Mx   Inclination of upper central incisors to the maxillary plane:
- The inclination of the upper incisor teeth can illustrate an existing compensation for a skeletal discrepancy. For example, class III cases can be associated with retroclined lower incisors and proclined upper incisors in the presence of a class III skeletal pattern. An increase in inclination of the upper incisors classifies the incisor position as being proclined. In clinical practice this may alter treatment mechanics based on the need to improve the inclination of the upper incisors. For example, in a case being treated with a functional appliance where the upper incisors are proclined, a labial bow may be incorporated in the appliance design to retrocline the upper incisors.
- When the upper incisors are of average inclination in the presence of a skeletal class II pattern, this may indicate the need for bodily retraction during treatment to avoid excessive retroclination.
- In class II cases where the upper incisors are retroclined (class II division 2 cases) this indicates a need for palatal root torque (which is anchorage demanding) during treatment.
- Where the upper incisors are retroclined in class III cases, this may indicate some scope to procline the upper incisors during treatment and camouflage the skeletal discrepancy.

LI Md   Antero-posterior position of the lower incisors is important during treatment planning

Changes in inclination of the lower incisors as a result of treatment are thought to affect stability

Lower incisor inclination can also reflect the presence of dento-alveolar compensation

A-Pog   Pleasing facial aesthetics

Stability of antero-posterior lower incisor position

Measuring jaw position in relation to the anterior cranial base can be problematic because alterations in the SN plane caused by erroneous positions of either sella or nasion can influence the SNA and SNB values. If the position of nasion is at fault, this will also influence ANB. The **Eastman correction** is available to overcome this:
- For every degree SNA is greater than 81 degrees, 0.5 degrees° should be subtracted from the ANB value
- For every degree SNA is less than 81 degrees, 0.5 degrees should be added to the ANB value.

This correction for ANB can only be applied for changes in the position of nasion, which is indicated by a SN–maxillary plane within the normal range of 8 ± 3 degrees.

An SN–maxillary plane value outside this range indicates that the position of sella is at fault. Because this affects the SNA and SNB values to the same extent, the ANB value does not require correction.

However, the Eastman correction is associated with some overestimation of the true values as nasion moves both anteriorly and posteriorly in relation to sella and therefore, should only be used as a very approximate guide (Kamaluddin *et al.*, 2011).

To avoid errors associated with discrepancies of the position of the cranial base within the skull it is advisable to carry out an additional analysis that is independent of this region. This is easily achieved by using the **Wits appraisal of jaw disharmony**. This relates the jaws to the functional occlusal plane (FOP, which passes through the occlusion of the first permanent molars and premolars) via perpendicular lines drawn from A point and B point (AO and BO, respectively):

- For boys, BO should lie 1 mm ahead of AO in a class I relationship
- For girls, BO and AO should be coincident in a class I relationship.

Thus, a class II relationship is associated with AO being positioned ahead of BO for both sexes. A class III relationship occurs in boys when BO is positioned greater than 1 mm ahead of AO, whilst for girls any position of BO ahead of AO is class III. It should be remembered however, that there is error associated with locating the functional occlusal plane, which can lead to some inaccuracy in assessing the jaw relationship using this method.

Vertical skeletal base relationship: The vertical relationship between maxilla and mandible can be assessed by angular measurement and in relation to the face using linear values.

The maxillary–mandibular planes angle (MMPA) provides a useful angular measurement of the vertical jaw relationship. The maxillary plane is represented by a line constructed through ANS–PNS, whilst the mandibular plane is constructed using a line through Go–Me. The mean value of the MMPA is 27 ± 5 degrees. An alternative value is the Frankfort–mandibular plane angle (FMPA), with the Frankfort plane constructed as a line through Or–Po and this should also be 27 ± 5 degrees.

The upper and lower anterior face heights provide a linear measurement of face height and their ratio provides an indication of vertical facial proportion. The total anterior face height (TAFH) is measured from nasion to menton (mean value = 119 mm). The upper anterior face height (UAFH) extends from nasion to ANS (mean value = 54 mm), whilst the lower anterior face height (LAFH) is measured from ANS to menton (mean value = 65 mm). The LAFH should be approximately 55 ± 2% of the TAFH when measured cephalometrically.

Dental analysis

The position of the upper and lower incisors can be measured on a cephalometric lateral skull radiograph, both in relation to the individual jaws, the lower third of the face and to each other.

Incisor inclination: The upper and lower incisor inclinations are measured to the maxillary plane (UI Mx = 109 ± 6 degrees) and mandibular plane (LI Md = 93 ± 6 degrees), respectively.

Lower incisor inclination can be influenced by the mandibular plane angle, with an increase in this value being associated with retroclination and a decrease with proclination. A simple compensation can be applied to obtain the ideal lower incisor inclination for a particular mandibular plane angle by subtracting the MMPA value from 120 degrees.

Lower incisors: The position of the mandibular incisors within the face is often used as an aid to treatment planning. A relatively quick and simple means of assessing this is provided by measuring the distance of the lower incisor tip to a line constructed from A point to pogonion (A-Pog). In a well-balanced face the lower incisor edge should be approximately 1 mm (±2) ahead of A-Pog.

Inter-incisal angle: The inter-incisal angulation (UI–LI) should also be measured and has a mean value of 133 ± 10 degrees.

Soft tissue analysis

A multitude of soft tissue analyses have been described but two useful and relatively simple measurements are provided by the naso-labial angle (NLA) and Ricketts' Esthetic-line (or E-line).

- The NLA is formed at the intersection of a line extending from the subnasale tangent to the columella of the nose and upper lip. The average value is 110 ± 10 degrees.
- The E-line extends from the nasal tip to the soft tissue pogonion. Both lips should be behind this line, the upper by around 4 mm and the lower 2 mm.

Both of these relationships can be unduly influenced by morphology of the nose. The distance of the lips to the E-line is age-related, with both tending to become more retrusive with age. However, together they provide a useful assessment of lip position within the facial profile and supplement the antero-posterior skeletal analysis.

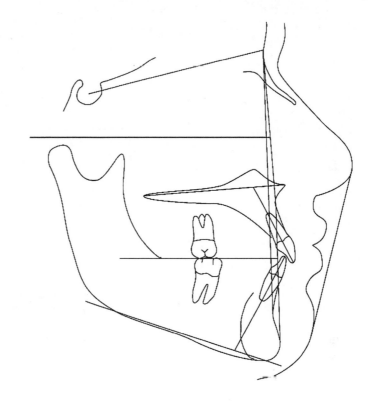

SNA	81
SNB	77
ANB	4
SN Mx	9
Wits Appraisal	1
FMA	18
MMPA	22
UI Mx	113
LI Md	100
Interincisor Angle	123
LI to APo	3
Upper lip E-plane	-4
Lower Lip E-Plane	-3
Nasolabial Angle	97
TAFH	135
UAFH	58
LAFH	76
% LAFH	56

Figure 1.20

Describe the essential features of the associated malocclusion in the cephalometric tracing in Figure 1.20

The maxilla and mandible are positioned normally in relation to the anterior cranial base (SNA and SNB are both normal) and the jaw relationship is class I because the ANB value is 4 degrees. Wits appraisal is +1 mm, which together with the ANB confirms a skeletal class I relationship.

Although MMPA and FMPA are reduced (MMPA = 22 degrees and FMPA = 18 degrees), the percentage LAFH is very slightly increased at 58%.

How is the dentition positioned within the face?

The dental relationship is characterized by a class I incisor relationship. The maxillary incisors are slightly proclined at 113 degrees, whilst the mandibular incisors are also proclined at 100 degrees and this is reflected in a reduced inter-incisal angle. The relationship of the mandibular incisor edge to the A-Pog line is +3 mm, which is essentially normal.

The naso-labial angle is reduced, almost certainly associated with quite a prominent upper lip morphology and both lips are situated behind the E-line, indicating a slightly retrusive facial profile.

Summary

A class I case on a skeletal class I base with average vertical proportions. The incisors are a little proclined and the profile is very slightly retrusive.

Describe the skeletal base relationship in Figure 1.21

The maxilla and mandible are positioned anteriorly in relation to the anterior skeletal base (SNA and SNB are both increased), but the jaw relationship is class II because the ANB value is increased (6 degrees). The anterior position of nasion can be corrected using the Eastman correction, and this reduces the ANB value to 2 degrees, making the jaw relationship class I. However, Wits appraisal is +6 mm, which together with the ANB is overall suggestive of a mild class II relationship.

The vertical jaw relationship is reduced (MMPA = 21 degrees and FMPA = 17 degrees), although the percentage LAFH is essentially normal at 54%.

How is the dentition positioned within the face?

The dental relationship is characterized by an increased overjet, with proclined maxillary incisors. The mandibular incisors are slightly retroclined and this is

SNA	89
SNB	83
ANB	6
SN Mx	3
Wits Appraisal	6
FMA	17
MMPA	21
UI Mx	126
LI Md	88
Interincisor Angle	124
LI to APo	-2
Upper lip E-plane	-0
Lower Lip E-Plane	-3
Nasolabial Angle	117
TAFH	106
UAFH	47
LAFH	58
% LAFH	54

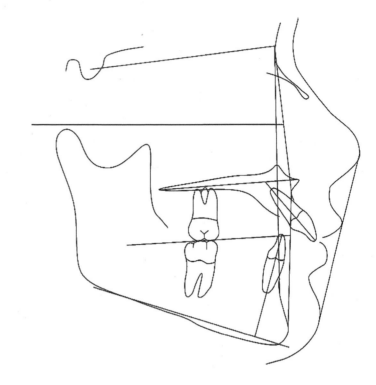

Figure 1.21

reflected in an increased inter-incisal angle. The relationship of the mandibular incisor edge to the A-Pog line is –2 mm, which is consistent with their slightly upright position.

The naso-labial angle is increased and the lower lip is situated behind the E-line, indicating a slightly retrusive facial profile.

Summary

A class II division 1 case on a moderate skeletal class II base with reduced vertical proportions. The upper incisors are proclined and the profile is slightly retrusive.

Describe the skeletal base relationship in Figure 1.22

In this example, the maxilla and mandible are set back in relation to the anterior skeletal base (SNA and SNB are both reduced quite significantly) and the ANB value is reduced, making this a skeletal class III base relationship with some bi-maxillary retrognathia. Whilst the low SNA value does suggest that the maxilla is set back within the face, it may also be due to a high or forward position of nasion or inferior position of sella. The SN–Mx value of 12 degrees means that it is likely to be an inferiorly positioned sella and the Eastman correction cannot be applied to the ANB value. A Wits

appraisal value of –3 mm confirms a mild class III jaw relationship.

The vertical jaw relationship is increased (MMPA and FMPA are both 36 degrees), although the percentage LAFH is only very slightly increased at 57%.

How is the dentition positioned within the face?

The dental relationship is characterized by a reduced overjet and overbite, with slight proclination of the maxillary incisors. The mandibular incisors appear retroclined, although if the increased MMPA value is taken into account, they are actually within the normal range (120 – 36 = 84 degrees) and the inter-incisal angle is increased. The relationship of the mandibular incisor edge to the A-Pog line is –2 mm, which is consistent with their slightly upright position.

The naso-labial angle is significantly increased and both lips are situated behind the E-line, indicating a slightly retrusive facial profile.

Summary

A class III case on a mild skeletal class III base with increased vertical proportions. The incisor relationship reflects this, with upper incisors that are slightly

SNA	72
SNB	71
ANB	1
SN Mx	12
Wits Appraisal	-3
FMA	36
MMPA	36
UI Mx	112
LI Md	88
Interincisor Angle	123
LI to APo	6
Upper lip E-plane	-3
Lower Lip E-Plane	-1
Nasolabial Angle	138
TAFH	120
UAFH	51
LAFH	69
% LAFH	57

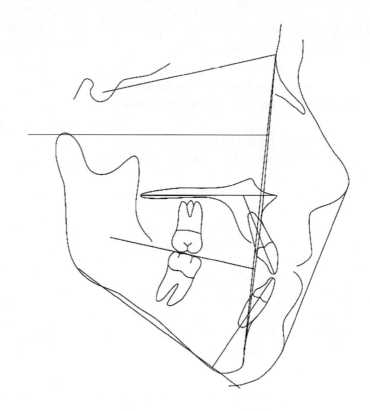

Figure 1.22

proclined, lower incisors that are retroclined and a reduced, incomplete overbite.

What technique has been carried out in Figure 1.23?

Structural superimposition of two cephalometric radiographs along the anterior cranial base. In this case SN has been used to represent the anterior cranial base and the radiographs have been registered at sella.

How accurate is this technique?

Neither S or N are completely stable structures in a growing individual and growth will influence their position, particularly vertical change at nasion.

Superimposition can also be done using the radiographic anatomy of the anterior cranial base, using either the method described by deCoster or a subsequent modification described by Björk and Skieller.

Which structures define the anterior cranial base according to Björk and Skieller's method?

- Anterior wall of sella turcica
- Cribriform plate of the ethmoid

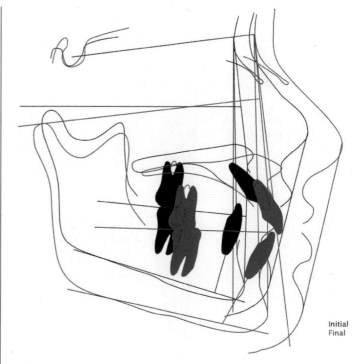

Initial
Final

Figure 1.23

- Fronto-ethmoidal crests
- Cerebral surface of the orbital roof

How does Ricketts' method differ from superimposition along the anterior cranial base?

Ricketts' method uses the entire length of the cranial base along a line constructed from nasion to basion (the point on the anterior margin of the foramen magnum where the mid-sagittal plane of the skull intersects the plane of the foramen magnum). For investigating mandibular changes, registration takes place at the CC point, which is the point of intersection of a line constructed from the pterygomaxillare (Pt) to gnathion (which represents the facial axis). For maxillary changes, registration takes place at nasion. Pterygomaxillare is supposed to represent the foramen rotundum, the point of exit of the maxillary branch of the trigeminal nerve from the intra-cranial cavity and to be a position of stability.

How would you summarize the changes that have taken place in Figure 1.23?

A class II division 1 malocclusion has been corrected and this has been achieved by skeletal and dento-alveolar changes. In particular, there has been downward and forward growth of the maxilla, forward and vertical growth of the mandible, retroclination of the maxillary incisors and proclination of the mandibular incisors. Overall, the initial skeletal class II pattern and retrognathia has improved.

What does the angle x represent in Figure 1.24? (where Na = nasion, Pog = pogonion and LS = upper lip)

x = the H-angle of Holdaway. This forms part of the Holdaway soft tissue analysis and is formed by the intersection of soft tissue nasion to soft tissue pogonion and a line tangent to the chin point and the upper lip (or Harmony (H) line). The H line measures the degree of upper lip prominence or soft tissue chin retrognathia. The desired value of the H angle is dependent upon the underlying skeletal convexity of the subject (measured as the distance from A point to the line Na–Pog). The greater the skeletal convexity, the larger the desired H angle. However, the normal range is 7–15 degrees (Holdaway, 1983; 1984).

References

Andrews LF (1972) The six keys to normal occlusion. *Am J Orthod* 62:296–309.

Arndt EM, Travis F, Lefebvre A, Niec A, Munro IR (1986) Beauty and the eye of the beholder: social consequences and personal adjustments for facial patients. *Br J Plast Surg* 39:81–84.

Arnett GW, Bergman RT (1993) Facial keys to orthodontic diagnosis and treatment planning: Part 1. *Am J Orthod Dentofacial Orthop* 10:299–312.

Ahlstedt S (1984) Penicillin allergy – can the incidence be reduced? *Allergy* 39:151–164.

Arias OR, Marquez-Orozco MC (2006) Aspirin, acetaminophen, and ibuprofen: their effects on orthodontic tooth movement. *Am J Orthod Dentofacial Orthop* 130:364–370.

Brook AH (1984) A unifying aetiological explanation for anomalies of human tooth number and size. *Arch Oral Biol* 29:373–378.

Brook PH, Shaw WC (1989) The development of an index of orthodontic treatment priority. *Eur J Orthod* 11:309–320.

Büyükyilmaz T, Zachrisson YO, Zachrisson BU (1995) Improving orthodontic bonding to gold alloy. *Am J Orthod Dentofacial Orthop* 108:510–518.

Egermark I, Carlsson GE, Magnusson T (2005) A prospective long-term study of signs and symptoms of temporomadibular disorders in patients who received orthodontic treatment in childhood. *Angle Orthod* 75:645–650.

Egermark-Eriksson I, Ingervall B, Carlsson GE (1983) The dependence of mandibular dysfunction in children on functional and morphologic malocclusion. *Am J Orthod* 83:187–194.

Fleming PS, Xavier GM, DiBiase AT, Cobourne MT (2010) Revisiting the supernumerary: the epidemiological

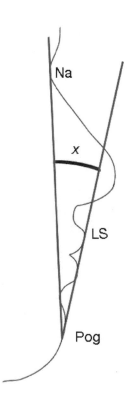

Figure 1.24

and molecular basis of extra teeth. *Br Dent J* 208: 25–30.

Frush JO, Fisher RD (1958) The disesthetic interpretation of the dentogenic concept. *J Prosthet Dent* 8:558.

Germane N, Staggers JA, Rubenstein L, Revere JT (1992) Arch length considerations due to the curve of Spee: a mathematical model. *Am J Orthod Dentofacial Orthop* 102:251–255.

Harris JE (1975) Genetic factors in the growth of the head: inheritance of the craniofacial complex and malocclusion. *Dent Clin North Am* 19:151–160.

Hirsch C (2009) No increased risk of temporomandibular disorders and bruxism in children and adolescents during orthodontic therapy. *J Orofac Orthop* 70:39–50.

Holdaway RA (1983) A soft-tissue cephalometric analysis and its use in orthodontic treatment planning. Part I. *Am J Orthod* 84:1–28.

Holdaway RA (1984) A soft-tissue cephalometric analysis and its use in orthodontic treatment planning. Part II. *Am J Orthod* 85:279–293.

Isiksal E, Hazar S, Akyalcin S (2006) Smile esthetics: perception and comparison of treated and untreated smiles *Am J Orthod Dentofacial Orthop* 129:8–16.

Kamaluddin JM, Cobourne MT, Sherriff M, Bister D (2011) Does the Eastman correction over- or under-adjust ANB for positional changes of N? *Eur J Orthod* [Epub ahead of print].

Kindelan SA, Day PF, Spencer JR, Duggal MS (2008) Dental trauma: an overview of its influence on the management of orthodontic treatment. Part 1. *J Orthod* 35:68–78.

Keene HJ (1963) Distribution of diastema in the dentition of man. *Am J Phys Anthrop* 21:437–441.

Kirschen RH, O'Higgins EA, Lee RT (2000a) The Royal London Space Planning: an integration of space analysis and treatment planning: Part I: Assessing the space required to meet treatment objectives. *Am J Orthod Dentofacial Orthop* 118:448–455.

Kirschen RH, O'Higgins EA, Lee RT (2000b) The Royal London Space Planning: an integration of space analysis and treatment planning: Part II: The effect of other treatment procedures on space. *Am J Orthod Dentofacial Orthop* 118:456–461.

Litton SF, Ackermann LV, Issacson R, Shapiro BL (1970) A genetic study of Class III malocclusion. *Am J Orthod* 58:565–577.

Luther F, Layton S, McDonald F (2010) Orthodontics for treating temporomandibular joint (TMJ) disorders. *Cochrane Database Syst Rev* 7:CD006541.

Mohlin B, Axelsson S, Paulin G, *et al.* (2007) TMD in relation to malocclusion and orthodontic treatment. *Angle Orthod* 77:542–548.

Mugonzibwa EA, Eskeli R, Laine-Alava MT, Kuijpers-Jagtman AM, Katsaros C (2008) Spacing and crowding among African and Caucasian children. *Orthod Craniofac Res* 11:82–89.

Murray AM (1989) Discontinuation of orthodontic treatment: a study of the contributing factors. *Br J Orthod* 16:1–7.

Nanda RS, Meng H, Kapila S, Goorhuis J (1990) Growth changes in the soft tissue facial profile. *Angle Orthod* 60:177–190.

NICE (2008) Short Clinical Guidelines Technical Team. Prophylaxis against infective endocarditis: Antimicrobial prophylaxis against Infective endocarditis in adults and children undergoing interventional procedures. London: National Institute for Health and Clinical Excellence.

Nielsen NH, Menne T (1993) Nickel sensitisation and ear piercing in an unselected Danish population. *Contact Dermatitis* 29:16–21.

O'Brien K, Wright J, Conboy F, *et al.* (2003) Effectiveness of early orthodontic treatment with the Twin-block appliance: a multicenter, randomised, controlled trial. Part 2: Psychosocial effects. *Am J Orthod Dentofac Orthoped* 129:488–494.

Patel A, Burden DJ, Sandler J (2009) Medical disorders and orthodontics. *J Orthod* 36:1–21.

Richardson ER, Malhotra SK, Henry M, Little RG, Coleman HT (1973) Biracial study of the maxillary midline diastema. *Angle Orthod* 43:438–443.

Richmond S, O'Brien KD, Roberts CT (1994) Dentists' variation in the determination of orthodontic treatment need. *Br J Orthod* 21:65–68.

Sarver DM (2001) The importance of incisor positioning in the esthetic smile: The smile arc. *Am J Orthod Dentofacial Orthop* 120:98–111.

Sarver DM, Weissman SM (1995) Nonsurgical treatment of open bite in nongrowing patients. *Am J Orthod Dentofacial Orthop* 108:651–659.

Seehra J, Fleming PS, Newton T, DiBiase AT (2011) Bullying in orthodontic patients and its relationship to malocclusion, self-esteem and oral health-related quality of life. *J Orthod* 38:274–286.

Shaw WC, Gabe MJ, Jones BM (1979) The expectations of orthodontic patients in South Wales and St. Louis, Missouri. *Br J Orthod* 6:203–205.

Shaw WC, Meek SC, Jones DS (1980) Nicknames, teasing, harassment and the salience of dental features among school children. *Br J Orthod* 7:75–80.

Shaw WC, O'Brien KD, Brook P (1991) Quality control in orthodontics: risk/ benefit considerations. *Br Dent J* 170:33–37.

Sheller B, Williams B (1996) Orthdontic management of patients with haematological malignancies. *Am J Orthod Dentofacial Orthop* 109:575–580.

van der Linden FP (1974) Theoretical and practical aspects of crowding in the human dentition. *J Am Dent Assoc* 89:139–153.

Watanabe M, Suda N, Ohyama K (2005) Mandibular prognathism in Japanese families ascertained through orthognathically treated patients. *Am J Orthod Dentofacial Orthop* 128:466–470.

Witcher TP, Brand S, Gwilliam JR, McDonald F (2010) Assessment of the anterior maxilla in orthodontic patients using upper anterior occlusal radiographs and dental panoramic tomography: a comparison. *Oral Surg Oral Med Oral Pathol Oral Radiol Endod* 109:765–774.

Zachrisson BU, Büyükyilmaz T, Zachrisson YO (1995) Improving orthodontic bonding to silver amalgam. *Angle Orthod* 65:35–42.

2

The Developing Dentition

Introduction

Human dental development consists of three stages: establishment of the primary dentition; the mixed dentition stage following eruption of the first permanent molars and incisors; and completion of the secondary (or permanent) dentition with eruption of the remaining permanent teeth, including the third molars if present.

Monitoring dental development with appropriate intervention (interceptive treatment) is an important aspect of orthodontics. Problems that can occur in either the primary or mixed dentitions are essentially anomalies in the developmental process, functional problems or early presentation of an underlying malocclusion, all of which may warrant early treatment. These include:
- Delay or failure of eruption of teeth
- Developmentally absent teeth (hypodontia)
- Supernumerary (extra) teeth
- Anomalous teeth (abnormal morphology)
- Early tooth loss due to dental trauma or caries (often resulting in space loss)
- Anterior and posterior crossbites with or without displacement
- Persistent habits such as digit sucking
- Early manifestation of tooth/arch size discrepancies (e.g. spacing or crowding)
- Early manifestation of skeletal discrepancies (moderate-to-severe class II and III cases).

Examples of interceptive treatment include:
- Elective extraction of primary teeth to encourage favourable eruption of permanent teeth, which may be ectopic in position; e.g. removal of maxillary primary canines to encourage an improvement in the position of ectopic maxillary canines.
- Elective extraction of first permanent molars of poor prognosis, with a view to encouraging the second permanent molars to erupt further forward in the arch.
- Space maintenance following early loss of primary teeth or for maintenance of the Leeway space.
- Treatment with removable or fixed appliances: to correct anterior or posterior crossbites associated with a significant displacement.
- Surgical exposure of impacted maxillary incisors, followed by removable or fixed appliances to apply traction to the impacted tooth or teeth, in order to facilitate eruption.
- Attempts at 'growth modification' may include functional appliances to address skeletal discrepancies in class II or class III cases, or the use of protraction headgear for management of maxillary hypoplasia, (with or without rapid maxillary expansion) in skeletal class III cases.

The merits of initiating orthodontics in the early mixed dentition has been debated and researched (Jolley et al., 2010). Generally, early or interceptive treatment should aim either to eliminate a problem or to simplify subsequent treatment. Focused aims and objectives avoid unnecessary or protracted treatment.

Advocates of early treatment claim that it optimizes growth potential when addressing skeletal problems, leads to better compliance, reduces risk of trauma in class II division 1 malocclusions, enhances

Clinical Cases in Orthodontics, First Edition. Martyn T. Cobourne, Padhraig S. Fleming, Andrew T. DiBiase, and Sofia Ahmad.
© 2012 Martyn T. Cobourne, Padhraig S. Fleming, Andrew T. DiBiase, and Sofia Ahmad. Published 2012 by Blackwell Publishing Ltd.

psychological wellbeing and limits or even eliminates the need for a second course of treatment in adolescence.

While all of these claims have merit and may be applicable to individual cases, the majority of orthodontic treatment can be successfully and efficiently carried out in the late mixed and early permanent dentition.

There is more positive evidence for early correction of some aspects of malocclusion than others. For example, it is generally accepted practice to correct an anterior or posterior crossbite early if there is a functional displacement. Maintenance of the Leeway space during the transition from the mixed to permanent dentition has also been shown to be an effective way of providing space to treat mild crowding (Little *et al.*, 1990; Brennan and Gianelly, 2000). Some early treatments are less widely accepted, e.g. there appears to be less evidence for early treatment designed to expand the dental arches in the mixed dentition to treat crowding.

The long-term results of early treatment for class II division 1 malocclusions are no better if treatment is started in the late mixed dentition in relation to growth or occlusal outcome. The only reported differences are the additional cost and duration of the treatment (Tulloch *et al.*, 2004).

Case 2.1

This is a 12-year-old child referred by her general dental practitioner (Figure 2.1). She is fit and well, but concerned about the prominence of her front teeth.

At what stage of development is her dentition in the clinical photographs?

She is in the early permanent dentition. The second permanent molars are unerupted, with the exception of the LL7, which is partially erupted.

What are the main features of her malocclusion?

- Class II division 1 incisor relationship with an increased overjet and increased overbite, which is complete to the palate

- Molar relationship is ½ unit class II on the right and class I on the left
- Centre lines are coincident
- Erupted supplemental UL2

Why is the molar relationship not the same on both sides?

The presence of an additional tooth in the upper left quadrant, but essentially coincident centre lines, means that the UL6 is positioned more distal than it would normally be – hence a class I relationship rather than class II.

How common are supernumerary teeth?

In the permanent dentition supernumerary teeth are seen in 0.1–3.2% of individuals. Caucasian males are more commonly affected than females in a ratio of 2:1 (Fleming *et al.*, 2010). The reported prevalence in the primary dentition ranges from 0.06% to 0.8% with no associated sexual dimorphism.

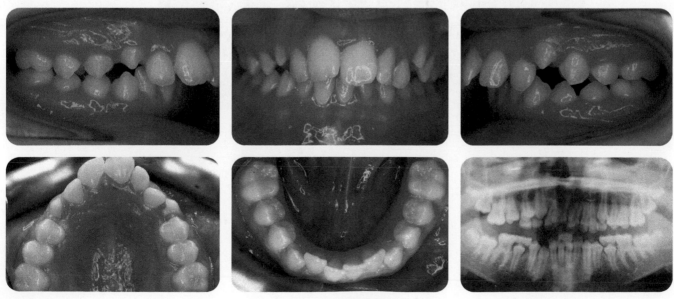

Figure 2.1

Where are supernumerary teeth most likely to be seen?

In the anterior maxilla.

What other forms of supernumerary teeth are seen in the permanent dentition?

The other forms are conical, tuberculate and odontome (complex and compound).

What consequences can supernumerary teeth have for the developing dentition?

If a supernumerary tooth erupts, it can cause localized crowding or spacing. If it remains unerupted, it can cause impaction or displacement of teeth, or occasionally may become cystic.

In the case described, what is the likeliest course of action?

The underlying malocclusion will require treatment to reduce the overjet and overbite, and align and co-ordinate the dental arches. To achieve this, the supernumerary tooth will require extraction; otherwise a tooth-size discrepancy would be present between the arches, making it impossible to achieve a co-ordinated class I occlusion.

When deciding which tooth to extract, generally the supernumerary tooth is chosen; however, the coronal and root anatomy of both the normal and supernumerary teeth should be evaluated carefully before making the final extraction decision. In this case the most distal (supplemental) lateral incisor was extracted. Following functional appliance treatment and fixed appliances the final occlusion is shown in Figure 2.2.

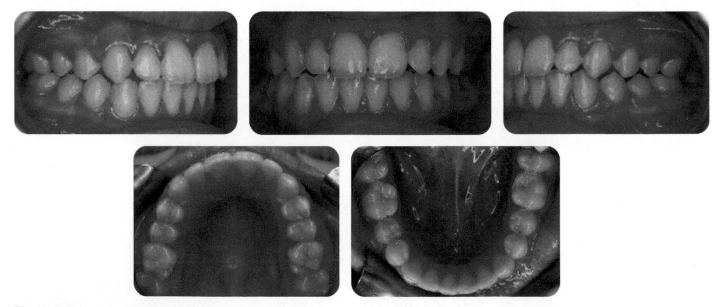

Figure 2.2

Case 2.2

This 9-year-old female was referred by her general dental practitioner as she was concerned about the large gap between her upper and lower teeth ("my teeth don't meet at the front").

Summary

A 9-year-old female presented in the mixed dentition with a class II division 1 malocclusion on a mild skeletal class II pattern with average vertical facial proportions (Figure 2.3).

What is the most likely cause of the anterior open bite?

The most likely cause is a persistent digit sucking habit.

Treatment Plan

- Stop the digit sucking habit
- Monitor further dental development and plan comprehensive treatment upon cessation of the habit

What are the typical effects of a digit sucking habit on the developing dentition?

- Increased maxillary and relative prognathism
- Increased maxillary length

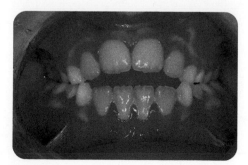

Figure 2.3

- Proclination of maxillary incisors
- Retroclination of mandibular incisors
- Increased overjet
- Reduced overbite
- Unilateral posterior crossbite

What factors influence the outcome of digit sucking?

The outcome of digit sucking is governed by the nature, frequency, intensity and duration of the habit (Larsson, 1987). A minimum threshold of 4–6 hours per day is believed to be required to produce a significant malocclusion. Specific effects are variable and often asymmetric, being mediated directly by the position of the digit or indirectly by alteration to tongue position.

What is the prevalence of digit sucking?

The prevalence of digit sucking is age-related. It has been reported as 12% of 9-year olds and 2% of 12-year olds (Brenchley, 1991).

What conservative techniques may be used to stop digit sucking?

Conservative methods of habit dissuasion are usually preferable to physical intervention in the first instance. Patient and parental education are instrumental (Levine, 1999). Non-invasive methods include:

- Positive reinforcement by reward and habit reversal where the child is taught to carry out an alternative activity when the urge to suck arises
- Use of plasters, gloves or bitter flavoured agents applied to the digit to make the habit less satisfying.

These non-invasive techniques should be attempted for 3–6 months and can be very successful in improving the occlusion.

What interceptive procedures may be performed to dissuade digit sucking?

Where the habit persists despite conservative measures, simple fixed orthodontic appliances including palatal arches, with one of a variety of projections (inverted goalposts, beads or cribs), may be used for 6–12 months. Use of removable orthodontic appliances may also be effective in these cases (Figures 2.4 and 2.5); however, they may be unsuccessful due to poor co-operation.

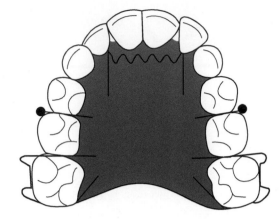

Figure 2.5

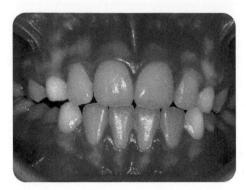

Figure 2.4

Case 2.3

This 12-year-old male was referred by his general dental practitioner because of a misplaced canine.

Summary

- Well-aligned arches in the late mixed dentition
- Retained, immobile maxillary primary canines
- Maxillary canines not palpable buccally

What Information does the panoramic radiograph provide (Figure 2.6)?

The UR3 is ectopic:

- Cusp tip of the UR3 crosses the UR2
- There is no evidence of root resorption of the URC
- There is no evidence of pathology.

Treatment Plan

- Extraction of both maxillary primary canines
- Review after 12 months

How common is impaction of the maxillary canine?

With the exception of the third molars, the maxillary canine is the most frequently impacted tooth with an incidence of 2–3% and a female predilection. The majority (up to 85%) lie palatal to the arch. Bilateral occurrence accounts for 8% of cases with ectopic maxillary canines (Ericson and Kurol, 1988).

The UR3 erupted 12 months after removal of the URC (Figure 2.7).

How useful is the interceptive removal of a primary maxillary canine in cases of maxillary permanent canine ectopia?

Interceptive removal of retained primary canines has been shown to promote favourable spontaneous alignment of the canine. In a prospective study, 78% of ectopic canines improved their position following removal of the upper primary canines in 10–13-year olds with well-aligned dental arches (Ericson and Kurol, 1988). The prognosis for spontaneous alignment reduces with greater mesial displacement of the canine tip (Ericson and Kurol, 1988; Power and Short, 1993). It is important to note that improvement in the eruption path of the permanent canine is unlikely to arise later than 12 months after the extraction of the primary canine.

How is maxillary canine ectopia diagnosed?

- Clinical inspection and palpation.
- Radiographs are a secondary measure. A survey of 505 Swedish schoolchildren has shown the

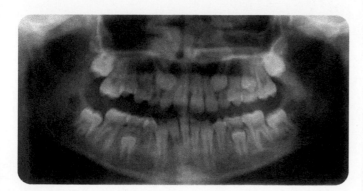

Figure 2.6

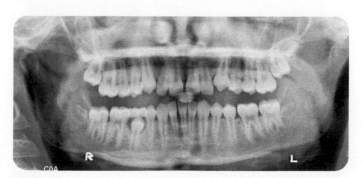

Figure 2.7

prevalence of non-palpable and unerupted canines where radiographic examination was necessary to be just 3% between 11 and 15 years (Ericson and Kurol, 1988).

What clinical features may be indicative of an ectopic maxillary canine?

- Non-palpable permanent canines in the buccal sulcus at 11–12 years of age
- Firm, immobile primary canine when the contra-lateral permanent canine has erupted 6 months earlier
- Significant displacement, including tipping and abnormal inclination of adjacent lateral incisors
- A palatal bulge in the presence of a firm retained primary canine
- Diminutive maxillary lateral incisors. Palatal impaction of canines is also associated with ectopic development, with 42% arising adjacent to diminutive or congenitally absent maxillary lateral incisors (Becker, 1984)

What other interceptive measures may be useful to encourage eruption while avoiding mechanical eruption?

Techniques, including expansion, space redistribution and distal molar movement, have all demonstrated higher levels of spontaneous eruption when compared with removal of primary canines in isolation (Baccetti et al., 2008; 2009).

Comment on the quality of evidence in relation to interceptive removal of primary canines and spontaneous eruption of canines

In a systematic literature review it has been suggested that the evidence in support of removal of primary canines to intercept ectopic development is unreliable (Parkin et al., 2009a). While a number of prospective studies have been published, the reviewers felt that they were poorly reported. Factors that should be considered when conducting trials in this area include: concealed random allocation, blind assessment, homogeneity of the groups at the beginning of the trial, correct statistical analysis taking into account clustering in patients with bilateral ectopic canines, and appropriate management of withdrawals.

Case 2.4

This case presented following referral from her general dental practitioner. She has a class I occlusion with minimal crowding and a grossly carious LL6, which the dentist has temporized. She has been having intermittent nocturnal pain associated with this tooth, which is now keeping her awake at night. An up-to-date panoramic radiograph was sent by the referring practitioner (Figure 2.8).

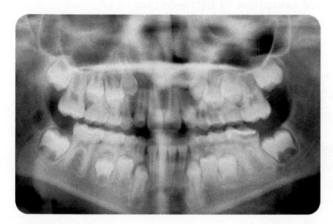

Figure 2.8

How old do you think she is?

Around 9–10 years of age.

Root development of the first molars is complete, which usually occurs around the age of 9.5 years.

What are the main features seen on the panoramic radiograph?

- Mixed dentition
- Incisors have erupted
- LL6 is grossly carious; there is evidence of periapical infection on the distal root and a temporary restoration is in place

- All the permanent teeth are present except the third molars (although there is some evidence of early follicular development of the LR8)
- Crown formation of the second molars is complete. In the mandibular arch, early development of the inter-radicular region has begun

The dentist does not believe the LL6 can be restored. What advice would you give?

Extract the LL6 and consider a compensating extraction of the UL6 to prevent over-eruption of this tooth. The lack of third molar development on the left side means that extraction of the UL6 is not ideal. However, there is early evidence of third molar development in the lower right quadrant and this, combined with the relatively young age of the patient, means that third molar development may well subsequently occur.

Alternatively, extraction of the UL6 might be delayed and the eruptive position monitored following extraction of the LL6.

The timing of extraction also needs to be considered, although in this case extraction should not be delayed because the patient is in pain. However, to ensure the best eruptive position for the lower second permanent molars, their development should be slightly more advanced and extraction of the LL6 carried out ideally in around 6 months' time. This is also dependent on the space requirement in the lower arch as if there is crowding that will require extractions to treat, it may be better to delay the extraction of the LL6 until the LL7 has erupted, so the space created can be used to relieve the crowding.

Other local problems

What dental abnormality is apparent in Figure 2.9?

Bilateral transposition of mandibular lateral incisors and canines.

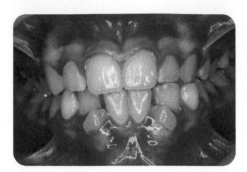

Figure 2.9

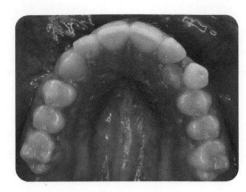

Figure 2.10

How is this anomaly classified?

Transpositions are classified by jaw of occurrence, tooth type and site. This bilateral transposition is classified as Mn.C.I2.

What is the difference between a true transposition and a pseudotransposition?

A true transposition involves both the crowns and roots of the affected teeth. A pseudotranspositon involves positional interchange of the crowns only.

What is the aetiology of dental transposition?

Transposition is a multifactorial disorder with both genetic and environmental contributions (Ely *et al.*, 2006).

Comment on the regional distribution of transpositions

Transpositions are most common in the maxillary arch and typically involve the canine. Involvement of the central incisors or molar teeth is uncommon. Bilateral transposition is less common than unilateral transposition in both arches. In bilateral cases, asymmetrical bilateral transposition is very rare.

Describe the appearance of the maxillary dental arch in Figure 2.10

A patient in the early permanent dentition with the UL3 erupted into a palatally-displaced position. The overlying ULC is retained. There is mild hypoplasia associated with the UR6.

What treatment is required?

Consideration should be given to removal of the primary canine as it is retained and likely to be displacing the permanent successor.

At what stage of root development do permanent teeth usually erupt?

A permanent tooth should erupt when approximately 75% of its root has formed.

What dental anomaly is apparent in Figure 2.11?

Infra-occlusion of the ULE and LLE.

How common is infra-occlusion?

Infra-occlusion most commonly affects primary molars with a prevalence of 5–11%.

How is the severity of infra-occlusion classified?

Infra-occlusion may be classified as mild, moderate or severe. It is diagnosed if the tooth had lost its vertical position relative to the neighbouring teeth. Moderately infra-occluded teeth lie below the level of adjacent contact points. Severely infra-occluded teeth are located at the level of or below the alveolar crest.

What two factors are most critical when planning treatment?

- Degree of infra-occlusion
- Presence of a permanent successor

If the permanent successor is present and the degree of infra-occlusion is mild, what treatment is usually required?

No active treatment is usually necessary, as the primary molar will normally exfoliate within the expected timeframe. Indications for removal of the involved primary tooth in such cases include severe infra-occlusion, beneath the adjacent contact points

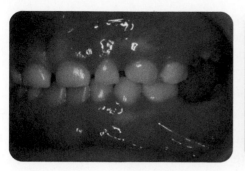

Figure 2.11

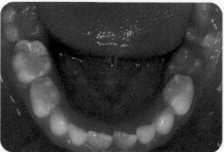

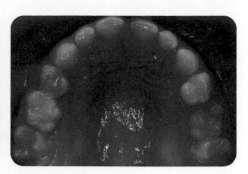

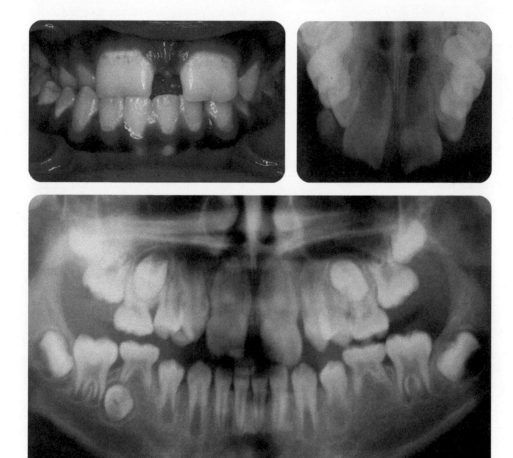

Figure 2.12

with a resultant risk of tipping of the adjacent teeth, and over-eruption of the opposing teeth.

Describe the dental features seen in this 15-year-old boy (Figure 2.12)

- Upper central and lateral incisors are double teeth
- LL5 is absent
- UL5, UR5 and LR5 are impacted
- LLE, ULE and LRE are retained

- Root formation associated with the canine and premolar dentitions is developmentally delayed

What is the difference between a double tooth and a megadont tooth?

A megadont tooth is one that is more than two standard deviations larger than the mean. It can be distinguished from a double tooth by an absence of coronal notching, relatively normal morphology and the presence of an appropriate number of teeth in the dental arch overall. Megadontia most commonly affects maxillary permanent central incisors and second premolars.

A double tooth occurs when there is hard tissue continuity between adjacent teeth.

Describe the dental features in Figure 2.13

- Primary dentition
- Class I incisor relationship
- Lower centre line displaced to the left
- Double tooth involving the LLB and LLC

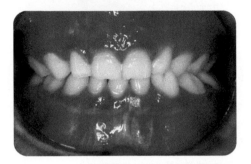

Figure 2.13

What is the condition seen in Figure 2.14?

Molar–incisor hypo-mineralization (MIH) – a condition associated with demarcated, qualitative defects of enamel of systemic origin affecting one or more permanent molars with or without involvement of the incisor teeth.

What is the cause of this condition?

The cause is currently unknown; however, there is some evidence to suggest that polychlorinated biphenyl/dioxin exposure is involved in the aetiology of MIH. Weaker evidence exists for the role of nutrition, birth and neonatal factors, and acute or chronic childhood illness/treatment; and there is very weak evidence to implicate fluoride or breastfeeding (Crombie et al., 2008).

How can MIH complicate future orthodontic treatment?

In severe cases:
- Difficulty bonding incisor teeth
- Need for first molar extraction (either enforced or elective).

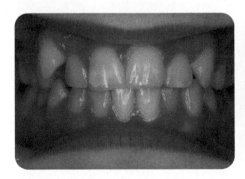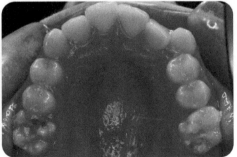

Figure 2.14

Case 2.5

A 10-year-old child was referred by her general dental practitioner concerning the appearance of the upper front teeth (Figure 2.15).

What are the main features of the occlusion?
- Mixed dentition
- Class II division 1 incisor relationship
- Absence of the UR1
- Crowding of the labial segments

What is the differential diagnosis?
- Impaction/failure of eruption of the UR1
- Previous loss of the UR1 following trauma
- Congenital absence of the UR1

What are the possible local causes of tooth impaction in the anterior maxilla?
- Supernumerary tooth
- Crowding
- Trauma and dilaceration
- Ectopic tooth germ position
- Retained primary teeth
- Local pathology

In this case, the UR1 was lost following trauma and avulsion. What potential problems are there in the long-term management of this malocclusion?
- There has been space loss in the anterior maxilla. This has occurred primarily by forward movement of the UR2 into the UR1 space, as the centre lines are coincident.
- Space could be regained at this stage with a simple fixed or removable appliance (possibly with extraction of the primary canines), followed by space maintenance with a removable retainer and pontic for the UR1. Definitive treatment could be undertaken in the permanent dentition with restoration of the UR1 space with a resin-retained bridge or dental implant.
- Alternatively, the space could be allowed to close spontaneously and the occlusion managed definitively in the early permanent dentition. This strategy has the advantage of maintaining alveolar bone height in the upper labial segment, which facilitates implant placement after space opening.
- In both strategies, extractions are likely to be required because of the underlying crowding.

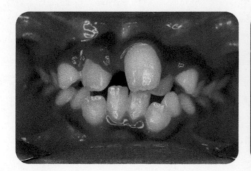
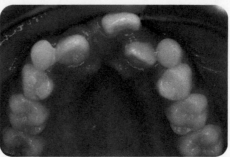

Figure 2.15

Case 2.6

This case is a 10-year-old boy referred by his general dental practitioner. He is fit and well, but the dentist is concerned about the appearance of his upper front teeth (Figure 2.16).

Summarize the main clinical features of this malocclusion

- A class III incisor relationship in the mixed dentition with a reduced and complete overbite
- Molar relationship is ½ unit class II bilaterally
- Upper centre line is displaced to the left
- UL1 is rotated mesio-palatally

Why is the molar relationship class II?

The lower Es are still present. These are larger in the mesio-distal dimension than the second premolars; consequently, the mandibular first molars are held in an artificial distal position.

What is the cause of the rotated UL1?

The UL1 has rotated due to the presence of an unerupted upper midline supernumerary tooth.

Comment on the morphology and position of the supernumerary tooth

This is an upper midline supernumerary. It is conical in morphology and is inverted. It is likely to be a mesiodens.

How should this case be managed?

Treatment will involve surgical removal of the supernumerary tooth. Fixed appliances will be required to de-rotate the UL1. Consideration will also need to be given to the removal of two upper premolars to relieve crowding and facilitate arch alignment. Following removal of the appliances, an upper bonded retainer will be necessary to prevent relapse of the rotational correction.

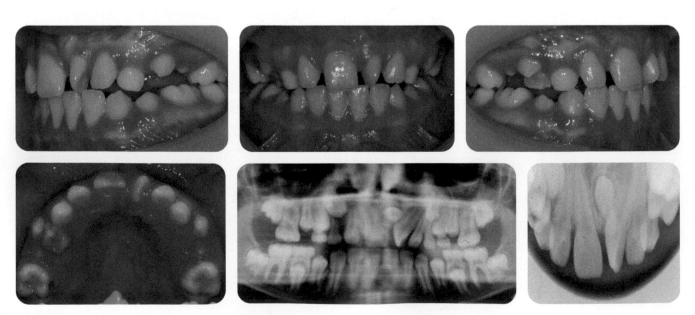

Figure 2.16

Case 2.7

This 8-year-old boy presented in the mixed dentition. His presenting occlusion is shown in the upper middle panel of Figure 2.17. His occlusion one year later is shown in the lower middle (labial view) and lower right panel (occlusal view) of Figure 2.17.

What has happened during this time?
The permanent lateral incisor teeth have erupted.

Describe the malocclusion
There is a class I incisor relationship, with the UR1 in crossbite. There is crowding in both arches, with the UR2 erupted palatally.

What are the advantages of correcting the crossbite at this stage?
- Removal of any mandibular displacement
- Prevention of any gingival recession occurring in association with the LR1

- Likely to be stable because of the presence of a positive overbite

What is the Dental Health Component of the Index of Orthodontic Treatment Need (IOTN) of this case?
It depends upon the size of the mandibular displacement between retruded contact position (RCP) and inter-cuspal position (ICP). In this case it was greater than 2 mm, which indicates an IOTN of 4.c. If it had been between 1 and 2 mm, the IOTN would have been 3.c, and if less than 1 mm, 2.c.

How would you manage this case?
With a removable appliance to procline the UR1 and correct the crossbite. A sectional fixed appliance or 2 × 4 appliance could also be used, but the position of the UR2 complicates this.

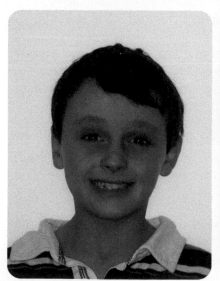
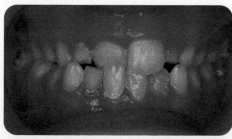
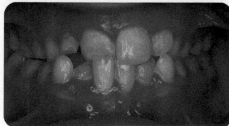
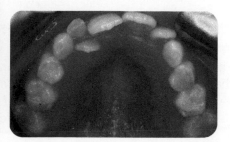

Figure 2.17

How would you design a removable appliance?

- Adams clasps for the <u>6D/D6</u> (or a double clasp for <u>6E/E6</u>) (0.7-mm stainless steel wire) for retention
- Z spring (0.5-mm stainless steel wire) to procline the UR1
- Acrylic base plate with posterior capping (to open the bite and allow movement of the UR1)

What is selective tooth agenesis?

Selective tooth agenesis (STHAG) is a failure of tooth development in either dentition. It has a number of alternative descriptors, with the most common being hypodontia, the precise definition of which is the developmental absence of six or fewer permanent teeth (not including the third molars).

What are the general characteristics of this condition in European populations?

- Prevalence is reported to be approximately 4–6% in the permanent dentition and 1–2% in the primary dentition.
- It is more common in females than males.
- Severity can vary from absence of one tooth to all the permanent teeth (anodontia), although this is rare.
- Severe hypodontia (oligodontia) is the term used where more than six permanent teeth (excluding third molars) are absent.
- The teeth reported as being most commonly absent are the mandibular second premolars, maxillary lateral incisors and maxillary second premolars. This has led to the term 'incisor–premolar' hypodontia being used.
- Hypodontia and microdontia (reduction in the size of teeth) are often associated. Generalized microdontia can occur in some cases and is often complicated by conical-shaped teeth, resulting in generalized spacing. In some cases microdontia only affects certain teeth, with diminutive (or peg-shaped) lateral incisors being most common.

What is the aetiological basis of this condition?

The aetiology of STHAG is still unclear. It is thought that both environmental and genetic factors may be involved (Cobourne, 2007; Parkin *et al.*, 2009b).

Two main forms of hypodontia have been identified:
- Non-syndromic (familial) STHAG
- Tooth agenesis associated with syndromic conditions.

How can familial (non-syndromic) STHAG be inherited?

The pattern of inheritance is variable, occurring as an autosomal dominant, autosomal recessive or sex-linked trait. STHAG can occur in the primary and permanent dentitions; however, it is more common in the permanent dentition. When occurring in the primary dentition, it often indicates the possibility of tooth agenesis in the permanent dentition.

Give some examples of syndromes associated with tooth agenesis

- Down syndrome
- Ectodermal dysplasia
- Incontinentia pigmenti
- Ellis–van Creveld syndrome

What are the main clinical features associated with severe STHAG (Figure 2.18)?

- Severe STHAG is often associated with a retrusive facial profile and reduced lower anterior face height. In cases where there are reduced vertical proportions, this often results in an increased overbite.
- The intra-oral features vary from mild cases where there is one congenitally absent tooth to more severe forms with more than six teeth missing. In severe cases there is often generalized spacing and retention of primary teeth.
- There is often an associated microdontia, either localized (peg-shaped lateral incisors) or generalized.
- Retained primary teeth can remain *in situ* until adulthood in many cases. Submerging primary molars are often an indication that the permanent successor may be absent.
- In cases where there are multiple teeth missing, the absence of a permanent successor results in underdevelopment of the alveolar bone with narrow alveolar ridges. This can occasionally manifest as lateral open bites.

What are the main options when treatment planning cases with tooth agenesis?

There are two main approaches to managing hypodontia:

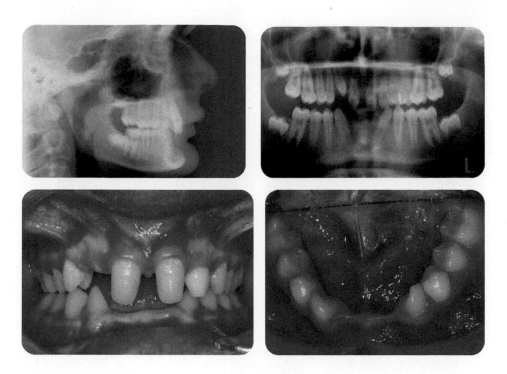

Figure 2.18

- Redistribution of space using orthodontics to allow restorative replacement of the missing teeth and restorative build-up of diminutive teeth
- Orthodontic space closure, which eliminates the need for restorations.

What factors can influence treatment planning decisions in cases with tooth agenesis?

- Underlying malocclusion.
- It is important to recognize that tooth agenesis can affect all malocclusions and the decision to open or close space will be influenced by the skeletal pattern, space requirements and anchorage demands of the case. In class II cases, where space is required for the reduction of an overjet to address crowding or to torque retroclined upper labial segments, space closure in the upper arch may be the favoured option.
- However, in class II cases where the antero-posterior discrepancy is managed by

growth modification with a functional appliance or orthognathic surgery (once growth is complete), space opening may still be an option.

- In class III cases: with a reverse overjet, space opening is often beneficial, as this helps maintain a class I incisor relationship by advancing the maxillary incisors.

What are the options for treatment in this class III case with a diminutive UL2, congenital absence of the UR2 and all second premolars, and retained second primary molars of poor prognosis (Figure 2.19)?

To manage the class III incisor relationship, a decision was made to open space for prosthetic replacement of the UR2 and build up the diminutive UL2. All of the infra-occluded second primary molars were removed with a view to closing the space.

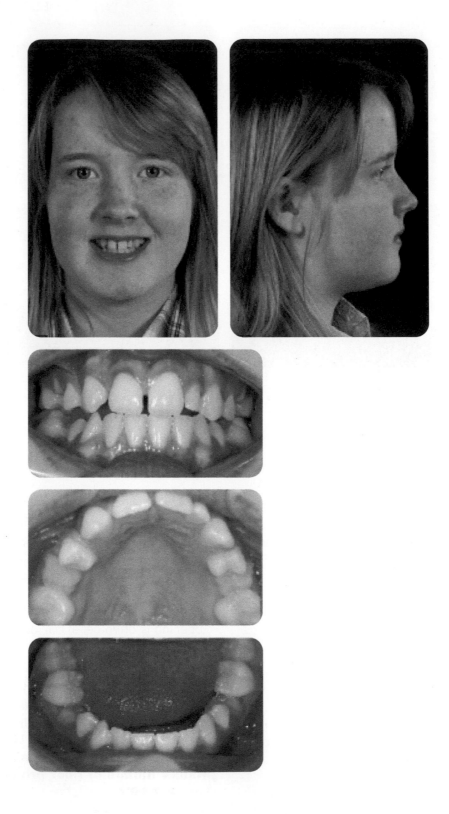

Figure 2.19

In cases where long-term maintenance of primary teeth is being considered, what factors indicate a poor prognosis?

- Presence of restorations or caries
- Poor root morphology (resorption)
- Mobility
- Evidence of submergence
- Ankylosis
- Pathology

The lack of a permanent successor often results in retention of primary teeth. Infra-occluded or submerged second primary molars are often seen when second premolars are missing and can be the first clinical indication of tooth agenesis.

Describe the appearance of the UL2 in Figure 2.20

The UL2 is peg-shaped or diminutive.

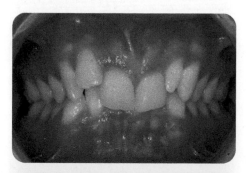

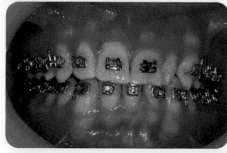

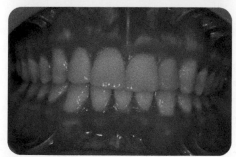

Figure 2.20

How is this problem managed?

Peg-shaped or diminutive lateral incisors result in a tooth-size discrepancy. In order to improve the aesthetics of diminutive teeth, orthodontic treatment planning often includes the creation of space around the diminutive teeth to allow build-up with composite resin.

The timing of restorative enlargement can vary. In cases where there is generalized spacing, it may be possible to restore the teeth prior to the start of orthodontic treatment. If teeth are rotated, it may be difficult to identify their long axis. In such cases, the build-up can either be performed on completion of the orthodontic treatment after or, ideally, prior to removal of appliances. The advantage of the latter approach is that the teeth can be built up to the ideal proportions with any residual space closed orthodontically. In the case shown, the diminutive UL2 was temporarily removed from the archwire after alignment to allow access for build-up with composite resin. Following the composite build-up, the tooth was rebonded and orthodontic treatment completed.

In cases where patients opt not to commit to the maintenance of composite restorations, it is important that they are aware that if all the space is closed around the diminutive teeth, occlusal and aesthetic compromise will result.

What treatment has been carried out in the case shown in Figure 2.21?

The UR2 is peg-shaped and the UL2 is absent. Due to the class III incisor relationship and lack of crowding, a decision was made to recreate space for the UL2 and build up the UR2. To improve the aesthetics in treatment and to help in space redistribution, the UR2 was built up and a prosthetic tooth ligated to the archwire to replace the UL2 prior to final space closure and completion of orthodontic treatment.

In the case shown in Figure 2.22 the UR2 is missing and the UR3 is unerupted and palatally displaced. What are the main options for the management of this situation?

The UR3 requires mechanical eruption and orthodontic alignment initially. After successful eruption, space opening or space closure may be considered for the absent UR2.

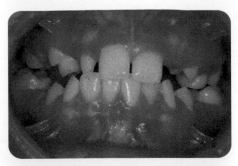

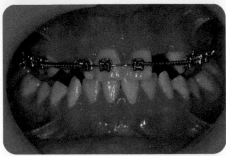

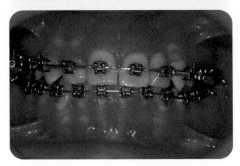

Figure 2.21

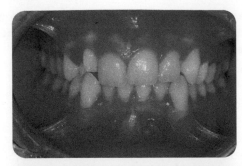

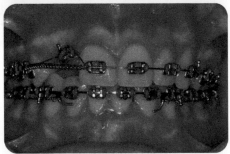

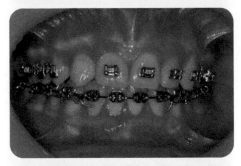

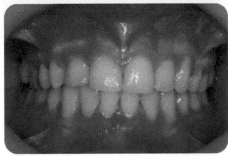

Figure 2.22

Treatment options are:
- Open space for restorative replacement of the UR2
- Space closure, with composite build-up of the UR3 to mimic the appearance of the UR2.

In the case shown, the second option was chosen as there was crowding in the lower arch which required premolar extractions to treat. As this was a crowded Class I malocclusion and the upper centre line was displaced to the right where the UR2 was missing, it was decided to extract the UL4, LR4 and LL4, and substitute the UR3 for the UR2.

How has the UR3 been modified to resemble the absent UR2?

The mesial edge has been built up with composite, whilst the tip has been smoothed down. Finally, localized bleaching has been carried out to whiten the UR3.

What factors influence the decision to open spaces, with a view to future restorative replacement of missing lateral incisors, or close spaces and accept the canine in the position of the lateral incisor?

- **Malocclusion and skeletal pattern:**
  - In class II cases where space is required for overjet reduction or relief of crowding, the decision to close lateral incisor spaces may be favoured. The aesthetics of space closure may be

better in cases of bilaterally absent lateral incisors due to symmetry.
  ○ In class III cases, space opening for absent maxillary lateral incisors may be preferable to facilitate correction of the incisor relationship.

- **Size, colour and shape of the canine tooth:** When considering space closure with a view to accepting the maxillary canines in the lateral incisor position, the size, colour and shape of the canines are important factors influencing aesthetics. Canine teeth have large, bulbous, conical and yellow crowns with a high gingival margin. In the presence of a low smile line, the gingival margin height is less of a concern. In cases where the maxillary canines are aesthetically unpleasing, the decision may be made to extract teeth in the buccal segments whilst opening space for the absent lateral incisors, with a view to restorative replacement.
- **Degree of crowding:** Malocclusions complicated by crowding may be suited to space closure where maxillary lateral incisors are absent. This approach reduces the need for restorative treatment and avoids extraction of sound teeth.
- **Appearance of the contra-lateral tooth:**
  ○ In cases of unilateral absence of the maxillary lateral incisor, the dimensions of the contra-lateral tooth are an indicator of the space required for restoration of the missing lateral incisor.
  ○ In cases where the contra-lateral incisor is diminutive or peg shaped, space will be required to build up this tooth to average dimensions.
  ○ If both lateral incisors are missing, symmetry contributes to the aesthetics of both treatment approaches.

What factors influence the timing of treatment for tooth agenesis?

In cases of severe hypodontia, particularly where there is an associated microdontia, patients are often concerned about spacing in the early mixed dentition. Whilst it may not be appropriate to start definitive orthodontic treatment at this stage, if the spacing is generalized, the appearance of the upper labial segment may be improved restoratively with composite build-up of diminutive incisors.

Restorative treatment is ideally carried out once the majority of growth is complete. Restorative provision of resin-bonded bridges may be carried out at the age of 15–16 years, whilst placement of implants is generally delayed until 18 years and older when facial growth can be expected to have ceased.

In view of this ideal timing for the restorative treatment, it may be appropriate to delay the start of the orthodontic treatment, to allow a smooth transition between the completion of the orthodontics and the definitive restorative management.

What factors influence orthodontic retention for tooth agenesis cases?

In cases of severe hypodontia, where a definitive treatment plan includes restorations, it is important to ensure adequate retention between completion of orthodontic treatment and definitive restorative treatment.

Patients should be provided with retainers to maintain the position of the teeth, with full-time wear required until definitive restorations are provided. If patients are treated early, many years before restorative treatment is planned, this commits them to a long period of full-time retention.

Where teeth are being restored, removable retainers should include pontics and metal stops to retain post-orthodontic spaces. In cases where posterior spaces are being retained, motivation to wear the retainers may vary. If retainers are not worn, this can result in movement of teeth (crowns or roots) and in some cases results in the need for a second course of orthodontic treatment prior to restorative treatment being carried out.

Case 2.8

This 12-year-old female presented with a class II division 2 malocclusion on a moderate skeletal class II base with a retrusive profile and agenesis (Figure 2.23).

Which teeth are present clinically?

654321/12 456
76E4321/1234567

Which teeth are absent?

Radiographic examination demonstrates the congenital absence of UL3 and LR5, and a retained LRE with a good long-term prognosis.

What are the main problems in this case?

- Class II incisor relationship
- Crowding of the UR5 and lower incisors
- Rotated upper first premolars
- Spacing labially in the upper arch
- Congenital absence of UL3 and LR5
- Retained LRE (although good prognosis)

What is the IOTN of this case?

5i – this is based on the impaction of the UR5.

Treatment Plan

- Upper and lower fixed appliances on a non-extraction basis
- Alignment of the teeth and correction of the incisor relationship
- Retain the LRE, with a view to restorative replacement, when lost in the future
- Redistribution of space to allow alignment of the UR5 and create space for restorative replacement of the UL3

What is the justification for this treatment plan?

This patient presented with a class II division 2 malocclusion, with an increased overbite and retrusive

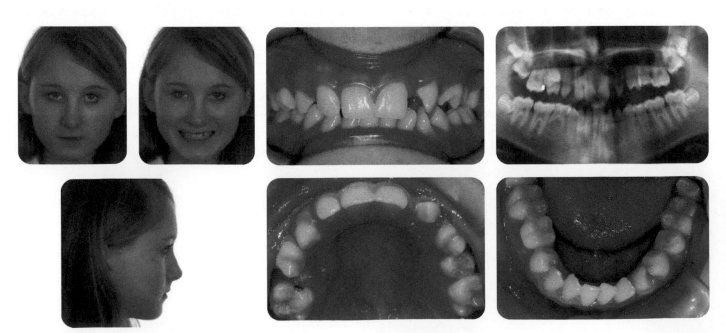

Figure 2.23

facial profile. It was felt that a non-extraction approach would be beneficial for aesthetics and would simplify overbite reduction.

In the lower arch the LRE has a good prognosis. This tooth has a reasonable root length, is unrestored, asymptomatic and immobile. In view of the favourable prognosis of the tooth, it was decided to retain it indefinitely.

In the upper arch, there was enough space to accommodate the impacted UR5 and to create space for the missing UL3. There was some spacing already present with the potential for additional space to be created by de-rotation of the UR4 and UL4, which were rotated through 90 degrees.

Why were some teeth in the lower arch not bonded at the time of the bond up (Figure 2.24)?

The LL2 and LL3 are rotated through almost 90 degrees and there is insufficient space present to de-rotate and align these teeth. It would be difficult to bond brackets to these teeth in the correct position and therefore, the decision was made to avoid including these teeth at the start of treatment. An elastomeric sleeve has been placed to support the archwire and minimize soft tissue irritation. Space will be created for these teeth later in treatment to allow their alignment.

Describe the mechanics that are being used in Figure 2.25

- A rigid 0.018-inch stainless steel archwire is in place.
- In the upper right quadrant, an open coil spring is being used to create space to accommodate both premolars.
- A lingual button has been bonded onto both premolars to allow the use of an elastomeric chain to aid de-rotation of these teeth.

- Elastomeric chain has also been attached to the UL6, UL5 and UL4 via palatal cleats to consolidate their position.
- The UL1, UR1 and UR2 have been ligated together into one unit and elastomeric chain is being used to move the UL2 into the correct position adjacent to the UL1, creating space for replacement of the UL3.

What options are there for replacement of the UL3?

The UL3 could be replaced with an adhesive bridge, an implant-retained crown or a denture.

What factors need to be considered in assessing the space requirements for this tooth?

The UR3 acts as a guide for the dimensions of the future restoration replacing the UL3. In order to achieve optimal aesthetics, best practice would be to aim to achieve symmetry, with both upper canines of the same width.

In cases where there is associated microdontia, it is important to recognise that achieving symmetry may make implant replacement difficult if the ideal restoration size is very narrow.

If an implant-retained crown is the preferred option for replacement, it may be possible to consider

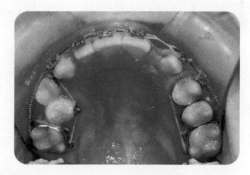

Figure 2.25

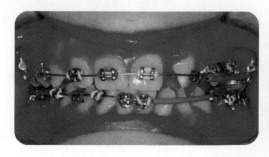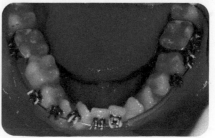

Figure 2.24

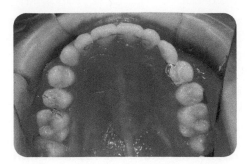

Figure 2.26

building up the contra-lateral tooth (with composite resin) to increase its dimensions in order to achieve the required aesthetics.

The UL3 has been replaced by a resin-bonded bridge (Figure 2.26). Discuss the design of this bridge

This is a cantilever-type bridge with a single metal wing palatal to the UL4. Cantilever type bridges (single abutments) are believed to give a better prognosis than double abutment designs. Double abutment designs have a higher failure rate. Undetected failures related to detachment of one wing may result in undetected caries of the abutment tooth. The UL4 was chosen as the abutment tooth as it has a greater palatal surface area than the slightly diminutive UL2. In addition, the effects of any 'shine through' of the metal wing would be less obvious in this position.

What is the rationale behind placing a bonded retainer in this case?

The UL2 was rotated at the start of treatment. Placement of a bonded retainer decreases the risk of relapse, as rotated teeth are thought to be at greater risk. The final occlusion is shown in Figure 2.27.

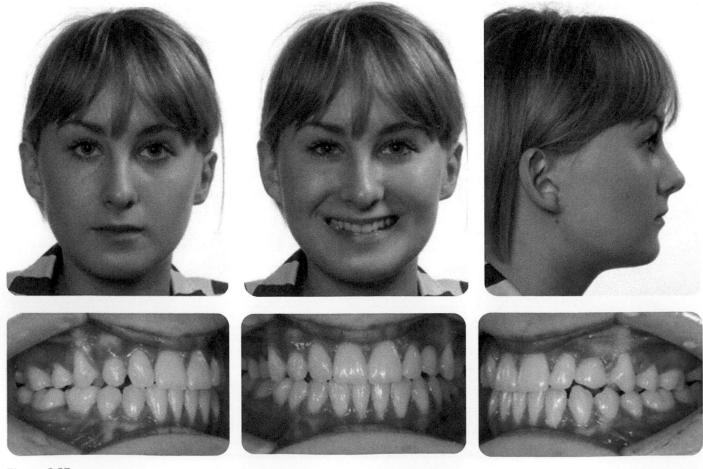

Figure 2.27

Case 2.9

This child presented with significant pain in his upper left dental quadrant. He has an overjet of 8 mm, a mild skeletal class II pattern and average vertical proportions, and is still sucking his thumb.

What features are revealed by the radiographic examination (Figure 2.28)?

- Teeth present: $\dfrac{\text{6EDC2 /12BCDE6}}{\text{6EDC21/12 CDE6}}$

- UR1 is absent
- Evidence of crown fracture to the UL1

- Large amalgam restorations in the: $\dfrac{\text{/DE}}{\text{6ED/DE6}}$

- Gross caries in the UL6

- Caries in the: $\dfrac{\text{6ED/E}}{\text{E /E}}$

The developing canines, premolars and second molars are all present and in a good position. There is no evidence of third molar development.

How old do you think this patient is?

Around 9 years of age. The bifurcations of the developing second permanent molars have still to begin calcifying and root development of the first permanent molars is almost complete.

What treatment is required in the short-term?

The UL6 requires extraction as it is grossly carious with pulpal involvement. The long-term prognosis for

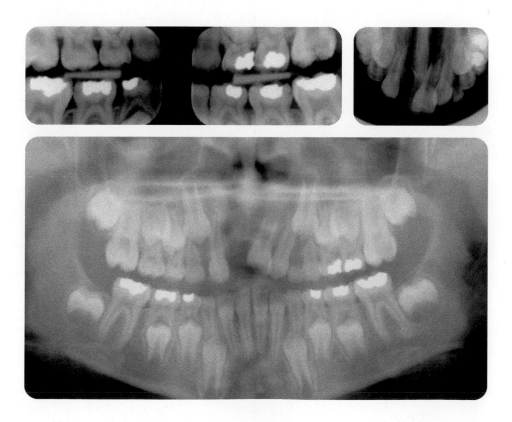

Figure 2.28

the lower first permanent molars needs to be assessed. However, the amalgam restorations in these teeth appear to be sound and, if at all possible, they should not be extracted. A lower compensating extraction for a first permanent molar is not indicated.

The caries in the primary molars should be treated as these teeth are required to act as space maintainers whilst the dentition continues to develop. If extractions are necessary, then consideration should be given to a space maintainer in the lower arch. In the upper arch, a space maintainer is required for the UL1 and if primary molar extractions are required here (ULD are ULE are possibilities), then eruption of the second molar should be monitored closely to avoid excessive space loss following extraction of ULD, ULE and UL6.

Case 2.10

This 13-year-old boy has been referred by his general dental practitioner for an orthodontic assessment. He has a history of previous primary tooth extractions due to caries. There is an overjet of 9 mm. He is not currently in any pain.

Summarize the clinical features of the malocclusion (Figure 2.29)

- This is a class II division 1 case on a skeletal class II base with increased vertical proportions
- Increased overjet (9 mm) and reduced overbite
- Buccal segment relationship ½ unit class II bilaterally
- Both centre lines are to the left of the face with the upper displaced 2 mm more than the lower
- Bilateral posterior crossbite

- Severe crowding in the upper labial segment and in all four buccal segments, with the upper left quadrant short of two units of space
- UL6, UR6 and LL6 are carious and LR4 hypoplastic. The UL5, UR5, LL4 and LR5 are unerupted and impacted
- Lower second molars are erupted
- Oral hygiene is poor

What are the main features on the panoramic radiograph (Figure 2.30)?

- UL6 and UR6 are grossly carious. The LL6 has a significant occlusal carious lesion. The LR6 also has early occlusal caries; a bitewing radiograph should be taken to confirm its extent.
- Severe crowding in the buccal segments, with all four second premolars present but short of space, particularly in the upper arch.
- Lower third molars are present but there is no evidence of upper third molar development.
- UL7 is potentially mesially impacted against the UL6.

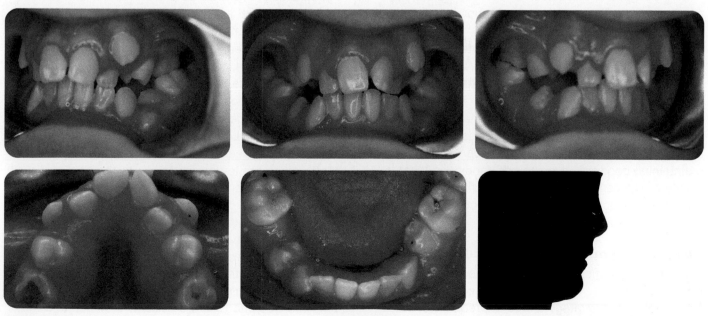

Figure 2.29

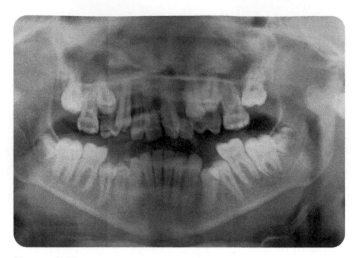

Figure 2.30

What are the main problems associated with this malocclusion?

The upper first permanent molars are grossly carious and have a poor long-term prognosis. The lower first permanent molars also have occlusal caries, the LL6 having a poor prognosis, but the LR6 is probably restorable. The upper third permanent molars have not developed and the UL7 appears to be mesially impacted against the UL6.

Early loss of primary molars has caused severe crowding in the buccal segments. The UL5 and UR5 are palatally impacted, the LL4 is buccally impacted and the UL3 is crowded buccally.

The overjet is increased to 9mm, the skeletal pattern is class II and the lower anterior face height is increased.

There is a bilateral posterior crossbite.

What factors contribute to the management of this malocclusion?

The successful management of this malocclusion is dependent upon excellent future co-operation with dental treatment, orthodontic appliance wear, maintaining good oral hygiene and modifying what is clearly a high-caries diet. If all these criteria are met, then this malocclusion could be corrected with orthodontic treatment.

How would you manage this malocclusion?

It would be beneficial to temporize the carious first permanent molars. The extent of the caries in these teeth makes this strategy a little unpredictable, but maintaining these teeth in the short-term would allow some space maintenance during the first phase of orthodontic treatment.

Following the temporization of these teeth, orthodontic treatment would begin with the provision of a twin-block functional appliance in conjunction with high-pull headgear. Maintaining the upper first permanent molars would also help with the retention of this appliance. The aim of this treatment phase would be to reduce the overjet, correct the crossbite and achieve some improvement in the overbite. If successful, this would take around 8–12 months and the overjet, crossbite and molar relationship would be corrected.

Correcting the sagittal discrepancy with a functional appliance makes subsequent treatment planning more straightforward, although this remains a challenging malocclusion. Following the functional appliance phase, fixed appliances would be required to align the teeth, co-ordinate the dental arches and maintain the sagittal correction achieved. It is this stage that is quite difficult and, as with many aspects of orthodontic treatment planning, there are several potential options.

In the lower arch, the LL6 should be extracted. At this time, a decision also needs to be made regarding management of the impacted LL4. With suitable anchorage support (a lingual arch), the extraction of the LL6 will provide enough space to retract the LL5 and align the LL4 using a fixed appliance. For convenience the LL4 could also be exposed at the time of LL6 extraction.

In the lower right quadrant, either the LR6 or the hypoplastic LR4 should be extracted. The amount of caries in the LR6 and any sensitivity associated with the LR4 will dictate the extraction decision. If the LR5 remains unerupted, it should also be exposed at this time. In this case, we are going to assume that the balance of factors has dictated extraction of the LR6. As already mentioned, a lingual arch can be fitted to provide anchorage for alignment of the LL4 (extending from the LL7 to LR7). Orthodontic treatment in the lower arch will require a fixed appliance to align the teeth, move the lower centre line to the right and close any residual space from the first molar extractions.

In the upper arch, both upper second permanent molars should have erupted by the end of the functional phase, and at this stage the UL6 and UR6 should be extracted (in conjunction with the LL6 and LR6). Space requirements are high in the upper arch, both the UL5 and UR5 are palatally crowded and the UL3 is buccally displaced. In addition, the upper centre line needs to be moved to the right. The space to align these teeth will come from extraction of the first molars, but anchorage reinforcement will be required. This can be provided by a palatal arch (with a Nance button) or more usefully, from continued wear of headgear via bands on the upper second molars.

A potential problem is the position of the upper second premolars. If these teeth remain unerupted, they will require exposure when the first molars are extracted. Second premolars in this position often erupt palatally. It would be important to monitor this during the functional phase, modifying the acrylic coverage of the appliance if the second premolars start to erupt. An upper fixed appliance will be used in conjunction with the lower to achieve the necessary tooth movements.

With this treatment plan, the potential exists to use all of the space created by extraction of the upper first permanent molars. However, the crowding is so severe in the upper left quadrant that a single molar unit will not necessarily provide enough space to align the impacted UL5 and buccally crowded UL3; therefore, some further distal movement of the UL7 may be required, which is why headgear is preferable to a palatal arch.

What happens if the UL7 has not erupted by the end of the functional appliance phase?

If the UL7 has not erupted by the time the UL6 is extracted, this will dictate a period of time waiting for it to erupt following the extraction. This is complicated by the fact that eruption of the UL7 will almost certainly be accompanied by space loss in the upper left quadrant, because it will erupt in a more mesial position. This will have implications for alignment in the upper left quadrant as there is already severe crowding, with both the UL5 and UL3 excluded. Therefore, with an unerupted UL7, the UL5 can also be extracted, which will then allow the buccally crowded UL3 to be aligned with fixed appliances. All things being equal, this strategy would also probably tip the balance in favour of extracting the impacted LL4. In the upper right quadrant there is also severe crowding, with the UR5 being palatally impacted. However, the UR3 is not as short of space as the UL3 and therefore, premolar extractions are probably not necessary in this quadrant. However, it should be borne in mind that the upper centre line will need to be moved to the right during treatment, which will require some additional space in this region.

What if the child is in pain?

The treatment plan outlined above relies upon preserving the first permanent molars and correcting the sagittal relationship first with a functional appliance. If preservation of these teeth is not possible and they need to be extracted immediately, then management of this malocclusion becomes more problematic.

It would still be desirable to attempt correction of the sagittal relationship at this stage with a functional appliance. In this scenario, an alternative functional appliance could be used (such as a bionator, which is not tooth-borne). However, loss of the first molars at this stage will lead to some space loss as the second permanent molars erupt, particularly in the upper arch where space is at a premium. This makes subsequent extraction of premolars more likely during the fixed appliance phase of treatment, which is not ideal (particularly in the upper arch where there is no sign of third molar development).

Case 2.11

This 12-year-old patient presents complaining of the appearance of his upper anterior teeth (Figure 2.31).

Summarize the clinical findings

This patient presents in the late mixed dentition with a class III incisor relationship. The malocclusion is complicated by a megadont UR1 and ectopic UL1, with severe crowding in the upper arch and mild crowding in the lower arch.

How would you describe the upper labial segment?

The upper labial segment is severely crowded with a megadont UR1 and ectopically positioned UL1 lying in the midline high in the buccal sulcus.

What is the difficulty with maintaining a megadont tooth?

Disproportion between the size of maxillary and mandibular teeth is described as a tooth-size discrepancy. In this case there is a clear tooth-size discrepancy with the UR1 having a greater than average mesio-distal width. It is not possible to achieve an ideal occlusion in the presence of a tooth-size discrepancy.

In some cases, if the dimensions of a megadont tooth are only slightly greater than average, enamel reduction (stripping) of the tooth to reduce its dimensions may be a suitable option. This was not appropriate in this case and a decision to extract the tooth was made.

What factors would you take into account when assessing the prognosis of the UL1?

- Position of the tooth (height, distance towards the midline)
- Evidence of ankylosis (sound on percussion)
- Space available in the upper arch

In this case, the UL1 is high in the buccal sulcus and appears to have erupted through unattached mucosa. This suggests that the gingival attachment of this tooth, if aligned, is likely to be poor, compromising the aesthetics. In view of the severe crowding and the ectopic position of the tooth, a decision was made to extract it.

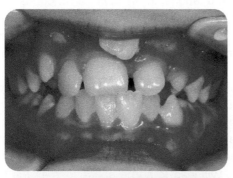

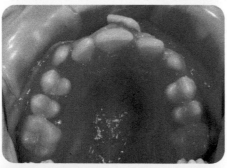

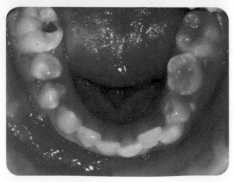

Figure 2.31

Case 2.12

This child is 10 years old (Figure 2.32).

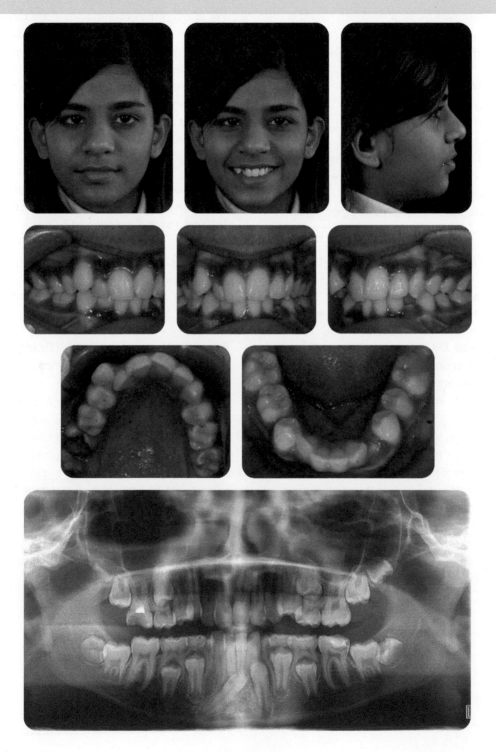

Figure 2.32

Summarize this malocclusion

- The patient presents with a class I malocclusion complicated by severe crowding of both dental arches, both lower canines are unerupted and impacted, and the UR3 is excluded buccally
- LR3 is ectopic in position
- UR6 and LL6 are heavily restored, and the UL6 is hypoplastic
- There is a retained, carious ULE
- Upper and lower dental centre lines are coincident but displaced to the right of the facial midline

What would your problem list be?

- Severe upper and lower arch crowding
- Buccally excluded UR3, impacted lower canines
- Ectopic and impacted LR3
- LR3 is excluded from the arch and ectopic in position, with its crown lying beneath the roots of the lower central incisors
- Potentially impacted LL3 due to insufficient space
- Heavily restored LL6 and UR6
- Hypoplastic UL6
- Upper and lower centre line shift to the right

An appropriate extraction pattern for this case would include extraction of the ectopic LR3, LL6, UL6, and retained upper Es. The lower Cs and lower Ds (seen radiographically) were lost prior to treatment planning. Justify this extraction pattern and discuss the potential difficulties associated with this approach

This class I malocclusion is complicated by severe crowding. Space to align the arches will need to be provided by extractions. The LR3 is lying beneath the roots of the lower central incisors. Attempts at aligning this tooth could risk damage to the roots of the lower incisors. In this case, having lost the LRC, there is no space to align this tooth, making the LR3 the tooth of choice for extraction in this quadrant.

In the lower left quadrant there is insufficient space to allow the LL3 to erupt. The LL6 is heavily restored, with possible caries beneath the restoration, encroaching on the pulp. This tooth is of relatively poor prognosis, and therefore would be an appropriate tooth for extraction. However, correction of the lower centre line is made more challenging by extraction of the LL6.

In the upper arch the UR6 is heavily restored with a large amalgam restoration approaching the pulp, and has a poor prognosis. Whilst the prognosis of the UL6 is reasonable, this tooth is hypoplastic and is the extraction of choice, as all other teeth in the upper left quadrant are unrestored. Extraction of the UL6 makes centre line correction in the upper arch more challenging.

When would be the appropriate time to arrange the extractions and start orthodontic treatment?

In order to have sufficient posterior anchorage it would be beneficial to delay the extractions until the lower second permanent molars have erupted, allowing alignment and correction of the centre lines with sufficient posterior anchorage.

What is the potential difficulty with space closure in cases where first permanent molars are extracted?

It is important to ensure space closure is carried out on rectangular stainless steel archwires to ensure there is appropriate torque in the buccal segments. There is a tendency for the lower second molars in particular to tip lingually. To avoid this, it would be appropriate to ensure a rectangular archwire is placed in the lower arch as soon as possible during treatment.

Case 2.13

This 14-year-old male was referred to his orthodontist with a class I occlusion complicated by mild crowding of the lower incisor teeth.

What has been carried out between the first (upper) and second (lower) radiograph in Figure 2.33?

All four second permanent molars have been extracted and the third molars have erupted into a good occlusion to replace the second molars at the back of

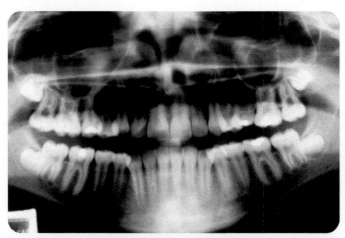

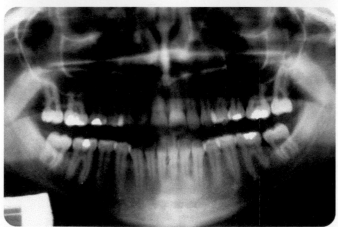

Figure 2.33

the dental arches (Huggins and McBride, 1978; Pearson, 1996; Richardson and Richardson, 1993).

What are the supposed advantages of extracting lower second permanent molars?

Advocates of this procedure suggest that it can provide space to relieve mild crowding, particularly for erupting second premolars, but also in the incisor region. In addition, it can help reduce the incidence of late lower incisor crowding. It also removes the potential for later problems associated with impacted wisdom teeth (assuming these teeth erupt into a good position). In this case, the second molars were extracted to relieve lower arch crowding.

What are the disadvantages?

The extractions can be quite difficult to perform under local anaesthetic, requiring excellent cooperation.

Timing of extraction is important to ensure the best possible chance of successful third molar extraction. However, predictable eruption of the third molar is not possible, even with optimum timing of extraction, and the third molar rarely provides a replacement that is as good as the original second molar (crown and root morphology of a third molar is variable, the eruptive position of the third molar is often mesially tipped or rolled lingually).

There is no firm evidence that this procedure provides any significant relief of crowding, particularly in the labial segments.

How would you rate the result in this case?

The eruptive position of the third molars is good. However, all four first permanent molars were restored when the decision was made to extract the four (unrestored) second permanent molars.

Is there an optimum time to extract lower second permanent molars to obtain the best eruptive position for the third molar?

The eruption of third molars is notoriously unpredictable. However, it has been suggested that extraction of the lower second molars should take place just as the bifurcation of the third molar root is beginning to calcify. In addition, third molars that are mesially inclined at around 45 degrees to the occlusal plane will erupt into the best position.

What are the indications for extracting a maxillary second permanent molar?

The extraction of this tooth can be useful during distalization of the first upper first molars using headgear. This procedure is also facilitated by the fact that the third molar usually erupts into a good position if it is unerupted at the time of second molar extraction. However, morphology of the third molar crown and root is also more variable than that seen in the second molar.

Case 2.14

This 12-year-old girl has been referred in relation to an increased overjet. She is concerned in relation to her dento-facial appearance and has been the subject of teasing.

What baseline information does the cephalometric radiograph (Figure 2.34) provide?

The skeletal pattern is moderate class II, primarily due to mandibular retrognathia. The lower anterior facial height is in proportion to the mid-facial height; however, the maxillary–mandibular planes angle (MMPA) appears to be reduced. The maxillary incisors are proclined considerably, whilst the mandibular incisors are upright.

What is the significance of these observations?

The cephalometric findings provide an indication of the aetiology of the presenting malocclusion; this can then be translated into treatment planning.

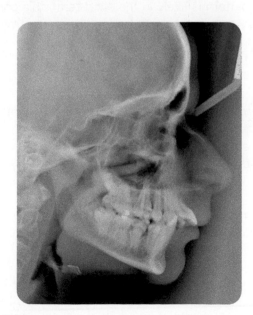

Figure 2.34

The moderate skeletal class II discrepancy is indicative that alteration in the sagittal skeletal base relationship may be beneficial both in improving the facial appearance and addressing the malocclusion. Hence, in a growing patient, functional appliance therapy could be considered. The normal antero-posterior position of the maxilla and absence of increased vertical proportions mean that headgear is probably not indicated.

In a non-growing individual, an alternative may include a combined orthodontic–surgical approach (mandibular advancement surgery), although orthodontic camouflage may also be considered.

The reduced MMPA has contributed to the increased overbite. It also indicates that this individual may have an anterior growth rotation pattern, which is generally beneficial for successful orthodontic treatment.

Dento-alveolar factors have also contributed to the increased overjet. The maxillary incisors are significantly proclined and the mandibular incisors upright. This implies that soft tissue pressures may be exacerbating the overjet. Hence, alteration in the resting position of the lips following treatment is a requirement for stable overjet reduction. In particular, achievement of lip competence with elimination of the lip trap is important.

The intra-oral records are shown in Figure 2.35. Summarize the presenting malocclusion

A 12-year-old female in the late mixed dentition with a class II division 1 incisor relationship on a moderate skeletal class II pattern with reduced MMPA. The malocclusion is complicated by:
- Increased overjet (12 mm)
- Increased and complete overbite
- Crowding of both arches
- Mild molar–incisor hypomineralization.

What are the relevant findings on the panoramic radiograph (Figure 2.36)?

The panoramic radiograph demonstrates the presence of all permanent teeth, including third molars, with the

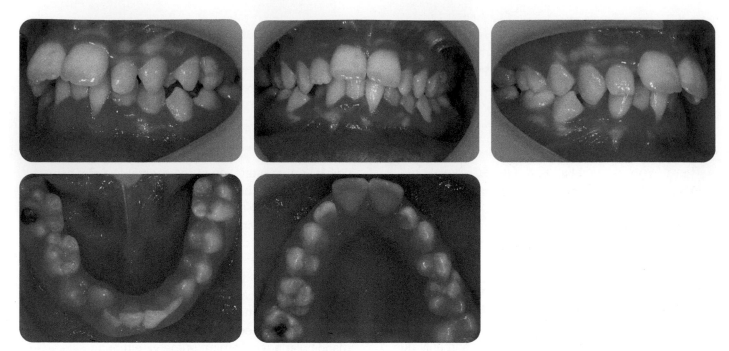

Figure 2.35

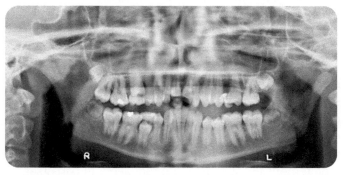

Figure 2.36

exception of the UL6 (this tooth was previously extracted). The remaining primary molars (URE, ULE, LRE) are nearing natural exfoliation. There are small restorations in the UR6 and LR6.

Is removal of the URE, ULE and LRE indicated at this point?

Extraction of these teeth would be inappropriate. All three primary molars have undergone considerable root resorption and will exfoliate naturally within a 3-month period. Removal of these teeth would subject the patient to unnecessary intervention.

How would you treat this malocclusion?

Successful treatment is reliant on patient co-operation and would be facilitated by favourable growth. In view of the large overjet and sagittal skeletal discrepancy,

functional appliance therapy could be considered in the first instance.

The aims of this treatment phase include:
- Overjet reduction
- Overbite reduction
- Elimination of the lip trap
- Correction of the buccal segment relationship.

Improvement in the skeletal pattern would be beneficial. However, while some normalization of the skeletal pattern is likely in the short-term, this change is unlikely to be sustained. Nevertheless, treatment should result in improvement of the facial profile due to retraction of the maxillary incisors and the establishment of a class I incisor relationship. An increase in lower anterior face height is also likely.

Following a functional appliance phase of treatment, the overjet should have diminished within 9–12 months and overcorrection should ideally achieve an edge-to-edge relationship. At this stage further records, including a second lateral cephalogram, are indicated. Consideration should then be given to arch alignment and levelling with optimization of the buccal occlusion. Treatment is likely to involve removal of four second premolars to relieve crowding in the mandibular arch, permitting arch alignment and levelling without excessive advancement of the lower anteriors as mandibular incisor proclination has been shown to be unstable in the long-term.

Do you feel it would be to remove the remaining first permanent molars in this instance?

Removal of first permanent molars could be considered in view of the molar–incisor hypomineralization. There are amalgam restorations in both right first permanent molars and hypoplastic defects, particularly in the LR6. However, the restorations are small and single surface; the degree of hypoplasia is minor; there is no evidence of caries and the oral hygiene is good. In addition, removal of first permanent molars is of little strategic benefit to addressing the malocclusion; their removal therefore would risk complicating and prolonging appliance therapy. A key factor in deciding on the extraction of these teeth is whether any of them is associated with sensitivity. If this is not the case, then the relatively minor hypomineralization would mean that they can be left *in situ*, possibly with replacement of the deficient amalgam restorations.

What are the potential orthodontic problems associated with removal of the first permanent molars?

Traditionally, it was believed that first molar extractions risked 'doubling the treatment time and halving the prognosis'. While this is not entirely accurate, particularly with the wider use of fixed appliances, there remains some truth in this statement. Space closure following extraction of first molars may be prolonged, particularly in the mandibular arch, adding approximately 6 months to the duration of treatment. Furthermore, closure of these spaces may be complicated by mesial tipping and mesio-lingual rotation of the second permanent molars as they are protracted. With large overjets, maxillary second molars provide little anchorage to effect overjet reduction. Consequently, augmentation of anchorage in the maxillary arch with transpalatal arches or temporary anchorage devices may be necessary.

What prescription should be used during the fixed appliance phase?

Following functional appliance therapy, a high torque prescription in the upper anterior region is sensible to enhance palatal root torque secondary to retroclination during the functional phase. If upper arch expansion was undertaken during the functional phase, additional buccal root torque is preferable. Furthermore, labial root torque in the lower anterior region is helpful to counteract lower incisor proclination during the functional phase. The MBT prescription satisfies these criteria.

Case 2.15

This 10-year-old class I case presents with pain from the hypoplastic and carious UR6 and LR6 (Figure 2.37). Although not associated with any discomfort, the LL6 and UL6 are also carious. A paediatric dental opinion is that the UR6 and LR6 require extraction and the LL6 is also likely to need extraction. An orthodontic opinion has been sought. The patient is in the mixed dentition and there is good alignment of the teeth. The maxillary canines are palpable buccally.

What suggestions would you make with regard to the management of this problem?

The panoramic radiograph demonstrates that all four third molars are developing, which is ideal if planned extraction of the first molars is being considered. In addition, the second molars are at the optimal developmental stage to extract and expect good eruption of these teeth into the first molar position with the inter-radicular region just beginning to

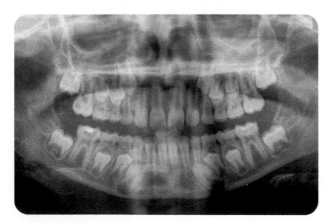

Figure 2.37

mineralize. This is particularly important for the lower second molars.

The absence of any significant malocclusion also favours immediate extraction of the first molars.

It is likely that extraction of all four first molars would be recommended, particularly as the long-term prognosis for the UR6 and LR6 is poor. With regard to the first molars on the left, the poor prognosis for the LL6 means that its enforced extraction is likely. In these circumstances the UR6 should be extracted as well, to prevent over-eruption of this tooth.

If the LL6 were sound, what should be done?

If the LL6 were sound, the UR6 and LR6 should still be extracted; however, a decision would need to be made regarding extraction of the UL6. This tooth is hypoplastic and has some caries, and therefore would be difficult to restore, making extraction a reasonable decision. Leaving a sound LL6 is reasonable, but if the UL6 is to be extracted, given the favourable prognostic indicators for extraction in this case, the LL6 could also be extracted as well.

How would the absence of third molar development affect the management of this case?

A radiographic absence of third molar development in a 10-year old does not mean that these teeth will not form, but it does make it less likely. In this case, an absence of third molar development does not significantly affect the management decisions, but the patient would need to be informed of the possibility that they would potentially only have a single molar in each quadrant. However, with a sound LL6 and no LL8 development, extraction of the LL6 might be avoided if done in conjunction with extraction of the UR6, LR6 and UL6.

Case 2.16

This 12-year-old boy was referred by his general dental practitioner because of the unusual position of the UR2.

How does his occlusion deviate from what is considered to be normal (Figure 2.38)?

- Class II division 2 incisor relationship
- Increased and incomplete overbite
- Centre line discrepancy (upper to right by 2 mm)
- Buccal segment relationship ½ unit class II bilaterally
- Bilateral posterior open bite and crossbite tendency
- Mild crowding of the upper labial segment
- Unerupted UR3, which appears to be transposed with the UR2

An upper anterior occlusal radiograph was taken (Figure 2.39). What does this show?

The UR3 is unerupted, palatally positioned and transposed with the UR2. It is mesially angulated and in close association with the root of the UR1, which appears to have undergone extensive resorption.

What investigation has been carried out in Figure 2.40?

A cone beam computed tomography (CT) scan has been undertaken of the UR1 region. This confirms the presence of resorption associated with the UR1 root.

What are the main problems associated with this case?

- There is a class II division 2 malocclusion with a posterior crossbite.
- The long-term prognosis for the UR1 is poor; however, this tooth can be replaced ultimately with a resin-retained bridge or implant.
- A more pressing problem is the impacted and transposed UR3, which ideally needs to be accommodated in the maxillary arch. Given the poor prognosis for the UR1, this makes it even more important to bring the canine down. Unfortunately, the position of the erupted UR2 makes alignment of the UR3 difficult.

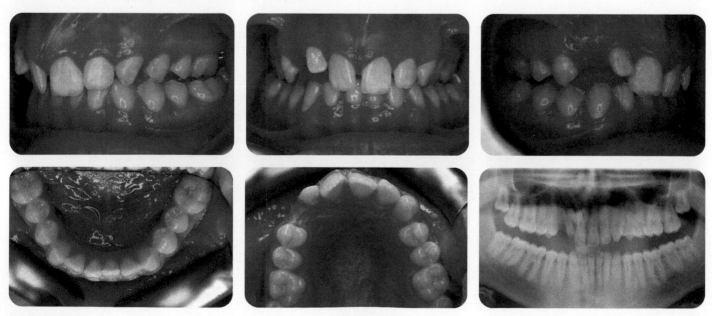

Figure 2.38

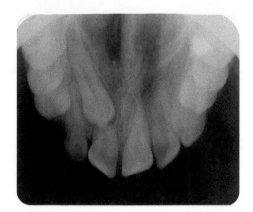

Figure 2.39

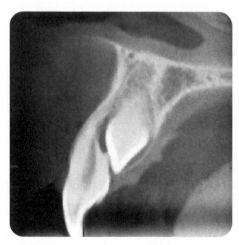

Figure 2.40

What are the options for treatment?

Considering the transposition first. One option would be to move the UR2 distally and bring the UR3 into the UR2 position; however, the lateral incisor is a poor substitute for a canine.

Alternatively, the UR3 could be transplanted into the correct position; however, the long-term prognosis for the canine may well be compromised with this approach, and it also makes correcting the malocclusion more difficult because orthodontic movement of a transplanted UR3 would be limited.

Finally, the UR2 could be extracted and the UR3 aligned following exposure and bonding. This is the option that was decided upon.

Treatment for the underlying malocclusion also needs to be planned. Given the fact that this case is a growing child with a well-aligned lower arch and only a mild class II division 2 malocclusion, it was decided to use headgear to correct the buccal segment relationship and molar crossbite. This could be used in conjunction with extraction of the UR2; exposure and bonding of the UR3 and fixed appliances to align UR3 co-ordinate the dental arches and correct the incisor relationship.

In the long-term, the UR2 and UR1 will be replaced with implant restorations or adhesive bridges. Getting the UR3 into the correct position in the arch simplifies resin-retained bridge replacement of the UR2, whilst the UL1 could be used as an abutment for an adhesive bridge replacing UR1. Following extraction of the UR2 and exposure of the UR3 a fixed appliance is being used to bring the UR3 into occlusion (Fig. 2.41).

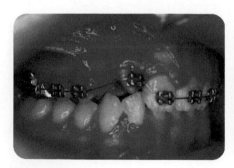
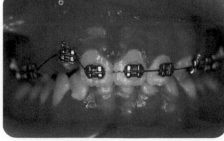
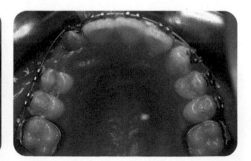

Figure 2.41

Case 2.17

A 13-year-old male presented with the malocclusion seen in Figure 2.42.

Summarize the findings from the panoramic radiograph

- The panoramic view confirms the presence of all teeth including the third molars
- UR3 is unerupted, slightly distally angulated and high, encroaching on the UR4 root
- UR3 has an open root apex
- Both mandibular second premolars are vertically impacted
- There is no evidence of pathology related to the unerupted teeth

At what age might you expect there to be radiographic evidence of development of third molars?

There is a significant age range within which third molar calcification becomes evident radiographically.

An age range of less than 6 years to 14 years has been demonstrated in a large Spanish sample (Bolaños et al., 2003). The initial development of maxillary third molars tends to be less clear and difficult to diagnose. There are also secular trends in relation to timing of development. Development of third molars in a Japanese group has been shown to be significantly slower than in a similar German sample (Olze et al., 2003).

The cephalometric radiograph is shown in Figure 2.43. Summarize the malocclusion

- A 13-year-old male with a class I malocclusion on a mild skeletal class II base with average vertical proportions.
- Molar relationship is class I bilaterally, the centre lines are coincident and the canine relationship is ½ class II bilaterally.
- Malocclusion is further complicated by:
  - Ectopic UR3
  - Impacted mandibular second premolars

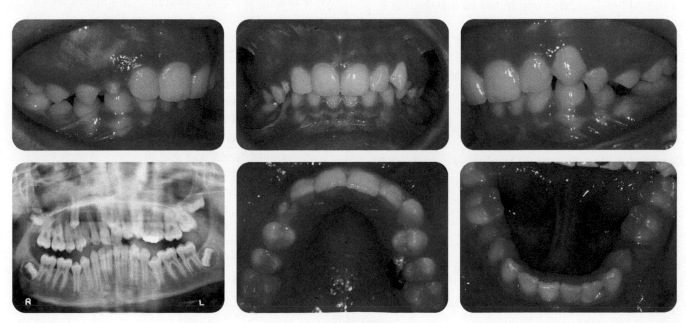

Figure 2.42

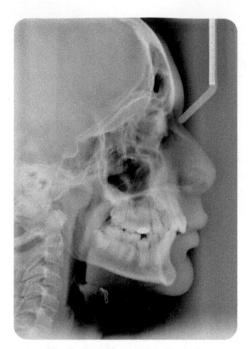

Figure 2.43

○ Increased overbite
○ Crowding of both arches.

What is the aetiology of the malocclusion?

- **Skeletal:** There is a mild skeletal class II discrepancy characterized by mandibular retrognathia. This has contributed to the ½ class II canine relationship.
- **Abnormal dental development:** The UR3 has developed ectopically. With further vertical eruption it is likely to become transposed with the UR4. A multifactorial aetiology involving both genetic and environmental factors has been implicated in unilateral transpositions (Ely *et al.*, 2006).
- **Dento-alveolar:** There is a tooth size-to-arch length discrepancy in both arches resulting in crowding, rotations of the lower anteriors, buccal displacement of the UL3 and lingual displacement of the mandibular second premolars.
- **Local factors:** Premature loss of the mandibular second primary molars may well have exacerbated the underlying dento-alveolar disproportion. This has led to impaction of LL5 and impeded eruption of the LR5.

Comment on the soft tissue profile and its relevance to treatment planning

The soft tissue profile is full. The naso-labial angle is between 90 and 110 degrees and the upper lip drapes slightly anteriorly, with fullness to the upper vermilion. The upper and lower lips are thick and robust. The labio-mental groove is relatively deep. Overall the soft tissue profile is acceptable and could withstand retraction subsequent to extractions.

What treatment would you suggest in this case?

The aims of treatment will include relief of crowding, arch alignment and levelling, overbite reduction and management of the impacted and ectopic teeth. While consideration could be given to alignment of the UR3, this tooth is in an unfavourable position and complex and prolonged orthodontics would be involved to address it. In addition, there is a space requirement in the maxillary arch to relieve crowding and to impart palatal root torque on the maxillary incisors. The canines are also ½ class II. Therefore, consideration could be given to loss of the UL3 in conjunction with the UL4 to maintain the integrity of the maxillary centerline. In the mandibular arch, consideration should be given to removal of either premolar units or possibly second molars bilaterally. In this case, it was decided to remove both mandibular second molars. Although removal of the second molars is potentially more difficult, loss of lower premolars would create excessive space to align the mandibular arch and would risk prolonged treatment. In addition, there would be a significant anchorage demand to maintain the molar relationship and correct the canine relationship to class I.

Which appliances could be used to facilitate eruption of the mandibular second premolars following extraction of the second permanent molars?

Possible options include use of a lingual arch to prevent mesial migration of the first molars or a lip bumper to encourage distal movement and tipping of the first molars. In addition a simple lower fixed appliance could be placed with coil spring to reopen space for eruption of the second premolars. This option is likely to lead to proclination and advancement of the mandibular incisors. In this instance, no active treatment was undertaken for 6 months following the extractions. The premolars erupted independently

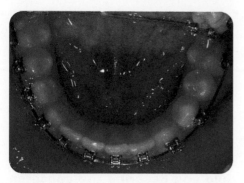

Figure 2.44

during this period due to uprighting and distal movement of the first molars (Figure 2.44).

What modifications should be made to the UR4 to simulate the appearance of the UR3?

The objectives for the UR4 are influenced by the position of the upper lip and display of the upper anterior teeth at rest and during function. In this instance the upper lip line was quite low with little incisal exposure at rest; therefore, disparity between gingival margin heights was not considered significant. As the first premolar is narrower mesio-distally than a canine, the bracket could be placed distally to encourage mesio-palatal rotation of the tooth. To extrude the premolar, the bracket could be placed slightly gingival to the centre of the clinical crown to harmonize the buccal cusp tip position with that of the canine on the opposing side. If extrusion results in premature occlusal contact, some reduction of the palatal cusp of the premolar could be undertaken.

If the smile line were higher, consideration could be given to intrusion of the first premolar or gingival surgery to equalize the gingival heights. The premolar could also be veneered to better simulate the appearance of a canine, recreating the appropriate vertical position of the cusp tip. The final occlusion is shown in Figure 2.45.

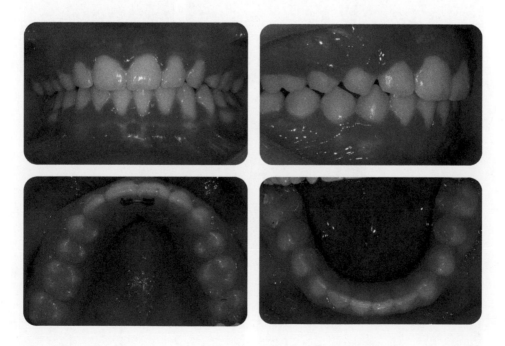

Figure 2.45

Case 2.18

This patient presents complaining of the appearance of his teeth, in particular the UR1 (Figure 2.46).

How would you describe the appearance of the upper right central incisor?

The UR1 is discoloured (grey in appearance) and appears intruded relative to the UL1.

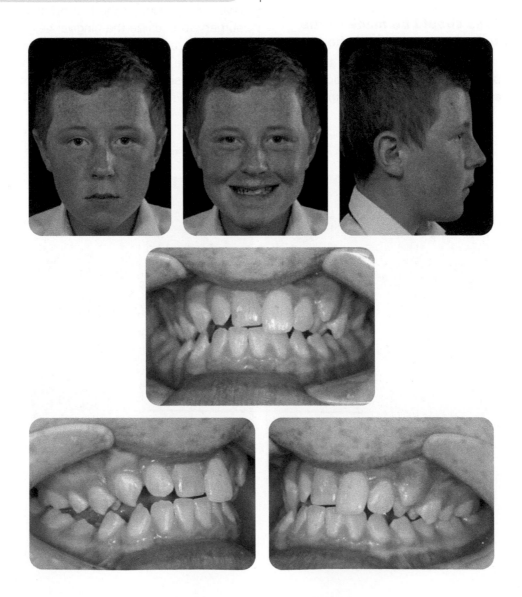

Figure 2.46

What is the likely aetiology of this problem?

The discolouration of this tooth is most likely the result of a loss of vitality. The most common cause of this is previous trauma to the tooth. It would be important to establish the timing and nature of the trauma and any subsequent treatment.

What additional investigation would be helpful?

During history taking it would be important to establish if the tooth is currently symptomatic.

Clinical and radiological examination would help confirm if the tooth has been previously root canal treated.

In this case the UR1 had been previously avulsed with subsequent re-implantation and splinting. This was followed by root canal treatment. In light of this information, what additional information could radiographic examination provide?

A long cone periapical radiograph would identify any external root resorption.

How would you expect external root resorption to manifest clinically?

External root resorption may manifest as mobility of the tooth. In some cases there may be replacement resorption (ankylosis). In cases where ankylosis has occurred, the tooth will often appear intruded relative to the contra-lateral tooth. Percussion of the tooth would reveal a high pitched or dulled sound. Orthodontic traction to the tooth would not be successful. Clinical and radiographic examination (Figure 2.47) in this case suggests that the UR1 is ankylosed.

What is the long-term prognosis for the UR1? How will this affect the management of this patient's malocclusion?

The long-term prognosis of this tooth is poor. Options for future replacement of this tooth will need to be discussed. Joint planning with a restorative colleague would be advisable.

Summarize the problem list for this case

- Discoloured, ankylosed UR1
- Mild skeletal class III pattern
- Increased vertical proportions
- Mild crowding in the upper and lower arches
- Evidence of dento-alveolar compensation in the lower arch, with a retroclined lower labial segment

What changes in the patient's malocclusion may occur with future growth?

In view of the patient's increased vertical proportions and possible downward and backward growth rotation, there is a tendency for development of an anterior open bite with further growth.

What implications does the potential future growth have on the timing of the patient's orthodontic treatment?

In view of the patient's age, it would be prudent to monitor his growth (in particular his overbite) prior to making any definitive decisions regarding his management.

Whilst monitoring the patient's developing malocclusion, how would you manage the ankylosed tooth?

The decision around the timing of removal of the ankylosed tooth is difficult. It is important to consider the relative advantages and disadvantages of removing the tooth earlier rather than later.

As the patient matures the relative infra-occlusion of the tooth will increase, which will result in a greater vertical bony defect when the tooth is removed in the future. Early removal of the tooth, however, will result in a greater buccal bony defect and the added disadvantage of the need for a removable prosthesis to maintain the space and restore the aesthetics.

In this case the decision was made to continue monitoring the tooth and the level of infra-occlusion during growth.

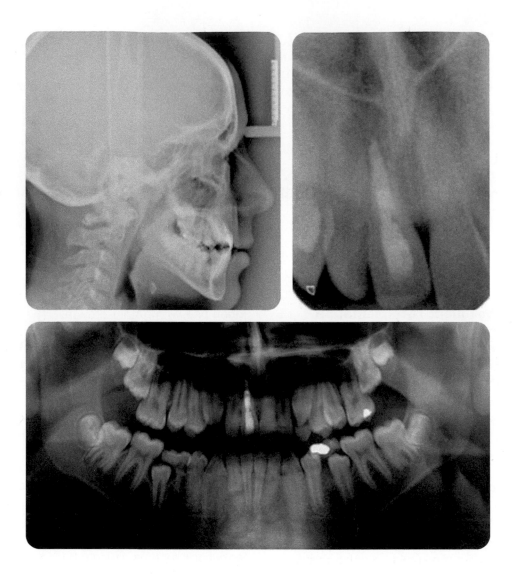

Figure 2.47

Case 2.19

This 11-year-old patient presents complaining of his prominent upper anterior teeth.

Discuss the relevance of the extra-oral and radiological examination in relation to treatment planning in this case (Figures 2.48 and 2.49)

Extra-oral examination of the patient allows skeletal and soft-tissue factors contributing to the malocclusion to be identified.

In this case the aetiology of the malocclusion is multi-factorial:

- Skeletal discrepancy both antero-posteriorly and vertically
- Skeletal class II pattern with increased lower anterior face height and Frankfort–mandibular planes angle.

Soft tissue examination reveals a short upper lip, which contributes to the increased incisor and gingival show at rest. There is a lower lip trap with the lower lip lying behind the upper incisors, increasing the overjet.

In treatment planning in growing individuals it is important to take into account future growth. Why is this?

It is important to identify patients in whom future growth may be unfavourable as this will affect the stability of any orthodontic treatment undertaken.

Patients identified as 'high angle class II cases' are often perceived to have challenging malocclusions. Why is this?

High angle cases are thought to have downward and backward growth rotations. In class II cases, this may result in an increase in the overjet and reduction in the overbite and a deterioration of facial aesthetics with further growth.

What type of appliance would be suitable to address the skeletal and soft tissue factors contributing to this patient's malocclusion?

As this patient is still growing, a modified functional appliance would be appropriate.

The mode of action of functional appliances is thought, in the main, to be dento-alveolar; however, there may also be minimal skeletal effects with limited potential for modification of growth.

In this case a modified twin-block appliance with occlusal coverage of the upper block will allow an intrusive force to be applied to address the vertical maxillary excess. High pull headgear applied to flying extra-oral traction (EOT) tubes to the upper block may potentially restrain vertical growth.

How do we assess the success of a functional appliance (Figure 2.50)?

Reduction of the overjet and correction of the molar relationship are the most commonly used outcome measures.

How do radiographs help with the confirmation of the changes (skeletal and dento-alveolar) that have occurred (Figure 2.50)?

Radiographic superimposition (of the post-functional cephalogram on the pre-treatment cephalogram) can demonstrate both dento-alveolar changes and growth.

treatment in a Medicaid population: interim results from a randomized clinical trial. *Am J Orthod Dentofacial Orthop* 137:324–333.

Larsson E (1987) The effect of finger-sucking on the occlusion: a review. *Eur J Orthod* 9:279–282.

Levine RS (1999). Briefing paper: oral aspects of dummy and digit sucking. *Br Dent J* 186:108.

Little RM, Reider RA, Stein A (1990) Mandibular arch length increase during the mixed dentition: postretention evaluation of stability and relapse. *Am J Orthod Dento Orthop*; 97:392–404.

Olze A, Taniguchi M, Schmeling A, *et al.* (2003) Comparative study on the chronology of third molar mineralization in a Japanese and a German population. *Leg Med (Tokyo)* 5:256–260.

Parkin N, Benson PE, Shah A, *et al.* (2009a) Extraction of primary (baby) teeth for unerupted palatally displaced permanent canine teeth in children. *Cochrane Database Syst Rev* CD004621.

Parkin N, Elcock C, Smith RN, Griffin RC, Brook AH (2009b) The aetiology of hypodontia: the prevalence, severity and location of hypodontia within families. *Arch Oral Biol* 54 (Suppl 1):S52–56.

Pearson MH (1996) The effects of extracting upper second permanent molars. *Br J Orthod* 23:378–379.

Power SM, Short MB (1993) An investigation into the response of palatally displaced canines to the removal of deciduous canines and an assessment of factors contributing to favourable eruption. *Br J Orthod* 20:215–223.

Richardson ME, Richardson A (1993) Lower third molar development subsequent to second molar extraction. *Am J Orthod Dentofacial Orthop* 104: 566–574.

Tulloch KF, Proffit WR, Phillips C (2004) Outcomes in a 2-phase randomized clinical trial of early Class II treatment. *Am J Orthod Dento Orthop* 125: 657–667.

3

Class I Malocclusion

Introduction

A class I malocclusion is associated with a class I incisor relationship and an Angle class I molar relationship. However, the molar relationship is not immutable; it can be affected by dental factors and may not truly represent the underlying skeletal relationship. The skeletal pattern is usually class I, with any variation from this being generally mild antero-posteriorly. In the vertical dimension a larger range of difference can be seen; from a slightly increased overbite to a frank anterior openbite with an associated increase in the lower face height. A markedly increased overbite is incompatible with the definition of a class I incisor relationship and is more in the domain of a class II division 1 or a class II division 2 malocclusion. Again, by definition, the overjet is within the normal range, although cases of bi-maxillary proclination can have a class I incisor relationship with an increased overjet or even slightly reduced overjet. The soft tissues in class I cases are generally favourable and rarely have a significant influence on the malocclusion, although an increased lower face height and anterior openbite is usually associated with lip incompetence and bi-maxillary proclination may occur in association with lip protrusion.

A spectrum of dento-alveolar problems can be seen in class I malocclusions, including dental crowding, crossbite and open bite. Crowding or dento-alveolar disproportion is one of the commonest manifestations of a class I malocclusion. Indeed, in developed countries crowding is endemic and has become more prevalent over the last century. There has been much speculation why this is the case. Lack of inter-proximal

attrition or jaw development as a result of a soft diet has been implicated (Begg, 1954; Varrela, 2006). However, compared to isolated communities, most Western societies represent significant genetic heterogeneity and as such, there is probably a large genetic component to the increased incidence of crowding that has been reported.

Transverse or vertical problems can have a variety of causes. An anterior open bite can be skeletal in origin, secondary to a hyper-divergent facial form, or due to failure of incisor eruption following a persistent non-nutritive sucking habit. An important part of diagnosis is therefore to define the aetiology, as this determines the treatment aims and mechanics. Posterior crossbites can be associated with digit sucking or a skeletal discrepancy and facial asymmetry. In the former, simple dental expansion is usually appropriate, but in the presence of skeletal discrepancy this is often inappropriate.

Treatment planning is influenced primarily by the dento-alveolar features of the malocclusion, as the skeletal pattern is generally class I:

- **Orthodontic treatment:** The treatment of crowding usually requires comprehensive upper and lower fixed appliance therapy with or without the extraction of permanent teeth. Mild crowding can usually be managed without extraction, space being created by distalization of arches, utilization of the Leeway space or inter-proximal reduction (Cetlin and Ten Hoeve, 1983; Sheridan, 1985; Brennan and Gianelly, 2000). Excessive lower arch expansion or proclination of the lower incisors should generally be avoided as this is inherently unstable (Ackerman and

Proffit, 1997). In severe crowding the extraction of teeth is usually required. The premolars are often the teeth of choice as they are close to the site of labial crowding and are of similar size and form in the maxillary and mandibular arch. A vocal minority has made much of the possible detrimental effects associated with elective orthodontic tooth extraction, particularly in relation to the effect on the soft tissue profile and as a cause of temporo-mandibular dysfunction. However, to date there is no evidence that the use of extractions, when appropriate and as part of a properly planned course of treatment, leads to any long-term problems. As such, extractions remain a valuable tool to address dento-alveolar disproportion (DiBiase and Sandler, 2001).

- **Orthodontics and surgery:** For those cases with a significant vertical skeletal component to their malocclusion, combined orthodontic–surgical treatment can be carried out. In growing patients, numerous techniques have been described to treat an anterior open bite, including extra-oral traction and repelling magnets designed to intrude the buccal dentition, all with limited success. More recently, mini-screws and plates have been introduced, which may in the long-term prove to be an effective alternative to surgery.

Case 3.1

This 13-year-old female was referred by her general dental practitioner complaining of crowding associated with her teeth. There was no relevant medical history and she was quite happy to wear braces.

Extra-oral

Skeletal relationship	
Antero-posterior	Mild skeletal class II
Vertical	FMPA: Average
	Lower face height: Average
Transverse	Facial asymmetry: None
Soft tissues	Lip competence: Competent
	Naso-labial angle: Obtuse
Upper incisor show	At rest: 4 mm
	Smiling: 9 mm
Temporo-mandibular joint	Healthy with good range and co-ordination of movement

Intra-oral

Teeth present	7654321/1234E67
	7654321/1234567
Dental health (restorations, caries)	Good
Oral hygiene – periodontal	Poor with gingival hyperplasia labial to UL2
Lower arch	Crowding: Mild
	Incisor inclination: Average
	Curve of Spee: Average
Upper arch	Crowding: Moderate
	Incisor inclination: Average
	Canine position: Buccally placed
Occlusion	Incisor relationship: Class I
	Overjet: 3 mm
	Overbite: Average and complete
	Molar relationship: ¼ unit class II bilaterally
	Canine relationship: ½ unit class II bilaterally
	Centre lines: upper centre line 1 mm to left
	Functional occlusion: Group function

Summary

A 13-year-old female presented with a class I malocclusion on a mild skeletal class II pattern with average vertical dimensions complicated by moderate upper arch crowding, palatal displacement of the UL2 and a localized crossbite (Figure 3.1).

Treatment Plan

- Occipital pull extra-oral traction to reinforce anchorage
- Upper and lower pre-adjusted edgewise appliances
- Long-term retention

Treatment Progress

Headgear compliance was poor. It was therefore decided to remove both maxillary second premolars to recreate space for maxillary arch alignment (Figure 3.2).

What options were there in this case in the absence of headgear wear?

The initial aim of this case was to achieve a class I incisor relationship with distal movement of the upper

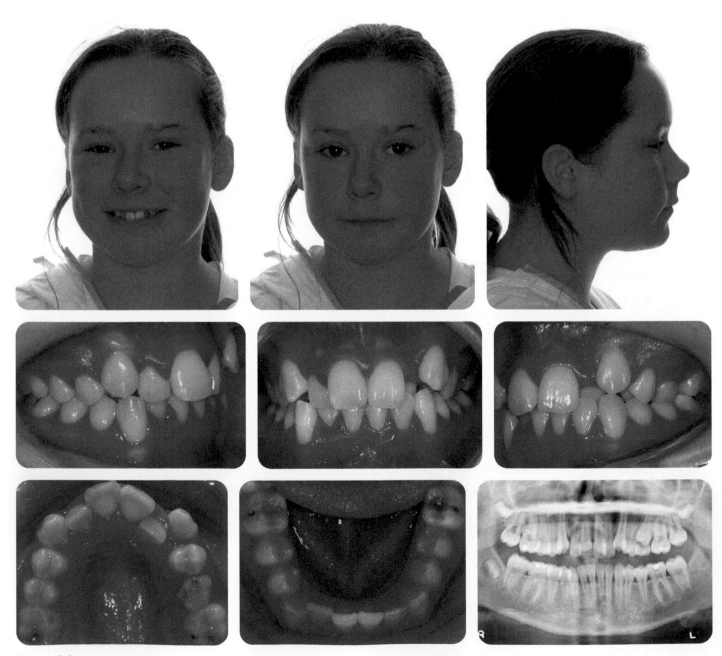

Figure 3.1

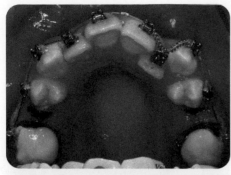

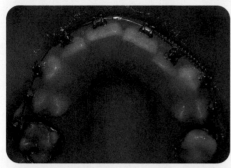

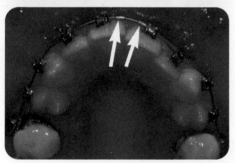

Figure 3.2

molars. Distal molar movement would have facilitated upper arch alignment by space recreation.
Consideration was given to use of a non-compliance class II corrector (Pendulum appliance, Forsus spring, Jasper jumper) to correct the molar relationship. However, it was decided to remove maxillary second premolars in view of the space and anchorage requirements.

Self-ligating brackets (SLBs) were used in this case. What are SLBs and what are the advantages of these systems?

SLBs are brackets that use a clip or slide mechanism to engage the archwire rather than the application of ligatures. SLBs have demonstrated marked reductions in frictional resistance in laboratory studies, which might be expected to accelerate tooth movement and reduce orthodontic treatment time. However, clinical studies have largely failed to confirm this (DiBiase *et al.*, 2011; Fleming *et al.*, 2009, 2010; Scott *et al.*, 2008). A slight advantage of SLBs is a possible reduction in chair-side time for the orthodontist (Turnbull and Birnie, 2007).

Describe what is happening in Figure 3.2

Both maxillary second premolars have been removed and the upper fixed appliance has been placed. An 0.013-inch nickel–titanium archwire is in place, with nickel–titanium coil spring being used between the UL1 and UL3 to recreate space and accommodate the UL2 in the arch. Simultaneously, elastomeric chain has been placed from the first molars to maxillary canines to aid retraction of these teeth. The UL2 has been ligated directly to the archwire to initiate labial movement of this tooth. Use of active mechanics on nickel–titanium archwires is traditionally not recommended due to the risk of loss of arch form, round tripping of teeth and unpredictable reactionary forces. However, some clinicians believe the secure ligation afforded by SLBs lends itself to this approach (Damon, 1998).

What are the arrows pointing to in Figure 3.2 (lower panel)?

These are small metal stops placed on the archwire to prevent its excessive sliding through the SLBs, which can be a problem during the early stages of treatment because of the reduced static friction associated with these appliances. Without the use of stops, the archwire can slide into the soft tissues behind the molar bands and cause trauma.

Why has glass ionomer cement been placed on the maxillary first molars?

This is done to disengage the occlusion, facilitating correction of the crossbite involving the UL2. Removable appliances and fixed bite raisers may be used as an alternative.

What is the final buccal segment relationship (Figure 3.3)?

The final canine relationship is class I; however, the molar relationship is class II because premolar units have been removed in the upper arch only.

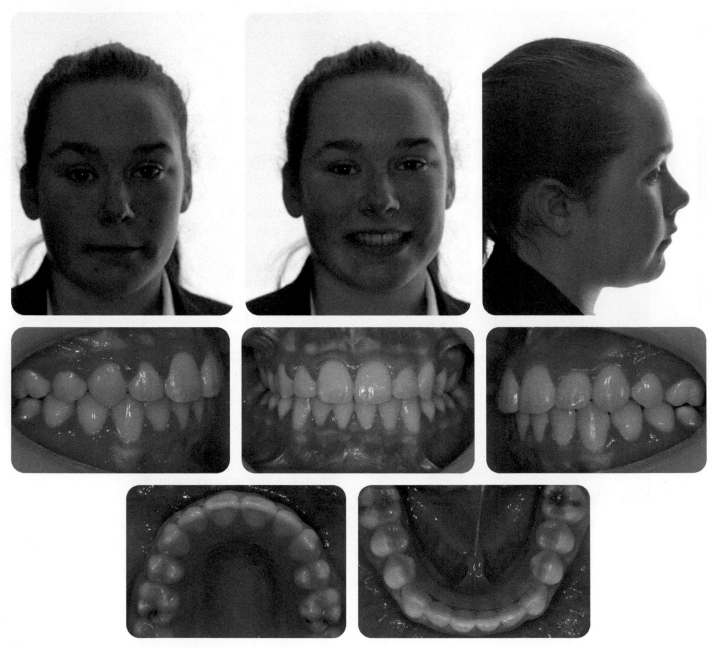

Figure 3.3

Case 3.2

This 13-year-old female was referred by her general dental practitioner concerned about her crooked teeth and misshapen incisor. There was no relevant medical history.

Extra-oral

Skeletal relationship
  Antero-posterior — Mild skeletal class II
  Vertical — FMPA: Average
                Lower face height: Average
  Transverse — Facial asymmetry: None
Soft tissues — Lip competence: Competent
                Naso-labial angle: Average
Upper incisor show — At rest: 4mm
                Smiling: 9mm
Temporo-mandibular joint — Healthy with good range and co-ordination of movement

Intra-oral

Teeth present

$$\frac{7654321/1234567}{76\ \ 4321/1234567}$$

Dental health (restorations, caries) — Good
UL2 is diminutive with abnormal coronal morphology
Oral hygiene – periodontal — Good
Lower arch — Crowding: Moderate
                Incisor inclination: Average
                Curve of Spee: Average
Upper arch — Crowding: Mild
                Incisor inclination: Average
                Canine position: Line of the arch
Occlusion — Incisor relationship: Class I
                Overjet: 3mm
                Overbite: Average and complete
                Molar relationship: Class I bilaterally
                Centre lines:
                    Upper centre line correct to mid-facial axis
                    Lower centre line deviated 3mm to right side
                Functional occlusion: Group function

What are the main radiographic findings (Figure 3.4)?

- LR5 is unerupted and distoangularly impacted against the LR6
- UL2 appears to be invaginated (dens in dente) with a short root form
- Upper third molars are absent but the lower third molars are developing

Summary

A 13-year-old female presented with a class I malocclusion on a mild skeletal class II pattern with average vertical dimensions complicated by impaction of the LR5 and an invaginated UL2 (Figure 3.4).

An opinion from a paediatric dentist suggested that the long-term prognosis for the UL2 was poor.

Treatment Plan

The moderate crowding in the lower arch was sufficient to indicate the need for extractions; in addition, the LR5 was impacted. Therefore, extraction of the LR5 and LL5 was indicated. Extraction in the lower arch dictated the need for extractions in the upper arch and, given the poor morphology associated with the UL2, a decision was made to extract this tooth. In the interests of symmetry, the UR2 was also extracted rather than a premolar in the upper right quadrant.

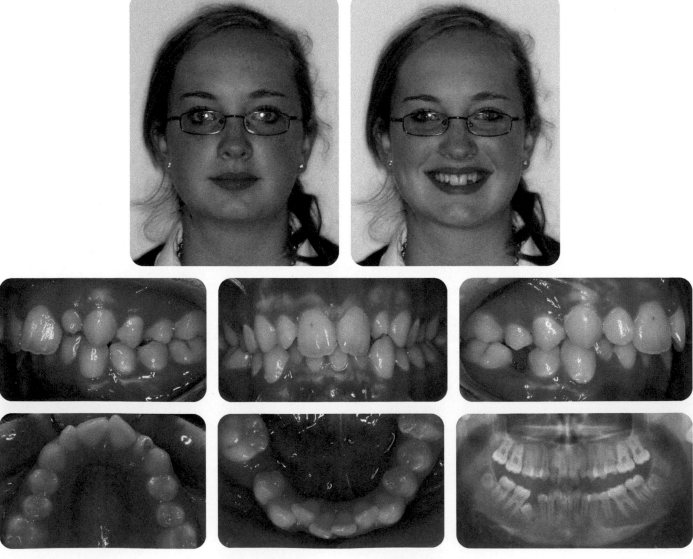

Figure 3.4

- Extraction of the UR2, UL2, LR5 and LL5
- Upper and lower pre-adjusted edgewise appliances
- Long-term retention

What factors need to be considered when substituting a maxillary canine for a lateral incisor?

Canine substitution may be performed to place a canine in the position of a maxillary lateral incisor. This can be achieved by orthodontic tooth movement, localized bleaching, reshaping and direct restorative build-ups. Orthodontic considerations include the mismatch in gingival heights and requirement for palatal root torque. Palatal root torque is enhanced by using bracket prescriptions that already incorporate this or inverting brackets with a labial root torque prescription (Figure 3.5) and by using large-dimension finishing wires (0.021 × 0.025 inch). Reshaping of cusp tips is performed incrementally to limit pulpal responses and sensitivity, and to avoid sclerosis or devitalization in the longer term (Thordarson *et al.*, 1991; Zachrisson and Mjor, 1975).

The archwire illustrated in Figure 3.6 is a heat-activated nickel–titanium wire. What properties make it a suitable initial aligning wire?

Archwires during initial alignment are required to have a large range, low stiffness and adequate strength to resist occlusal forces (Kusy, 1997). Nickel–titanium archwires demonstrate all of these features in addition to a property called shape memory, which in conjunction with their high flexibility permits alignment of grossly-displaced and rotated teeth. Nickel–titanium wires are also claimed to display superelastic properties, with constant levels of force delivered at varying deflections.

What are the alternatives to nickel–titanium wires during initial alignment?

- Multiloop stainless steel wires
- Co-axial or braided stainless steel wires

The flexibility of these steel wires is based on increasing the length of wire; however, their usability is poor, being susceptible to permanent deformation when fully engaged in teeth with more severe crowding.

Is there any evidence to suggest that orthodontic alignment is accelerated with nickel–titanium wires?

No. A recent systematic review considered seven randomized controlled trials comparing nickel–titanium wires and multi-strand stainless steel wires of varying dimensions. No differences in relation to the efficiency of alignment, root resorption and subjective pain experience were found (Wang *et al.*, 2010).

How have the canines been modified following appliance removal (Figure 3.7)?

The mesial tips have been built up with composite.

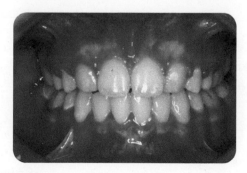

Figure 3.7

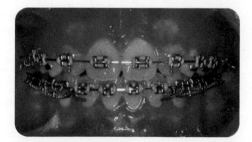

Figure 3.5

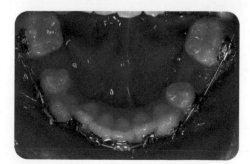

Figure 3.6

Case 3.3

This 13-year-old male was referred by his orthodontic specialist concerned about his ectopic canine teeth. There was no relevant medical history.

Extra-oral

Skeletal relationship
  Antero-posterior   Skeletal class I
  Vertical   FMPA: Average
                            Lower face height: Average
  Transverse   Facial asymmetry: None
Soft tissues   Lip competence: Competent
                            Naso-labial angle: Average
Upper incisor show   At rest: 3mm
                            Smiling: 6mm
Temporo-mandibular joint   Healthy with good range and co-ordination of movement

Intra-oral

Teeth present   7654 21/1234567
                            7654321/1234567

Dental health (restorations, caries)   Good
Oral hygiene – periodontal Good
Lower arch   Crowding: Severe
                            Incisor inclination: Average
                            Curve of Spee: Average
Upper arch   Crowding: Moderate
                            Incisor inclination: Average
                            Canine position: Palatal on right side; erupted on left
Occlusion   Incisor relationship: Class I
                            Overjet: 3mm
                            Overbite: Average and complete
                            Molar relationship: Class I on right side; ½ unit
                            class II on left
                            Centre lines:
                                Upper 2mm to right
                                Lower 2mm to left of facial midline
                            Functional occlusion: Group function

Radiographic Findings (Figure 3.8)

- UR3 is ectopic and mesially-angulated
- Cusp tip overlies the lateral incisor and has a favourable prognosis for mechanical eruption
- No evidence of associated pathology
- All third molars are developing

Summary

A 14-year-old male presented with a class I malocclusion on a skeletal class I base with average vertical dimensions complicated by an ectopic UR3, crowding of both arches and centre line discrepancies (Figure 3.8).

Treatment Plan

- Extraction of the UR5, UL4, LR5 and LL5
- Open surgical exposure of the UR3
- Trans-palatal arch
- Upper and lower pre-adjusted edgewise appliances
- Long-term retention

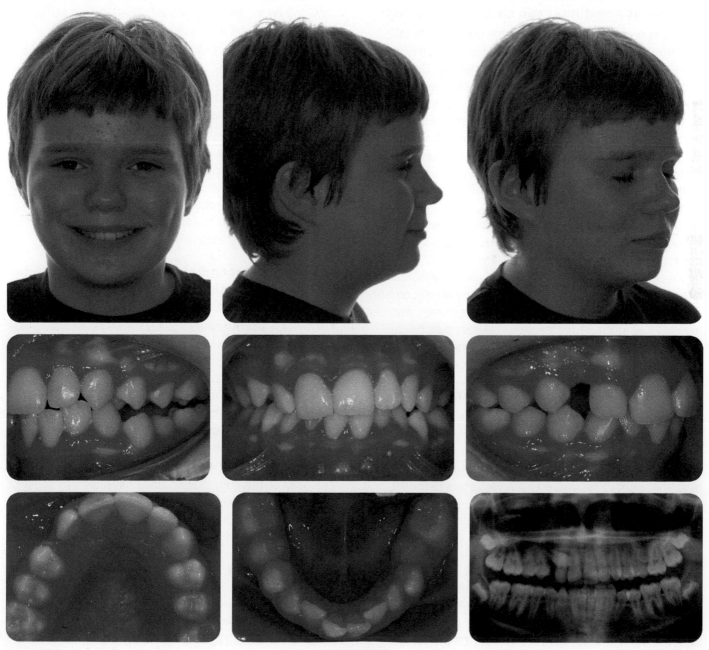

Figure 3.8

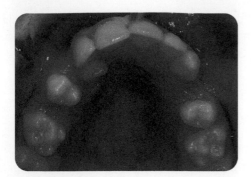

Figure 3.9

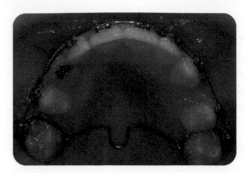

Figure 3.10

What are the common causes of a centre line discrepancy and how can they be corrected?

Centre line discrepancies may arise due to skeletal asymmetries, particularly mandibular asymmetry, or more commonly due to dental asymmetries. Dental causes include asymmetric crowding, early loss of primary teeth, tooth-size discrepancies, hypodontia, supernumerary teeth, localized impactions and other pathology (Holmes *et al.*, 1989). A mandibular deviation on closing (secondary to an anterior or posterior crossbite) can also cause a centre line discrepancy due to the displaced position of the mandible in the intercuspal position.

Centre line deviations of dental origin may be treated with unilateral or asymmetric extraction patterns, asymmetric mechanics (asymmetric headgear, push–pull mechanics and asymmetric inter-arch elastics) and elimination of any displacement. Centre line discrepancies of skeletal origin may also be masked using these techniques; however, significant asymmetries may warrant a combined orthodontic–surgical approach to permit complete correction.

What has happened in Figure 3.9?

An open surgical exposure of the UR3 has taken place. The tooth has subsequently been allowed to erupt for 3 months. Advocates of open surgical exposures favour this approach as it may permit autonomous eruption without recourse to active forces (Schmidt and Kokich, 2007).

What mechanics are being used in Figure 3.10?

An open nickel–titanium coil spring has been used on an 0.018-inch stainless steel archwire to recreate space for alignment of the UR3. The UR4 has been moved distally and the UR2 has been moved mesially to facilitate correction of the maxillary centre line. Elastomeric traction is also being used to move the

UR3 buccally and distally. Anchorage support is provided by a trans-palatal arch. The UR2 and UR4 have been ligated with stainless steel ligatures to maintain rotational control of these teeth as space is created for the UR3.

Why is 0.018-inch stainless steel favoured as a base archwire during this treatment phase?

Stainless steel arch wires have sufficient rigidity to provide anchorage and resist unwanted reactionary forces to the elastomeric traction (such as loss of arch form). Round steel wire also has relatively low frictional resistance; therefore sliding mechanics can be performed easily to recreate the space required to accommodate the canine in the arch.

Mandibular second molars were also included in the fixed appliance. What are the advantages of this?

- Provide vertical anchorage facilitating overbite reduction
- Prevent mesial tipping of first molars during space closure
- Alignment of the second molars

Nickel–titanium closing coils are being used for space closure (Figure 3.11). Is there any evidence to support their use?

Yes. Nickel–titanium closing coils have proven superior to elastomeric chains during space closure (Dixon *et al.*, 2002; Nightingale and Jones, 2003; Samuels *et al.*, 1998). However, their additional cost makes their use over alternative methods of space closure (elastomerics) less clear-cut.

What force level should be used during space closure with nickel–titanium closing coils?

Force levels of approximately 150 g are considered ideal (Samuels *et al.*, 1998). Lower levels result in

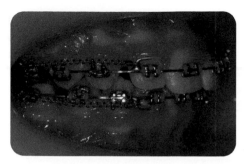

Figure 3.11

slower tooth movement. Higher force levels do not increase the rate of tooth movement but may predispose to greater pain levels, undermining resorption and root resorption.

Figure 3.12 shows the final occlusion.

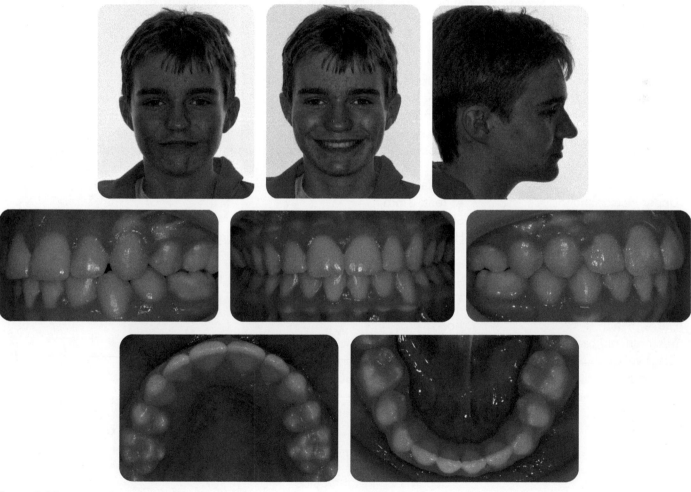

Figure 3.12

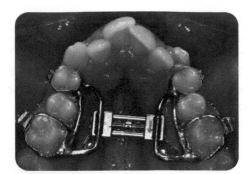

Figure 3.14

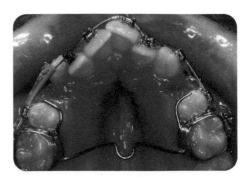

Figure 3.15

What is the biological basis of rapid maxillary expansion?

Rapid maxillary expansion (RME) is a form of palatal expansion used during adolescence. It relies on the presence of the mid-palatal suture, which in autopsy studies has been shown to remain patent until 15 years at least (Melsen, 1975). Appliances may be banded (usually on first premolars and first molars) or bonded to the buccal segment teeth. Expansion usually occurs at a rate of 0.5–1 mm per day, while slow expansion with removable appliances is usually undertaken at 0.25–0.5 mm per week. Over-expansion is usually desirable to allow for some relapse during fixed appliance therapy. The RME is usually left *in situ* for 3 months following the active phase of treatment to help maintain the expansion. Alternatively, a modified palatal arch can be fitted with palatal arms to maintain the expansion, which is a little less obtrusive than leaving the RME appliance in place.

How is arch expansion generally achieved?

Arch expansion arises through a combination of bodily tooth movement and tipping. Tipping movements are likely to be unstable and may have bite-opening effects with inferior movement of supporting cusps resulting in a decrease of overbite. Tipping and bodily movements occur in a ratio of almost 1:1 with rapid expansion, while tipping movements predominate with more gradual forms of expansion, including removable appliances and quadhelices (Frank and Engel, 1982). Banded rapid expansion designs are commonly used; however, bonded designs may limit bite opening due to occlusal coverage posteriorly (Reed *et al.*, 1999).

What were the main options to achieve maxillary arch expansion in this case?
- Removable appliances
- Fixed appliances:
  - Quadhelix
  - Bonded or banded RME

Why was RME used?
- Greater than 4 mm of expansion was required.
- Patient was of a suitable age and likely to have a patent mid-palatal suture.
- RME offers greater potential bodily movement, which would mean any likely bite opening effect may be less marked. This is important in this case because of the reduced overbite.

What is the role of the cemented appliance in Figure 3.15?

This is a modified trans-palatal arch. Its purpose is to retain the expansion generated with RME following removal of the active appliance. It is discarded when rigid stainless steel wires are engaged in the fixed appliance. The modification involves extending rigid wires from the first molar band to the second premolars.

Why were mandibular second premolars extracted as part of the treatment plan in this case?
- Relief of crowding
- Transverse constriction of the mandibular arch
- Maintain a positive overbite

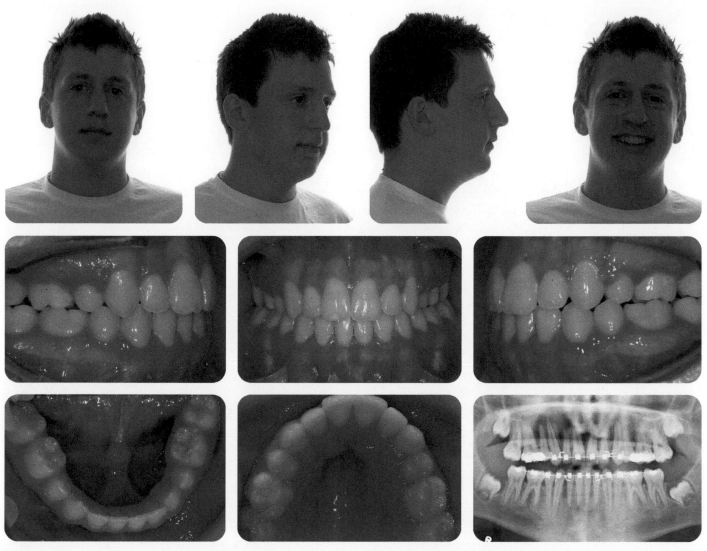

Figure 3.16

The final result is shown in Figure 3.16. Is crossbite correction likely to be stable?

Maxillary arch expansion is inherently unstable. Prolonged follow-up suggests that significant reductions in transverse skeletal and dental dimensions occur following therapy (Lagravere *et al.*, 2005a,b).

Consequently, prolonged retention is necessary to maintain transverse increases, with rigid Hawley-type retainers recommended for this purpose. Removal of mandibular second premolars and transverse constriction is likely to be more stable and may contribute to the stability of crossbite correction.

Case 3.5

This 16-year-old female was referred by her general dental practitioner because she did not like the gaps between her teeth. There was no relevant medical history.

Extra-oral

Skeletal relationship	
Antero-posterior	Skeletal class I
Vertical	FMPA: Average
	Lower face height: Average
Transverse	Facial symmetry: None
Soft tissues	Lip competence: Competent
	Naso-labial angle: Average
Upper incisor show	At rest: 4 mm
	Smiling: 8 mm
Temporo-mandibular joint	Healthy with good range and co-ordination of movement

Intra-oral

Teeth present

$$\frac{76E\ \ 3\ \ 1/123\ \ E67}{76ED321/123DE67}$$

Dental health (restorations, caries)	Good
	No active caries and good oral hygiene
Lower arch	Well aligned
	Lower primary molars infra-occluded
	Second molars partially erupted and mesioangually impacted
	Incisor inclination: Upright
Upper arch	Spaced
	Upper second primary molars infra-occluded
	Incisor inclination: Upright
	Canine position: Both in the line of the arch
Occlusion	Incisor relationship: Class I
	Overjet: 3 mm
	Overbite: Average and complete
	Upper centre line to right by approximately 3 mm
	Molar relationship: ½ unit class II bilaterally
	Lateral open bites left and right

Summary

A 16-year-old female presented with a class I malocclusion on a skeletal class I base with average lower face height, severe permanent tooth agenesis (oligodontia), generalized spacing, infra-occlusion of primary molars and impaction of the lower second permanent molars (Figure 3.17).

Which teeth are congenitally absent according to the panoramic radiograph (Figure 3.18)?

LR8, LR5, LR4, LL4, LL5, UL8, UL5, UL4, UR2, UR4, UR5, UR8.

The LR7 and LL7 are mesially impacted.

Treatment Plan

The patient was assessed initially on a combined clinic.

- Treatment was aimed at consolidation of space in the upper labial segment for prosthetic replacement of the UR2 and build up of the UL2.

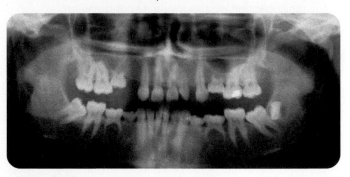

Figure 3.18

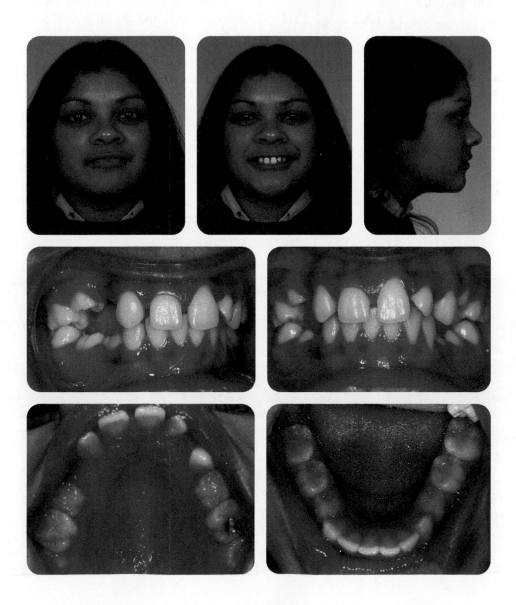

Figure 3.17

- In the buccal segments, the aim was also to consolidate space for prosthetic replacement of, ideally, one premolar unit per quadrant. In the lower arch this would be achieved by mesial movement of the lower first molars which would also create space for disimpaction of the lower second molars.
- The lower second primary molars were extracted, but the remaining primary teeth were retained to maintain bone.

A pre-adjusted edgewise fixed appliance was placed with initial nickel–titanium aligning archwires. The initial working archwires were 0.018-inch stainless steel in the upper arch and 0.019 × 0.025-inch stainless steel in the lower arch.

How was space created for the UR2 (Figure 3.19, upper panel)?

Space was recreated for the UR2 using compressed nickel–titanium push coil between the UR1 and UR3.

What mechanics are being used in Figure 3.19 (lower panel)?

In the lower arch, spacing anteriorly has been consolidated and space closed in the buccal segments using intra-arch mechanics supported by inter-arch class II elastics. Anterior anchorage was also reinforced by placing labial crown torque in the lower rectangular steel archwire anteriorly to prevent lingual movement of the lower incisors.

Once some space had been created, the lower second molars were bonded and aligned using nickel–titanium wires (Figure 3.20). Once space for the UR2 was acceptable, the remaining upper primary molars were removed and final space closure in the upper buccal segments was undertaken on a rectangular stainless steel archwire. A prosthetic tooth was placed on the archwire to replace the UR2 and improve aesthetics.

On debond the patient was provided with upper and lower Hawley retainers incorporating prosthetic teeth, which the patient was instructed to wear full time (Figure 3.21). Despite maintaining the primary molars for as long as possible, the patient needed augmentation of bone in the upper right quadrant to allow for implant placement.

Following this, the missing teeth were replaced with implants and the UL2 was built up with composite (Figure 3.22).

What specific problems are there in treating severe hypodontia?

Severe hypodontia can present a real challenge to the orthodontist and prosthodontist in achieving both an aesthetically good and functionally stable outcome. This challenge depends on the number of teeth missing, the size and shape of the teeth present, the position of these teeth and the underlying malocclusion. There appears to be an association

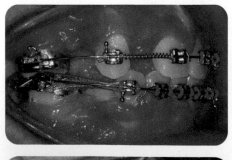
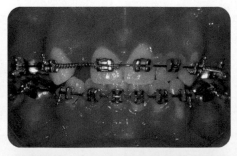
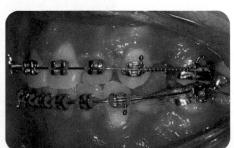
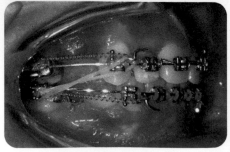
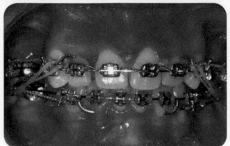
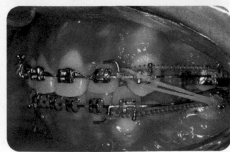

Figure 3.19

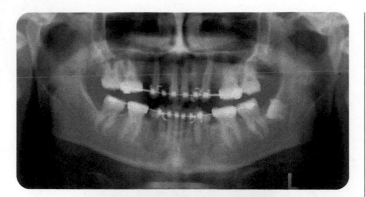

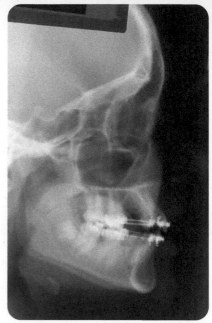

Figure 3.20

of the lower molars, to close space down in the mandibular buccal segments, was aided by increasing the anchorage value of the lower labial segment by placing labial crown torque in the lower archwire and the use of class II elastics. In the upper arch, space was created for the UR2 by using compressed push coil and reciprocal anchorage, avoiding anchorage loss associated with the maxillary molars.

What other techniques are available to facilitate space closure from behind?

- Protraction headgear
- Temporary anchorage devices
- Self-ligating brackets on individual teeth

What are the different options for replacing missing teeth?

Initially, removable retainers can be used that incorporate prosthetic teeth, but whilst these may be acceptable in the short-term, they do not provide a long-term solution. Therefore, once periodontal re-organization has occurred, more permanent solutions are often sought. The main choice is between bridges and implants. In a growing patient, implants are contra-indicated due to the risk of infra-occlusion with continued vertical facial growth. Therefore bridges can be used as a semi-permanent solution. Due to the destructive nature of traditional fixed–fixed bridges, adhesive bridges are increasingly favoured. These have very good aesthetics, and can be placed in areas with inadequate alveolar bone for implants and also where there is insufficient space between the teeth. The biggest drawback with these types of bridges is their higher failure rate when compared to implants.

Whilst infra-occlusion can occur in adults, implants are generally the treatment of choice in patients past their adolescent growth. The problem, particularly with patients affected by severe hypodontia, is the lack of bone to allow implant placement. Bone can be generated by orthodontic tooth movement or alternatively by augmenting the area with autogenous grafting of bone or synthetic bone substitutes.

between severe hypodontia and microdontia. This is most evident in patients with ectodermal dysplasia (see Figure 11.5). Therefore, treatment involves not only replacing missing teeth, but also reshaping or building up the natural teeth that are present. In this case the diminutive UL2 was built up to restore normal shape and size.

Another problem is the lack of potential anchorage in these cases for correct tooth movement, which worsens with the increasing number of missing teeth. Mechanically there are certain techniques that can be used to overcome this. In this case, mesial movement

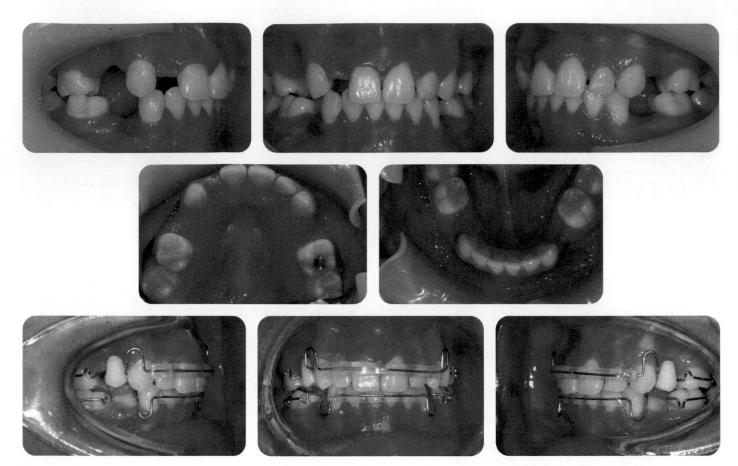

Figure 3.21

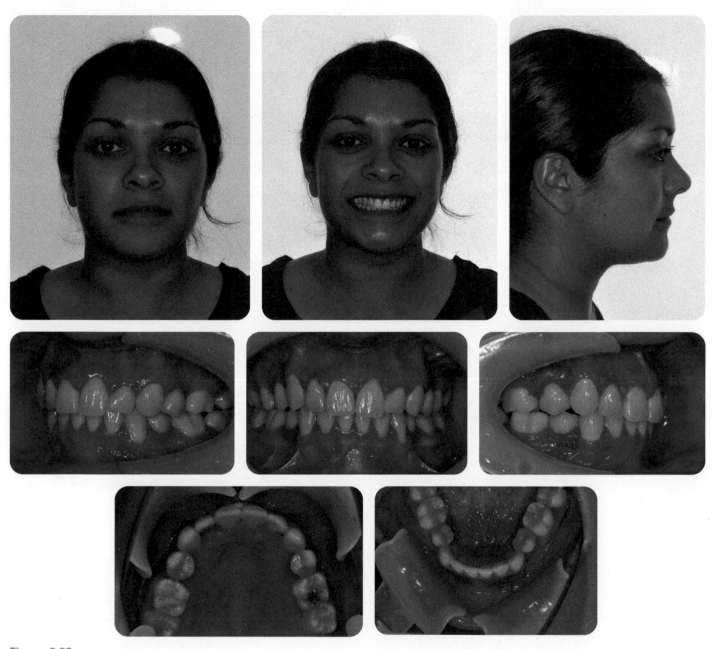

Figure 3.22

Case 3.6

This 15-year-old female patient was referred by her general dental practitioner concerned with delayed dental development. There was no relevant medical history.

Extra-oral

Skeletal relationship
   Antero-posterior   Skeletal class I
   Vertical   FMPA: Average
                            Lower face height: Average
   Transverse   Facial asymmetry: None
Soft tissues   Lip competence: Competent
                            Naso-labial angle: Average
Upper incisor show   At rest: 3 mm
                            Smiling: 8 mm
Temporo-mandibular joint   Healthy with good range and co-ordination of movement

Intra-oral

Teeth present

$$\frac{76ED\ 21/1234567}{7654321/12C4567}$$

Dental health
(restorations, caries)
Large occlusal restoration in the LL6
Small occlusal restorations in the LR6 and LR7
URDE restored and carious
UR1 crown fracture with evidence of pulpal access (this tooth had been traumatized with pulpal exposure and a superficial pulpotomy carried out by the general dental practitioner 6 months previously)
Extensive white spot lesions along the cervical margin of all four first permanent molars

Oral hygiene – periodontal   Below average

Lower arch
Crowding:
   Severe
   LL3 unerupted (in this case palpable buccally)
Incisor inclination: Average
Curve of Spee: Average

Upper arch
Crowding: Severe
Incisor inclination: Average
Canine position:
   UL3 mesially angulated and erupted
   UR3 unerupted and palatal

Occlusion
Incisor relationship: Class I (UL2 in crossbite)
Overjet: 2 mm
Overbite: Reduced and complete
Molar relationship: Class I bilaterally
Centre lines: Upper centre line 3 mm to right and lower 1 mm to left of facial midline
Posterior crossbite tendency (the retained URDE are in crossbite, but the first molars are edge-to-edge)
Functional occlusion: Group function

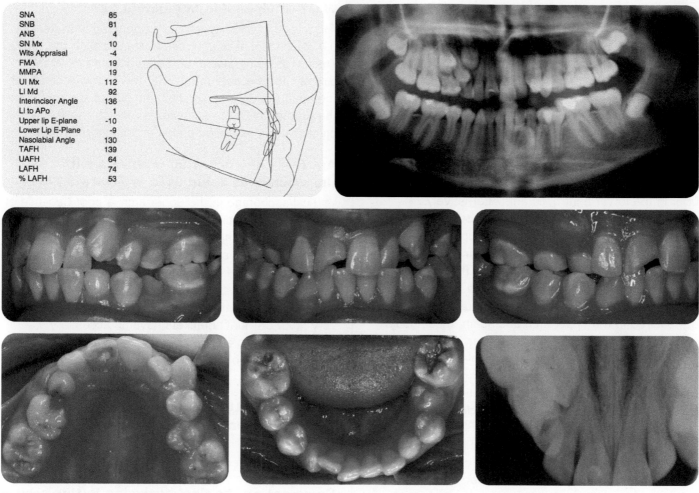

SNA	85
SNB	81
ANB	4
SN Mx	10
Wits Appraisal	-4
FMA	19
MMPA	19
UI Mx	112
Li Md	92
Interincisor Angle	136
LI to APo	1
Upper lip E-plane	-10
Lower Lip E-Plane	-9
Nasolabial Angle	130
TAFH	139
UAFH	64
LAFH	74
% LAFH	53

Figure 3.23

Radiographic Findings (Figure 3.23)

- UR3 is ectopic and on the palatal side of the arch
- Crowding associated with the unerupted UR3, UR4 and UR5
- LL3 is unerupted and vertically positioned UR1 has a crown fracture, evidence of an access cavity, but no root canal treatment
- UR1 has a crown fracture, evidence of an access cavity, but no root canal treatment

Summary

A 15-year-old female presented with a class I malocclusion on a skeletal class I base with average vertical dimensions complicated by severe crowding, ectopic UR3 and LL3, retained primary teeth and a traumatized UR1 (Figure 3.23).

What is the Index of Orthodontic Treatment Need (IOTN) of this malocclusion?

5i, based upon impeded eruption of the UR3 and LL3.

What are the main problems associated with this malocclusion?

- Poor dental health (restorations in the lower first molars, trauma to the UR1, early cervical decalcification in the lower first permanent molars)
- Severe crowding in both arches
- Ectopic UR3 (palatal) and LL3 (in line of the arch)
- UL2 in crossbite
- Retained primary teeth
- Patient now 15 years of age

How would you manage this patient?

- Improve the oral hygiene
- Obtain a specialist opinion regarding the UR1

At 15 years of age, this patient has impacted permanent teeth, retained primary teeth and dental arch crowding. Her problems need to be addressed sooner rather than later and need to be co-ordinated into a coherent and logical treatment plan. However, the oral hygiene should be improved and the UR1 temporized before any orthodontic treatment commences. The prognosis for the UR1 was good following endodontic temporization.

In the lower arch, the crowding will dictate a need for extractions. The LL3 is impacted and therefore is a candidate for extraction (particularly as the patient is nearly 16 years old) along with a premolar (or even the LR3) in the lower right quadrant. Alternatively, premolar extractions could be carried out and the LL3 exposed (it is in a good position to erupt favourably, particularly with orthodontic traction). In the upper arch, there is also severe crowding in the upper right quadrant and an ectopic UR3, which is quite high and palatal. The UR5 is also impacted. Extractions will also be required in the upper arch and again, these could involve canines or premolars; however, a decision was made to extract the upper first premolars and expose/bond the UR3.

The patient was referred for extraction of the LLC, URD, URE, LL4, LR4, UL4 and UR4, closed exposure and bonding with gold chain of the UR3 and open exposure of the LL3. This was carried out under a general anaesthetic in a single procedure.

Once these procedures were carried out, a trans-palatal arch was fitted to reinforce anchorage in the upper arch and a pre-adjusted edgewise fixed appliance system placed to align the teeth, co-ordinate the dental arches and produce a functional class I occlusion. The UR5 rapidly erupted unaided, but traction was required for the UR3 and LL3.

What is happening in Figure 3.24?

A Damon3 bracket system is being used with flexible 0.014-inch nickel–titanium archwires to align the teeth. Traction is being placed on both impacted canines directly; for the unerupted UR3, the archwire has been threaded through a gold chain bonded to the tooth; for the erupted LL3, the archwire is running through a bracket that has been bonded directly to this tooth.

Are there any potential problems with the mechanics being used in Figure 3.24?

Vertical anchorage in the upper arch is poor because of the archwire flexibility. If the UR3 does not move, the remaining teeth can intrude. This can be circumvented by running a rigid stainless steel archwire and a piggy-back flexible nickel–titanium archwire to erupt the UR3. However, this is difficult with a Damon3 self-ligating bracket because the bracket slot is very rigid. DamonQ brackets have an accessory horizontal slot to aid the use of a piggy-back (these brackets were not available when this patient was treated).

How has the UR1 been restored following the completion of orthodontic treatment (Figure 3.24)?

This tooth has been built up with composite resin.

Comment on the final occlusion in this case (Figure 3.25)

The upper and lower centre lines are not quite co-incident and the overbite is a little tenuous. The centre line discrepancy is partially related to the loss of some coronal tissue on the UR1.

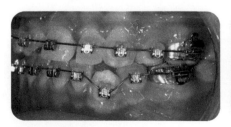
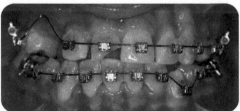
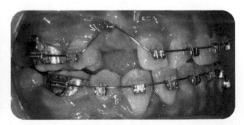

Figure 3.24

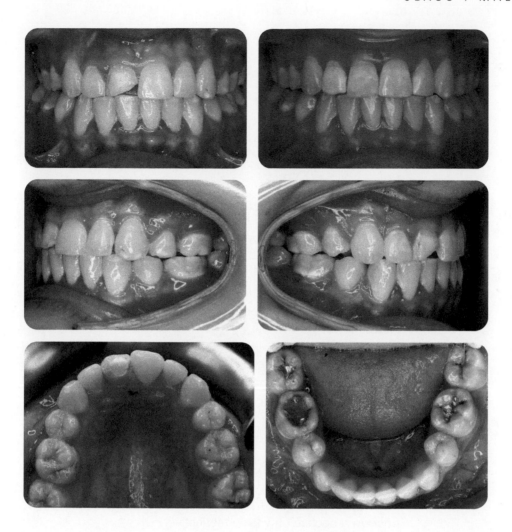

Figure 3.25

Case 3.7

This 12-year-old male was referred by his general dental practitioner with crowding. The patient did not like his crooked teeth. There was a history of trauma to the upper labial segment.

Extra-oral

Skeletal relationship
  Antero-posterior   Mild skeletal class II
  Vertical   Average FMPA and lower face height
  Transverse   No asymmetry
Soft tissues   Lips competent
                              Naso-labial angle: Average
Upper incisor show   Rest: 4mm
                              Smiling: 9mm

Intra-oral

Teeth present

$$\frac{7654321/1234567}{7654321/1234567}$$

Dental health   Good
(restorations, caries)   Uncomplicated crown fracture UL1 (tooth asymptomatic and positive response on vitality testing)

Lower arch   Crowding: Mild
                              Incisor inclination: Proclined
                              Curve of Spee: Normal
                              Canines: Distally angulated

Upper arch   Crowding: Mild
                              Incisor inclination: Average
                              Canines:
                                 Buccally displaced
                                 Upper right distally angulated

Occlusion   Incisor relationship: Class I
                              Overjet: increased (4mm to the UR1)
                              Overbite: Average and complete
                              Molar relationship: Angle class I bilaterally

                              Canine relationship: ½ unit class II bilaterally
                              Centre lines: Central and coincident
                              Functional occlusion: Group function left and right

Summary

A 12-year-old male presented with a class I malocclusion on a mild skeletal class II base with average vertical dimensions, complicated by mild crowding and history of trauma to the upper labial segment (Figure 3.26).

What are the aims of treatment?

The aims of treatment were to relieve the crowding, and level and align the arches to provide a class I incisor and buccal segment relationship.

As the crowding was mild, it was decided to treat on a non-extraction basis, creating space by inter-proximal reduction in the lower labial segment. To facilitate this, a self-ligating bracket system was used. According to the philosophy of the system, using light-force nickel–titanium wires will not overcome the soft tissue forces, thereby preventing over-expansion of the dental arches (Figure 3.27). Despite this, space was primarily created to align the dentition by proclination of the labial segments (Figure 3.28). As this is inherently unstable, particularly in the lower labial segment, permanent retention was necessitated in the form of a lower bonded retainer and upper and lower removable vacuum form retainers worn at night. Following treatment, the patient's general dental practitioner was asked to restore the upper left central incisor, which remained asymptomatic.

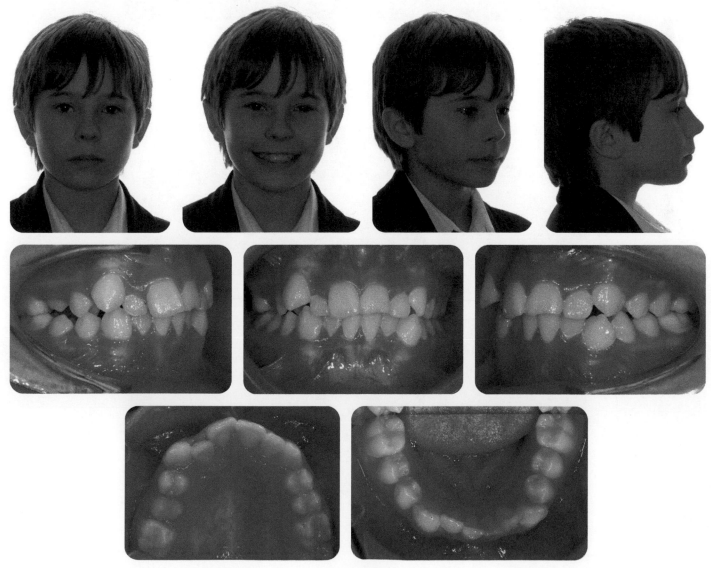

Figure 3.26

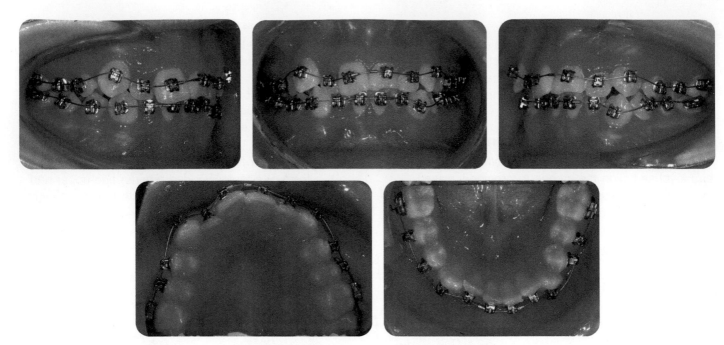

Figure 3.27

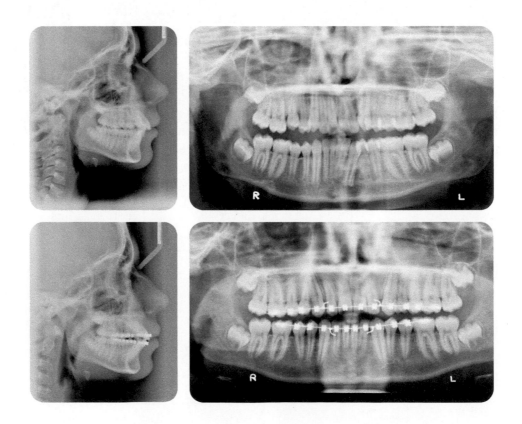

Figure 3.28

What are the advantages of using a self-ligating bracket system in this case?

A self-ligating bracket system was used in this case to facilitate treatment without extraction of teeth. Self-ligating brackets are either active or passive, depending on how closely they engage the teeth. Damon brackets used in this case are passive and treatment involves the use of primarily light nickel–titanium wires. When engaged these result in light forces that theoretically do not overcome the periodontium or the soft tissues, resulting in faster tooth movement and preventing proclination of the labial segments, whilst allowing physiological adaptation and expansion in the buccal segments (Damon, 1998). In reality there is no evidence that this type of bracket either moves teeth quicker or aligns them differently (Wright et al., 2011; Fleming and Johal, 2010).

During alignment, teeth will take the path of least resistance. In this case, as the crowding presented in the labial segments, the result was proclination of the incisors as no space was created for them further back in the arch by loss of teeth. Inter-proximal reduction was carried out later in treatment in an attempt to recapture this, but the labial segments were still left proclined at the end of treatment.

In what alternative ways could the patient be treated?

Non-extraction treatment resulted in excessive proclination of the labial segments. Therefore, to avoid this, four premolars could have been removed for relief of crowding and retraction of the incisors. Considering that the soft tissue profile was full at the start of treatment, there was certainly no risk of retracting the lips excessively if teeth had been extracted. One contra-indication to extraction is the history of dento-alveolar trauma, making it sensible practice to avoid excessive movement of the traumatized tooth and to avoid a protracted course of treatment to reduce the risk of iatrogenic damage.

What are the risks when orthodontically moving traumatized teeth?

Traumatic injuries to the dentition are extremely common in childhood, particularly in relation to an increase in overjet (Todd and Dodd, 1985; Bauss et al., 2008). There appears to be a greater risk when treating teeth with a history of trauma and loss of vitality and root resorption (Linge and Linge, 1991; Bauss et al., 2009).

What steps can be taken to reduce these risks?

If the trauma is sustained during or just prior to orthodontic treatment, a rest or observation period is recommended to allow the tooth and supporting structures to recover. The duration of this varies from 3 months for subluxated teeth or those sustaining an uncomplicated crown fracture, as in this case, to 24 months for more serious injuries such as root fractures (Atack, 1999). See Table 1.1.

During active treatment, light forces should be used and excessive movement of the traumatized tooth avoided, particularly in relation to root contact with the cortical bone which has been associated with root resorption. The tooth should be vitality tested if appropriate every 3 months and radiographs repeated 6–9 months into active treatment. If a radiograph shows evidence of root resorption, a pause in active treatment is recommended for 3 months (Levander et al., 1994).

Similarly, if teeth are traumatized during orthodontic treatment, an observation period is recommended during which active forces are suspended. If vitality is lost, necessitating root canal therapy, it is sensible practice to temporize the root canal with calcium hydroxide until the end of active orthodontics when a definitive root filling can be placed. However, for teeth that are devitalized prior to orthodontics, a definitive root filling should be placed before appliances are placed, as prolonged use of a calcium hydroxide dressing increases the risk of root fracture.

Case 3.8

This 15-year-old patient presented with a class I malocclusion. He was unhappy with the appearance of his upper front teeth.

What aspect of his teeth do you think he might have been unhappy with (Figure 3.29)?

He has quite a marked upper centre line shift over to the right of his facial midline. This is not necessarily something that a patient would notice; however, in this case it is quite obvious as the upper centre line is displaced by a full tooth width to the right.

What is the cause of this problem?

This case has a congenitally absent UR2, resulting in the upper centre line shift to the right.

Discuss a treatment plan to address the centre line shift

To correct the centre line, upper and lower pre-adjusted edgewise appliances would be required as well as space creation in the upper left quadrant. Space can be generated by unilaterally distalizing the UL6 or tooth extraction.

Distalizing the UL6 would be difficult. Headgear is not really practical in this case for several reasons. The UL6 would need to be distalized a full unit of space unilaterally, which is mechanically difficult. Asymmetric headgear can be used for this, but moving a first molar a full unit distally in this way is very ambitious and would require excellent co-operation. Realistically, the headgear would need to be supplemented with a distalizing appliance (e.g. a Ten Hoeve appliance), with extraction of the UL7 also likely to be required. The age of the patient means that compliance with headgear would be an issue and the lack of growth would make it very difficult to move the first molar more than a unit of space. A fixed anchorage device or fixed anchorage-supported appliance could be used

instead of headgear, but even with fixed anchorage, moving the UL6 the required amount would be problematic.

Alternatively, a tooth could be extracted in the upper left quadrant. This would either be a premolar tooth (usually the UL4, which provides the most accessible space for moving the upper centre line to the left) or, as in this case, the diminutive UL2, which helps to provide aesthetic symmetry.

Correction of the upper centre line will be anchorage demanding. How can this be managed?

Re-enforcement of the anchorage during centre line correction will be required. This can be achieved by the placement of a Nance palatal arch at the start of treatment. Alternatively, the placement of a mini-screw between the roots of the UL5 and UL6 would provide skeletal anchorage. Placement of a laceback at the time of the appliance placement in the upper left quadrant would prevent the tip in the UL3 bracket from being expressed. In order to reduce friction, correction of the centre line can be started on a round stainless steel archwire, once alignment has been achieved. The anchorage demands may be further reduced by moving the upper central incisor teeth individually to the left. The use of asymmetric elastics will also aid centre line correction.

Extraction of the UL2 will introduce a tooth-size discrepancy. What does this mean and what are the potential implications of this?

The loss of two incisor teeth in the upper arch in this case will mean the upper buccal segments finish with a bilateral class II relationship. The total tooth-size ratio between the upper and lower arches will be different, which sometimes means that closure of all space in the arch (in this case the upper dental arch) missing the teeth can be difficult. A diagnostic or Kesling set-up of the final planned tooth positions can be carried out on a stone model in advance to predict how well the two arches will fit together.

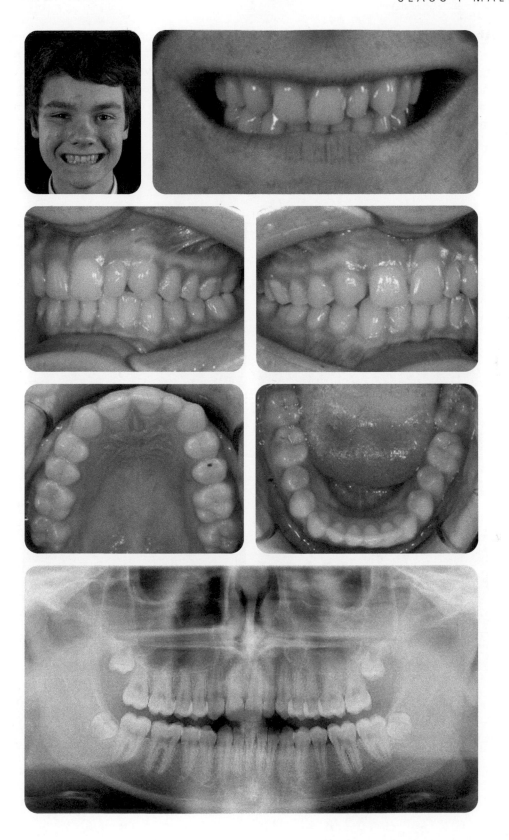

Figure 3.29

Are there any other implications of extracting the UL2 only?

A further factor to consider in this case is arch coordination. The incisor relationship is class I but has a class III tendency and the overbite is reduced. Extracting the UL2 and correcting the centre line, whilst maintaining an intact lower arch, might make the maintenance of a class I incisor relationship quite difficult. However, the lower arch is well aligned and extractions here would demand a lot of time to close the space. The mid treatment occlusion is shown in Figure 3.30.

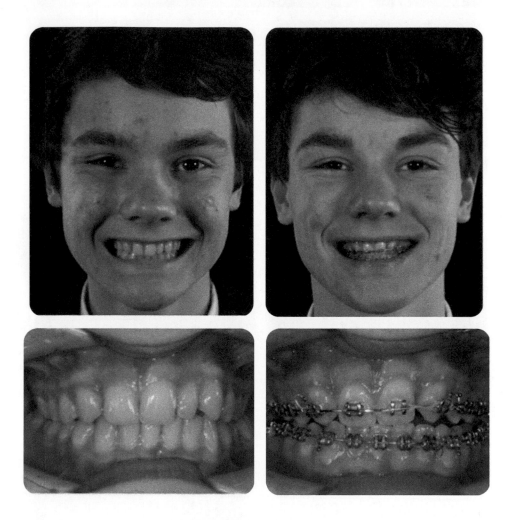

Figure 3.30

Case 3.9

This 10-year-old boy presented in the mixed dentition following referral from his dental practitioner.

Summarize the malocclusion shown in Figure 3.31

A class I incisor relationship on a skeletal class I pattern with average vertical dimensions complicated by:

- Impacted second premolars in all quadrants
- Class II molar relationship bilaterally
- Increased overbite
- Rotated mandibular first premolars
- Evidence of vitality loss to the UL1.

What treatment options would you consider?

There is crowding in both arches, which is severe in the upper arch. In order to align the upper arch, premolar extractions would be required in conjunction with headgear to reinforce anchorage. In the lower arch, premolar extractions should also be considered to relieve the crowding. Treatment would then involve upper and lower fixed appliances.

However, the lower arch could be treated on a non-extraction basis, recreating space for eruption of both lower second premolars. In this instance, the upper first premolars were removed under local anaesthetic and space created in the lower arch to treat the crowding with a non-extraction approach. This avoided extraction of the lower second premolars, which would have necessitated surgical extraction and a general anaesthetic. However, space needed to be maintained in the upper arch until the second premolars erupted.

What is the likely cause of the impacted second premolars in this case?

The impacted second premolars are likely to be related to premature loss of the second primary molars with resultant mesial migration (and rotation in the upper arch) of the first permanent molars, resulting in space loss. The second primary molars were likely to have been lost due to caries; the first permanent molars have had fissure sealants and are unrestored.

If further development of the second premolars occurred without space creation where would you expect the second premolars to erupt?

The second premolars are likely to have erupted palatally and lingually to the line of the upper and lower arches, respectively.

What appliance is shown in Figure 3.32, and what is its mode of action?

This is a lower lip bumper.

The lip bumper has an acrylic shield labial to the mandibular incisors. There is also a U-loop mesial to the first molar; this is activated and ligated to the first molar teeth. The muscular forces generated by the lip place a distal force on the acrylic shield, which is transferred to the first molars. Ultimately, this force may result in distal movement and tipping of the first permanent molars, generating sufficient space for eruption of the mandibular second premolars (Figure 3.33).

What are the disadvantages of using a lip bumper?

Any distal movement of the buccal dentition usually takes place in conjunction with mandibular incisor proclination (Davidovich et al., 2001), which can be unstable. Increases in arch width, particularly inter-canine and primary inter-molar and premolar distances are also likely to relapse (Hashish and Mostafa, 2009). Moreover, these appliances can be quite difficult to tolerate and are prone to fracture. Distalization of the mandibular first molars can also result in impaction of the second molars.

What are the loops in Figure 3.33?

These are Sandusky closing loops. They obviate dependence on sliding mechanics, with the force

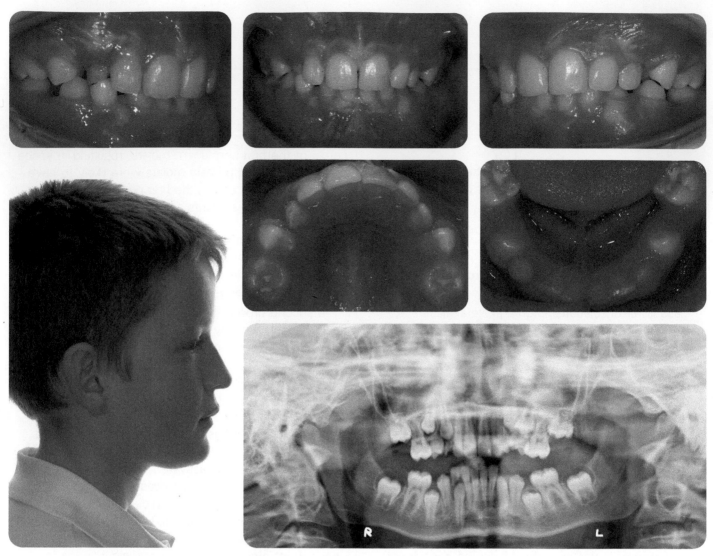

Figure 3.31

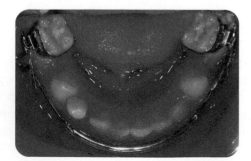

Figure 3.32

promoting space closure stored in the loop. By increasing the vertical arm of the loop, the horizontal flexibility of the wire increases, reducing the force levels.

The final occlusion is shown in Figure 3.34.

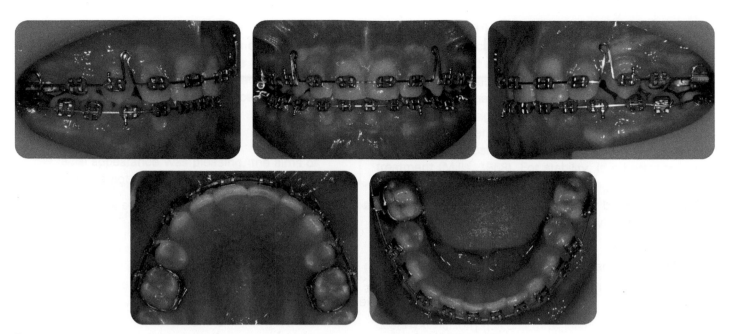

Figure 3.33

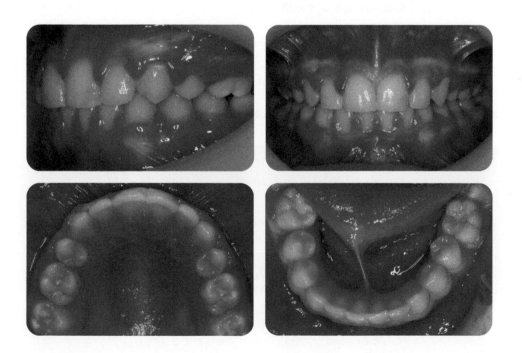

Figure 3.34

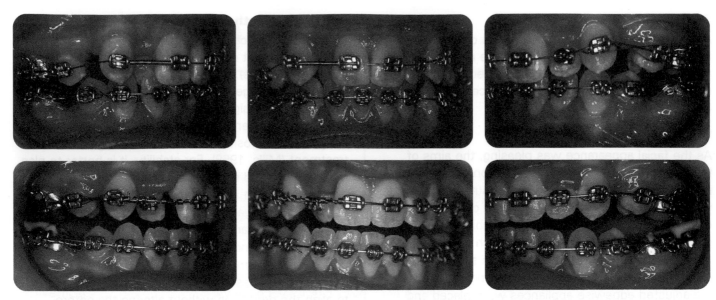

Figure 3.36

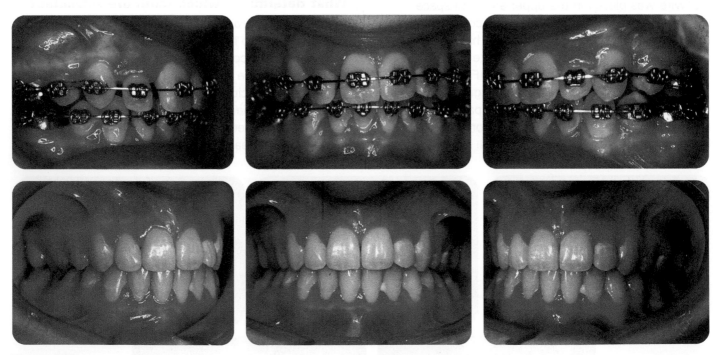

Figure 3.37

heavily restored. All teeth were of normal size and form.

In the lower arch the crowding was mild, the aim was not to retract the lower incisors and as such, the anchorage demand was minimal. Therefore, lower second premolars were extracted.

In the upper arch the crowding was severe and the upper canines were distally angulated. The anchorage demand was therefore moderate, resulting in a decision to extract upper first premolars. As the molar relationship was ½ unit class II bilaterally, an added benefit of this extraction pattern was that it would allow greater mesial movement of the lower molars than the uppers if anchorage were correctly managed during treatment, and this would help facilitate the correction of the buccal segments.

How were the dental centre lines corrected in this case?

The deviation of the centre lines in this case was primarily due to the asymmetry of the crowding. Correction of the centre lines started during the alignment stage with asymmetric use of lacebacks (see Figure 3.36). Lacebacks are figure-of-eight under-ties used from the first molar to the canine during the alignment phase of treatment. They are thought to prevent proclination of the incisors, particularly when the canines are distally angulated. In this case, the UL3 was distally angulated and therefore a laceback

was placed in the upper left quadrant. In the lower arch, although both canines were mesially angulated, the lower centre line was to the left and therefore a laceback was placed in the lower right quadrant. Although lacebacks are routinely used by many practitioners, their proposed benefits remain unproven (Usmani et al., 2002; Irvine et al., 2004).

Following initial alignment an upper round stainless steel archwire was placed and compressed nickel–titanium push coil was used to re-create space for the palatally displaced UR2. The advantages of using these types of mechanics is that they place minimal strain on posterior anchorage and aid in upper centre line correction.

How was the anterior crossbite corrected?

Once space had been created for the blocked out UR2, a bracket was placed on it and a piggy-back nickel–titanium archwire placed under the stainless steel wire to align it (Sandler et al., 1999). This was facilitated by the use of a fixed posterior bite plane, which was created by temporarily placing glass ionomer cement on the lower molars as the tooth was moved over the bite. The bracket was placed upside down on the lateral incisor, which has the effect of reversing the torque in the bracket base, in this case creating labial root torque to ensure that as the crown of the tooth was aligned the root was not left palatally.

Case 3.11

Describe her malocclusion (Figures 3.38 and 3.39)

There is a class I incisor relationship on a skeletal class I base with average vertical proportions. The soft tissues appear normal at both rest and in function.

This girl is in the late mixed dentition, with the following teeth present clinically:

76E4321/1 C4E67
76E4321/1234567

The LL5 has an enlarged, elongated and unusually shaped crown.

The oral hygiene is good and there is no evidence of caries or previous restorative work.

The lower arch has only very mild crowding in the labial segment, with upright canines. The buccal segments are essentially well aligned, although the LL5 is slightly crowded and rotated.

The upper arch has mild crowding in the labial segment, with the UR2 rotated mesio-labially. There is a midline diastema between the central incisors and the UL2 is not present clinically. The UR3 is mesially angulated but the UL3 is unerupted, with the ULC retained. The buccal segments are well aligned.

In occlusion, there is a class I incisor relationship with a slightly reduced but complete overbite. There is a centre line discrepancy of around 3 mm (½ tooth unit), with the upper centre line almost certainly displaced to the left of the facial midline because of the absent UL2 and unerupted UL3, and the lower centre line possibly displaced over to the right of the facial midline because of the enlarged LL5 (although the LRE is present). The molar relationship is class I bilaterally; however, the right canine relationship is ½ unit class II.

What information does the panoramic radiograph provide (Figure 3.39)?

The panoramic radiograph confirms that the UL2 is congenitally absent. It also shows that the UL3 is present and close to erupting. The position of this tooth is favourable for eruption. The remaining primary second molars are being resorbed normally. Root morphology of the enlarged LL5 appears normal.

What is the problem list for this patient?

- Congenital absence of the UL2
- Unerupted UL3 and retained ULC
- Centre line discrepancy
- Midline diastema
- Mild crowding
- Abnormally shaped LL5

What are the key considerations when planning treatment in this case?

A key decision in this case is how to manage the congenital absence of the UL2. Although the UL3 is unerupted, this tooth is likely to erupt fairly soon, and if it does not, then it is relatively simple to expose and apply traction.

How would you manage treatment to create space for prosthetic replacement of the UL2?

If a decision is made to open up space for the UL2, then treatment is likely to be carried out on a non-extraction basis. In this scenario, anchorage reinforcement would be required to establish and maintain a class I buccal segment relationship. It would be useful to institute headgear wear for 12–14 hours per day, prior to loss of the upper second primary molars. This would allow use of the leeway space to maintain the upper first molars in a good class I position. Fixed appliances could then be used to align the UL3 and correct the centre line relationship by opening up space for prosthetic replacement of the UL2. Once orthodontic treatment was complete, the UL2 could be replaced with a resin-retained bridge or implant (once the patient had ceased growing).

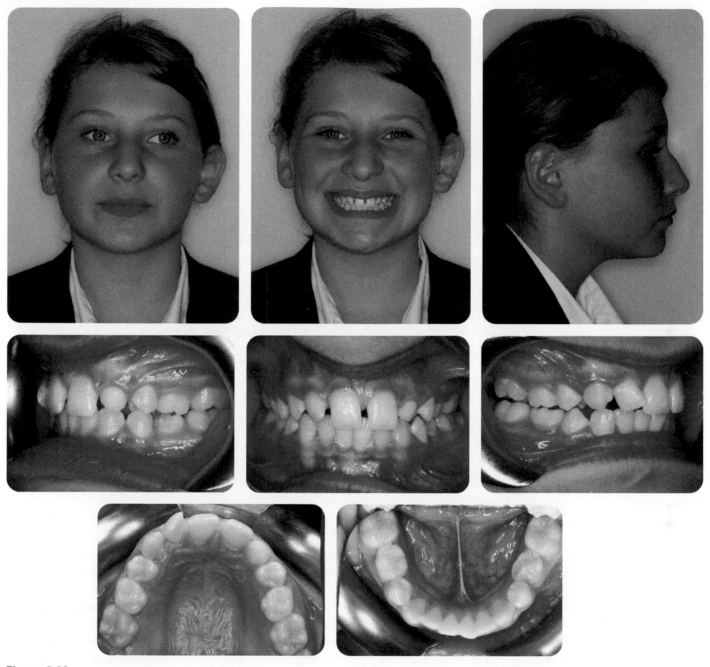

Figure 3.38

What are the problems associated with this approach?

This approach requires headgear wear by the patient, which is compliance-dependent. It also means that there will be a life-long reliance upon a prosthesis for the UL2. A further problem is created by retaining the enlarged LL5, as a potential tooth-size discrepancy will exist. This might make centre line correction difficult.

What is the alternative treatment plan?

An alternative plan would be to close space for the absent UL2 and carry out treatment on an extraction basis. In this case, a decision would need to be made regarding which teeth should be extracted.

The lower arch has only very mild crowding and minimal space requirements, therefore extractions could be carried out in the upper arch only. However,

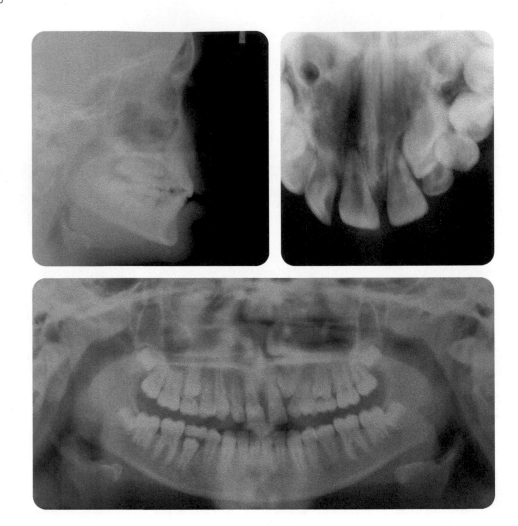

Figure 3.39

some inter-proximal reduction of crown size for the LL5 may be required to prevent a tooth-size discrepancy. A problem with extracting in the upper arch only would be the need to close excess space from behind. Maintenance of a class I incisor relationship might be quite difficult having corrected the centre line because residual space would need to be closed and a class II molar relationship established.

Another solution would be to extract one tooth unit from the lower left, lower right and upper right quadrants, respectively. Extractions in the lower arch would almost certainly involve the second premolars, which would remove the problem of the enlarged LL5 and allow a class I molar relationship to be maintained following treatment. There would be a lot of space to close in the lower arch, but maintaining a class I incisor relationship and correcting the centre lines would be more straightforward.

Once a decision has been made regarding which teeth to extract in the lower arch, the final decision is

which tooth to extract in the upper right quadrant. This choice is really whether to extract the UR2 or the UR4 or UR5. The main advantage of extracting the UR2 is that it will maintain symmetry in the upper labial segment, by ultimately having both canines in the lateral incisor positions. Extracting the UR4 or UR5 premolar introduces a potential tooth-size discrepancy and means that the UL3 will need to match the UR2 rather than the UR3.

What also needs to be considered if a decision is made to close space in the upper arch?

Canine morphology and colour is also important. In this case there is a problem in assessing this because the UL3 is unerupted; however, the UR3 is not too dark and has a good morphology to facilitate minor occlusal grinding or build-up to make this tooth more incisor-like once treatment is completed.

A decision was made to extract the lower second premolars and UR2. Then fixed appliances were to be used to correct the underlying malocclusion and to have the upper canines in the lateral incisor positions. How could this be managed practically?

Currently, the LRE, ULE, URE and ULC are retained, but all of these teeth are close to being exfoliated. As this patient is only 12-years old, she could be seen again in 6 months and treatment started once these teeth have been lost (and the LR5, UL5, UR5 and UL3 have erupted). Alternatively, these teeth could be extracted under local anaesthetic immediately to encourage eruption of the permanent teeth. If the UL3 fails to erupt, then this tooth could be surgically exposed if necessary.

Case 3.12

This 15-year-old female was referred by her dentist with a gap between her top and bottom teeth. There was no relevant medical history.

Extra-oral

Skeletal relationship	
Antero-posterior	Mild skeletal class II
Vertical	Increased FMPA and lower face height
Transverse	No asymmetry
Soft tissues	Lips competent
	Naso-labial angle: Average
Upper incisor show	Rest: 2 mm
	Smiling: 9 mm
Temporo-mandibular joint	No signs/symptoms
	Good range of movements

Intra-oral

Teeth present	7654321/1234567
	7654321/1234567
Dental health	Good
(restorations/caries)	Heavily restored LR7
Lower arch	Crowding: Mild
	Incisor inclination: Proclined
	Curve of Spee: Reduced
	Canines: Upright
Upper arch	Crowding: Mild
	Incisor inclination: Proclined
	Canines: Upright
Occlusion	Incisor relationship: Class I
	Overjet: 3 mm
	Overbite: Reduced and incomplete with a 3 mm anterior open bite extending from maxillary canines forward
	Molar relationship: Angle class I bilaterally
	Canine relationship: Class I bilaterally
	Centre lines: Lower to right by 1 mm
	Unilateral posterior mandibular buccal crossbite on right side with displacement from RCP to ICP
	Functional occlusion: Group function left and right

Summary

A 15-year-old female presented with a class I malocclusion on a mild skeletal class II base with increased vertical dimensions complicated by mild crowding, a unilateral posterior crossbite with displacement and an anterior open bite (Figures 3.40 and 3.41).

Treatment Plan

The aims of treatment were to relieve the crowding, level and align the arches, correct the crossbite and anterior openbite, to achieve a class I buccal segment and incisor relationship. The crossbite was initially corrected using an upper removable appliance with a midline expansion screw. Buccal posterior capping was prescribed to prevent worsening of the anterior open bite as the maxillary arch was expanded. Once the crossbite had been corrected, all four second molars were removed and a modified intrusion splint was cemented to the occlusal surfaces of the maxillary buccal dentition, again with capping, and two palatal arches were set away from the palate. A single micro-screw was placed under local anaesthetic bilaterally between the roots of the second premolar and first molar buccally (Absoanchor® 7 mm × 1.3 mm). An intrusive force was applied to the teeth using an activated nickel–titanium coil spring attached to the micro-screw (Figure 3.42). The micro-screw on the right side failed and was replaced with a second screw (Infinitas® 9 mm × 1.5 mm). Once adequate intrusion

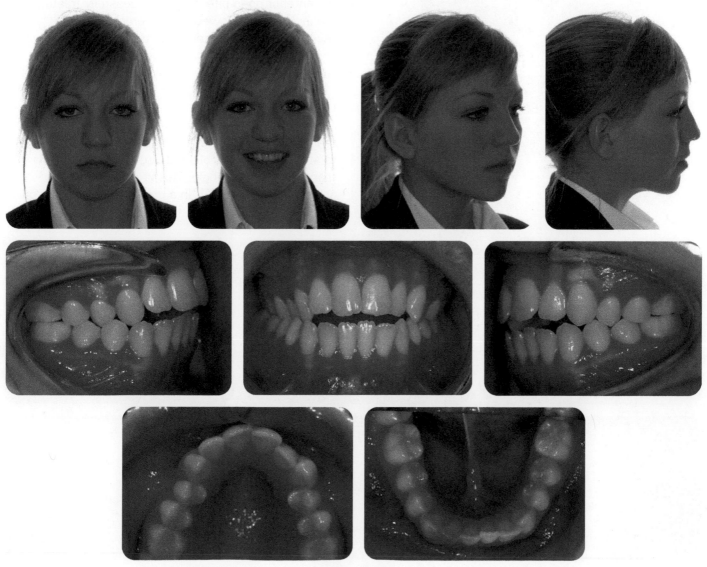

Figure 3.40

had been achieved, the intrusion splint was removed and an upper and lower pre-adjusted edgewise appliance system placed (Figure 3.43). The teeth were levelled and aligned, and a positive overbite and overjet were obtained. On removal of the fixed appliance, a lower bonded retainer was placed and supplemented with occlusal coverage vacuum formed retainers that the patient was instructed to wear at night (Figures 3.44 and 3.45).

What is the aetiology of the anterior open bite?

In this case the anterior open bite was in part due to the history of digit sucking, which had also caused narrowing of the maxillary arch and the posterior crossbite. The patient also presented with a hyper-divergent skeletal pattern and an increased maxillary–mandibular planes angle, indicating that a skeletal element was also involved. This is important because the aetiology of an anterior open bite will dictate the modality of treatment and will determine the stability of correction. If it is due to a physical obstruction preventing full eruption of the labial dentition, such as a thumb or finger, the obstruction can be removed and the anterior open bite can be successfully treated as the incisors are allowed to fully erupt. However, in the case of a hyper-divergent growth pattern, the aetiology is often primarily skeletal and the incisors are at the limit of their eruptive potential. Any orthodontic treatment aimed at extruding them further will be unstable.

Treatment should therefore be aimed at reducing the posterior dental height, resulting in an anterior rotation of the mandible and closure of the maxillary–mandibular planes angle. This is very difficult to achieve orthodontically. In a growing patient high pull

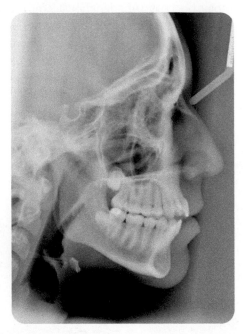

Figure 3.41

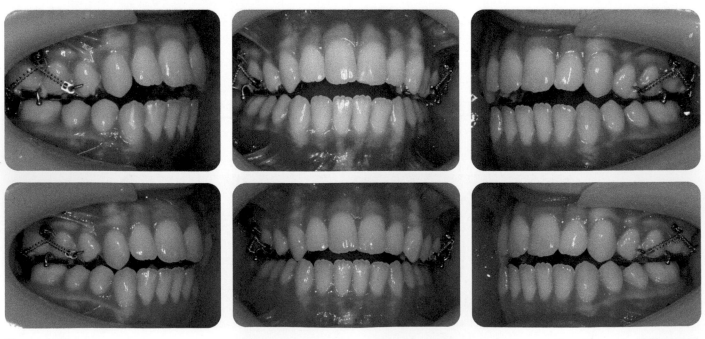

Figure 3.42

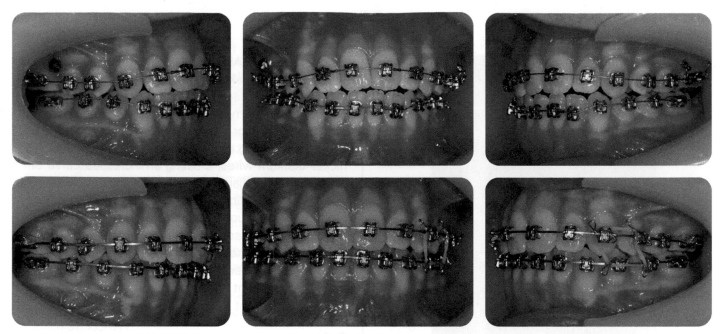

Figure 3.43

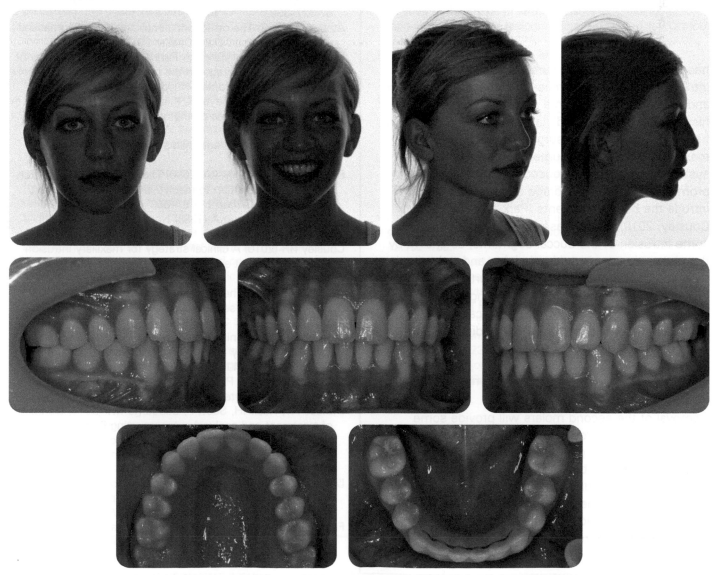

Figure 3.44

4

Class II Division 1 Malocclusion

Introduction

A class II division 1 malocclusion is defined by the presence of a class II incisor relationship with an increased overjet, and either proclined or normally inclined upper incisors. It is the most prevalent arch malrelationship in Caucasian populations, seen in between 15% and 27% of this population (Helm, 1968; Foster and Day, 1974; Proffit *et al.*, 1998). The molar relationship is usually Angle class II, but an increased overjet can occur in the presence of class I molars if the upper incisors are proclined or, rarely, with a class III molar relationship. Molar relationships are usually symmetrical but may be asymmetrical with alterations influenced by local factors. Therefore, a class II division 1 malocclusion should be defined primarily by the incisor relationship.

The skeletal pattern is usually class II secondary to mandibular retrognathia, with the extent of this discrepancy often dictating the severity of the malocclusion (McNamara, 1981). In the vertical dimension, variation across the whole spectrum can be seen, from a hypodivergent facial form with reduced lower face height and increased overbite to hyperdivergent with increased lower face height and reduced overbite or anterior open bite, depending on the extent of the disharmony. Malocclusions associated with an increased Frankfort–mandibular planes angle are generally more challenging to treat orthodontically because of the associated unfavourable downward and backward pattern of mandibular growth and unfavourable soft tissue pattern.

The soft tissues can play a role in the aetiology of a class II division 1 incisor relationship, particularly if the upper incisors rest on or are in front of the lower lip. This is known as a lip trap and can result in proclination of the upper incisors and retroclination of the lower incisors worsening the overjet. If the lower lip is particularly active, resulting in significant retroclination of the lower labial segment, it is described as 'strap-like'. Proclination of the upper incisors can also lead to protrusion of the upper lip.

In low or average angle cases, the resting position of the lower lip behind the upper incisors reflects lip incompetence. In this situation the lip relationship is sometimes described as potentially competent as it is only the position of teeth that prevents the patient from achieving lip competence without strain. In high angle cases, lip incompetence is usually due to the skeletal lower face height being greater than the lip length; muscular effort is required to achieve competence. The vertical growth pattern is also important in the long-term stability following overjet reduction in these cases. Stability is more likely if the lower lip rests in front of the upper incisors after treatment, which is more likely if the Frankfort–mandibular angle is average or low, with an associated anterior growth rotation. In high angle cases with a backward growth rotation and increased lower face height, even if the overjet is successfully reduced, the lower lip is likely to rest below the upper incisors, which is another reason why high angle class II division 1 malocclusions are difficult to treat.

While the overjet is increased, the overbite can range in depth, but is often incomplete due to the presence of an adaptive pattern of swallowing, secondary to the increased overjet. Dental crowding is also typical, particularly in the lower labial segment if it is retroclined. The maxillary incisors are often proclined and spaced due to the resting position of the lower lip in the presence of a lip trap.

As already outlined, the aetiology of a class II division 1 incisor relationship is often skeletal due to mandibular retrognathia, but can be related to lip position in the presence of a skeletal class I or rarely a class III pattern. It can also be due to a digit sucking habit that persists beyond eruption of the permanent maxillary incisors. An increased overjet can have negative psychosocial implications and is also associated with an increased risk of trauma to the upper labial segment, particularly in children, both of which are indications for treatment (Nguyen et al., 1999).

Treatment is influenced primarily by the extent of the skeletal discrepancy and the dento-alveolar contribution to the overjet. There are essentially three main approaches to the correction of a class II division 1 malocclusion:

- **Growth modification:** In a growing patient attempts can be made to correct the underlying skeletal discrepancy by utilizing or modifying growth, either with headgear, a functional appliance or a combination of the two. Success is determined by the patient's co-operation with what can be quite demanding treatment and the direction and extent of growth. Both of these variables are very difficult to predict.

- **Orthodontic camouflage:** The skeletal discrepancy is accepted and the overjet is corrected by orthodontic tooth movement, primarily uprighting, or retracting the upper incisors and proclining the lower incisors. Space is usually required in the upper arch to do this and can be created by either distalization of the maxillary buccal segments or extraction of maxillary premolars. This is appropriate treatment for a class II division 1 malocclusion on a skeletal class I or mild-to-moderate skeletal class II base in a non-growing individual, but may not be suitable for more severe skeletal class II discrepancies due to the potential negative effects on the soft tissue profile.

- **Combined orthodontic–surgical treatment:** For those cases with a significant antero-posterior or vertical skeletal component to their malocclusion, where camouflage treatment is not an option, combined orthodontic–surgical treatment is often carried out, with surgical repositioning of the jaws allowing definitive correction of the skeletal discrepancy as part of the treatment plan.

Case 4.1

This 12-year-old female was referred by her orthodontic specialist because she was concerned about her crowded and prominent upper front teeth and was being teased at school in relation to her dento-facial appearance. There was no relevant medical history.

Extra-oral

Skeletal relationship

Antero-posterior	Moderate skeletal class II
Vertical:	FMPA: Increased
	Lower face height: Increased
Transverse	Facial symmetry: None
Soft tissues	Lip competence: Incompetent with lower lip acting palatally to maxillary incisors
	Naso-labial angle: Obtuse
Upper incisor show	At rest: 6mm
	Smiling: 12mm
Temporo-mandibular joint	Healthy with good range and co-ordination of movement

Intra-oral

Teeth present:	7654321/1234567
	7654321/1234567
Dental health (restorations, caries)	Good
	No restorations or active caries
Oral hygiene – periodontal	Moderate with marginal gingivitis in the upper anterior region
Occlusion	Incisor relationship: Class II division 1
	Overjet: 12mm
	Overbite: Average and incomplete
	Molar relationship: Class II bilaterally
	Canine relationship: Class II bilaterally
	Centre lines: Coincident
	Functional occlusion: Group function
Lower arch	Crowding: Mild
	Incisor inclination: Average
Upper arch	Crowding: Mild
	Incisor inclination: Proclined
	Canine position: Line of the arch

Summary

A 12-year-old female presented with a class II division 1 malocclusion on a moderate skeletal class II pattern, with increased vertical dimensions complicated by an increased overjet (12 mm), crowding of both dental arches and teasing in relation to her dento-facial appearance (Figure 4.1).

Why is the skeletal pattern described as moderate?

An ANB value of 7 degrees and a Wits value of +2 mm

Treatment Plan

- Improve oral hygiene
- Functional appliance therapy with occipital-pull headgear
- Upper and lower pre-adjusted edgewise appliances with extraction of four second premolars
- Long-term retention

Is there a relationship between malocclusion and teasing/bullying?

Teeth have been reported as the fourth most common feature to provoke unfavourable social responses, including bullying. Increased overjet is linked with teasing (Shaw et al., 1980) and reduced self-concept. It is also associated with reduced levels of oral health-related quality of life (Johal et al., 2007; Marques et al., 2009). Some improvement in self-concept has been demonstrated in subjects undergoing early overjet reduction (O'Brien et al., 2003). However, prolonged follow-up has failed to show a sustained effect; self-concept is influenced by an array of features.

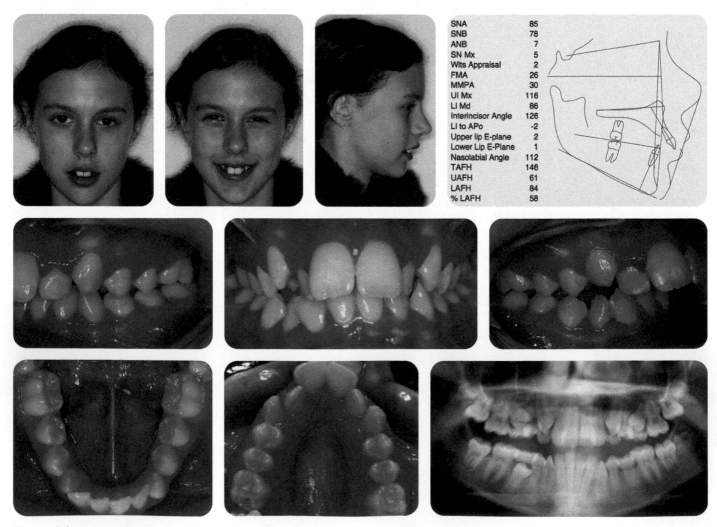

SNA	85
SNB	78
ANB	7
SN Mx	5
Wits Appraisal	2
FMA	26
MMPA	30
UI Mx	116
LI Md	86
Interincisor Angle	126
LI to APo	-2
Upper lip E-plane	2
Lower Lip E-Plane	1
Nasolabial Angle	112
TAFH	146
UAFH	61
LAFH	84
% LAFH	58

Figure 4.1

What are the short-term effects of functional appliances?

Short-term effects of functional appliance therapy are both skeletal and dento-alveolar in nature; but dental effects predominate. In particular, retroclination of maxillary incisors and proclination of mandibular incisors contribute to correction of the incisor relationship (O'Brien *et al.*, 2003). Maxillary restraint and acceleration of mandibular growth are also important in the short-term.

How do these changes contrast with the long-term effects?

Prospective research suggests that prolonged growth modification may not be achievable. These studies have confirmed that skeletal modification is instrumental in producing favourable occlusal change, including overjet reduction and molar correction; however, medium-term follow-up indicates that this growth enhancement may disappear with further maturation (O'Brien *et al.*, 2003; 2009). It appears that mandibular growth potential is largely pre-determined and that our capacity to permanently alter growth of this bone is limited. Nevertheless, occlusal correction tends to be effective and stable.

Why was this patient treated with a functional appliance?

- Growing adolescent
- Skeletal class II pattern
- Increased overjet (12 mm)

What type of functional appliance was used, how does this differ from other functional appliances and what are the potential advantages? (Figure 4.2)?

The appliance is a Dynamax appliance developed by Neville Bass (Bass and Bass, 2003).

This appliance consists of an upper removable component, which incorporates Adams cribs on the first molars and first premolars, a midline coffin spring and anterior torque spring on the maxillary central incisors. Mandibular posture is achieved using a lower fixed lingual arch, which has shoulders that project horizontally. As the patient closes, two vertical springs, which project from the upper appliance, ensure anterior posturing of the mandible through avoiding interference with the lower lingual arch. The appliance can be reactivated by adjusting the springs on the upper appliance.

The reported advantages include:

- Simple incremental advancement
- Simultaneous use of a lower fixed appliance
- Control of incisor inclination
- Restriction of vertical facial development.

A recent randomized controlled trial has demonstrated that the Twin Block is a more effective functional appliance than the Dynamax when overjet reduction is evaluated, with a significant increase in the incidence of adverse effects seen with the Dynamax (Thiruvenkatachari *et al.*, 2010).

What factors influence the need for headgear in association with functional appliance therapy?

The more severe the class II discrepancy, the more useful headgear support can be. Cases with maxillary excess, either antero-posterior or vertical will also benefit from the use of headgear with a functional appliance. In this case, occipital-pull headgear facilitated overjet reduction by restraining maxillary forward growth. The pre-treatment SNA value of 85 degrees was suggestive of a forward position of the maxilla. Also, the use of headgear, particularly when combined with torqueing spurs, will help prevent

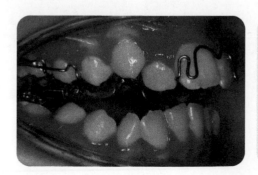

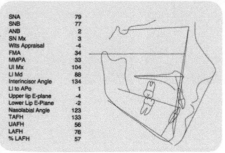

SNA	79
SNB	77
ANB	2
SN Mx	3
Wits Appraisal	-4
FMA	34
MMPA	33
UI Mx	104
LI Md	88
Interincisor Angle	134
LI to APo	1
Upper lip E-plane	-4
Lower Lip E-Plane	-2
Nasolabial Angle	123
TAFH	133
UAFH	56
LAFH	76
% LAFH	57

Figure 4.2

tipping of the maxillary incisors and a backwards and downwards rotation of the maxilla, a common side effect of functional appliances. By stabilizing the maxilla, theoretically there is greater chance of antero-posterior mandibular positioning, which is desirable, particularly in a high angle case, as opposed to vertical or rotational change, which is not.

How do functional appliances work?

Functional appliances harness the forces generated by the oral and facial musculature to produce tooth movement. The principle movements are maxillary incisor retroclination, mandibular incisor proclination and guidance of eruption of the posterior dentitions (distal in the maxilla and mesial in the mandible). Some favourable skeletal change can also occur (maxillary restraint, forward mandibular growth), although these effects are small in comparison to the dento-alveolar changes.

What types of functional appliances are there?

There are a number of classifications for functional appliances; however, the simplest is to categorize them according to basic design:
- Fixed (e.g. Herbst appliance)
- Removable (e.g. Twin Block, Bionator, Medium Opening Activator)
- Hybrid (e.g. Dynamax appliance).

What are the advantages and disadvantages of fixed functional appliances?

- Guaranteed wear of the appliance
- Improved compliance and completion rate

However, these advantages are tempered by:
- Greater onus on oral hygiene
- Increased cost
- Greater chair-side manipulation
- Higher breakage rate.

What factors influence the choice of a specific functional appliance?

- Anticipated compliance
- Vertical skeletal pattern

Fixed functional appliances are preferable where co-operation is likely to be poor. Patients with increased lower anterior face height may benefit from restraint of vertical maxillary growth; the addition of high pull headgear and use of specific functional appliances (Teuscher, van Beek, Dynamax) have been proposed to address this problem. Conversely, with a reduced lower anterior face height, the expression of vertical facial growth and posterior tooth eruption can be more favourable; consequently, specific appliances, including the Medium Opening Activators and Modified Twin Block, are useful.

Why were fixed appliances used in this case (Figure 4.3)?

Fixed appliances were used after the functional phase of treatment to align the arches, finish and detail the occlusion. Removal of four second premolars was considered necessary to alleviate the dental crowding. Consequently, fixed appliances were also required to close the remaining extraction spaces after alignment. Achievement of good buccal segment inter-digitation makes prolonged stability of class II correction more likely (Pancherz, 1991) (Figure 4.4).

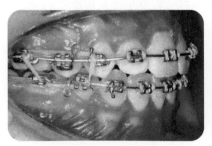 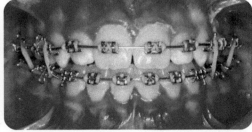 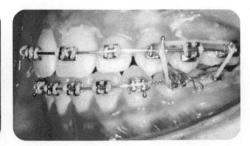

Figure 4.3

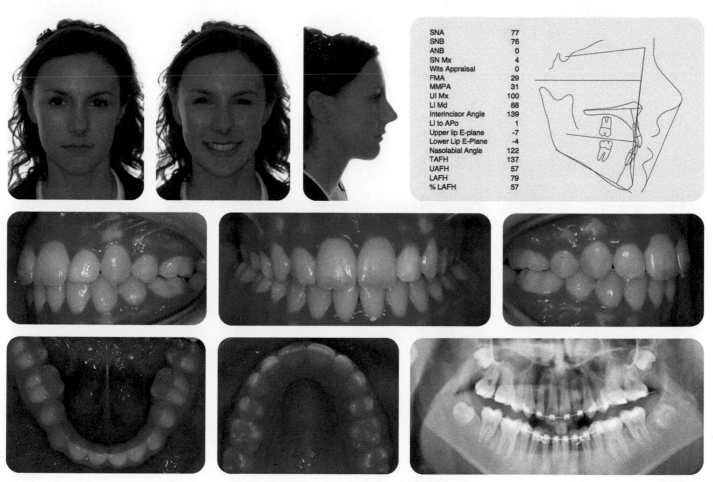

SNA	77
SNB	76
ANB	0
SN Mx	4
Wits Appraisal	0
FMA	29
MMPA	31
UI Mx	100
LI Md	88
Interincisor Angle	139
LI to APo	1
Upper lip E-plane	-7
Lower Lip E-Plane	-4
Nasolabial Angle	122
TAFH	137
UAFH	57
LAFH	79
% LAFH	57

Figure 4.4

Case 4.2

This 11-year-old female was referred by her dental practitioner because she was concerned by her generalized spacing and increased overjet. There was no relevant medical history.

Extra-oral

Skeletal relationship

Antero-posterior	Moderate skeletal class II
Vertical	FMPA: Reduced
	Lower face height: Reduced
Transverse	Facial symmetry: None
Soft tissues	Lip competence: Incompetent with lower lip resting palatally to maxillary incisors
	Upper lip length: 17 mm
	Naso-labial angle: Average
Upper incisor show	At rest: 3 mm
	Smiling: 8 mm
Temporo-mandibular joint	Healthy with good range and co-ordination of movement

Intra-oral

Teeth present:

$$\frac{7654321/1234567}{7654321/1234567}$$

Dental health (restorations, caries)	Good
	No restorations or active caries
Oral hygiene	Good
Occlusion	Incisor relationship: Class II division 1
	Overjet: 11 mm
	Overbite: Increased and complete
	Molar relationship: Class II bilaterally
	Canine relationship: Class II bilaterally
	Centre lines: Coincident with each other and the facial midline
	Functional occlusion: Group function
Lower arch	Spaced
	Incisor inclination: Proclined
	Curve of Spee: Increased
Upper arch	Spaced
	Incisor inclination: Proclined

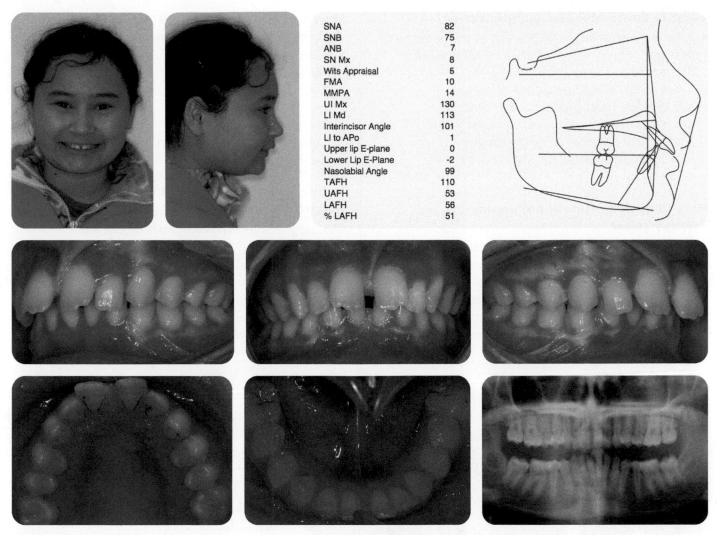

SNA	82
SNB	75
ANB	7
SN Mx	8
Wits Appraisal	5
FMA	10
MMPA	14
UI Mx	130
LI Md	113
Interincisor Angle	101
LI to APo	1
Upper lip E-plane	0
Lower Lip E-Plane	-2
Nasolabial Angle	99
TAFH	110
UAFH	53
LAFH	56
% LAFH	51

Figure 4.5

Summary

An 11-year-old female presented with a class II division 1 malocclusion on a moderate skeletal class II pattern with reduced vertical dimensions complicated by an increased overjet (11 mm), increased overbite, generalized spacing and bi-maxillary proclination (Figure 4.5).

Treatment Plan

- Modified Twin Block functional appliance with sectional lower fixed appliance
- Upper and lower pre-adjusted edgewise appliances
- Long-term retention
  The final result of treatment is shown in Figure 4.6.

What is the likely aetiology of this malocclusion?

The aetiology of this malocclusion is multi-factorial. The moderate skeletal class II discrepancy resulted in an increased overjet and class II molar relationship. The overjet was exacerbated by the presence of a lower lip trap. The generalized spacing was a result of an underlying dento-alveolar disproportion. This was compounded by bi-maxillary proclination, which arose due to resting soft tissue pressures and dento-alveolar compensation.

Why was a lower fixed appliance placed in conjunction with the functional appliance?

- To correct the inclination of the mandibular incisors
- To facilitate optimum skeletal changes with functional appliance therapy
- Consolidation of lower arch space

What is dento-alveolar compensation?

- A natural alteration in the position of the dentition to limit the occlusal effect of an underlying skeletal discrepancy.
- It can occur in all three planes of space.
- It is typically most pronounced in class III malocclusion with retroclination of mandibular incisors and proclination of the maxillary incisors compensating for a skeletal class III discrepancy.

How long does functional appliance therapy take?

At this stage there is no evidenced-based answer to this question, with treatment time being dictated by operator preferences and the individual response of patients to treatment. However, it usually takes around 6–12 months. Shorter periods of appliance wear are likely to be less stable than longer courses of treatment.

How can the transition between functional and fixed appliances be managed?

- Integration of functional and fixed appliances (e.g. Herbst appliance)
- Continuation of functional appliance wear at night only
- Use of headgear
- Inter-arch class II elastic traction following fixed appliance placement

Is this treatment result likely to be stable (Figure 4.6)?

The prognosis for long-term stability of class II correction is good in this case, as the new maxillary incisor position will be controlled by the lower lip following the achievement of lip competence. Prolonged compliance with the retention regimen will be required to maintain intra-arch alignment, particularly in view of the pre-treatment spacing and bi-maxillary proclination.

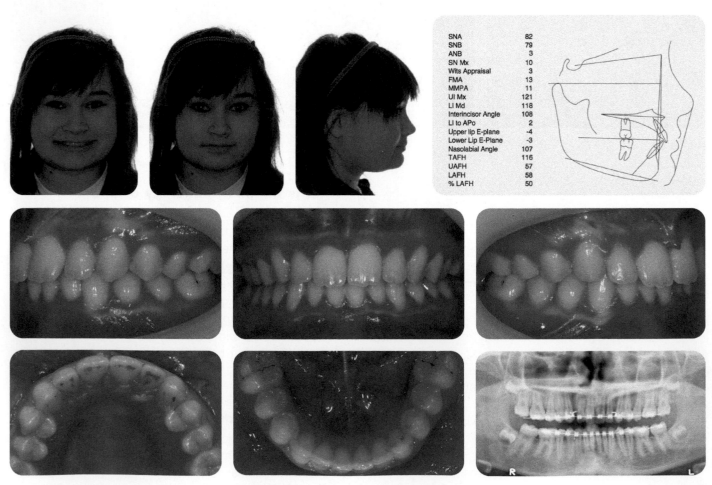

SNA	82
SNB	79
ANB	3
SN Mx	10
Wits Appraisal	3
FMA	13
MMPA	11
UI Mx	121
LI Md	118
Interincisor Angle	108
LI to APo	2
Upper lip E-plane	-4
Lower Lip E-Plane	-3
Nasolabial Angle	107
TAFH	116
UAFH	57
LAFH	58
% LAFH	50

Figure 4.6

Case 4.3

This 12-year-old male was referred by his dental practitioner as he was concerned by the space between his teeth. There was no relevant medical history.

Extra-oral

Skeletal relationship

Antero-posterior	Moderate skeletal class II
Vertical	FMPA: Average
	Lower face height: Average
Transverse	Facial symmetry: None
Soft tissues	Lip competence: Incompetent with lower lip acting palatally to maxillary incisors
	Upper lip length: 18 mm
	Naso-labial angle: Obtuse
Upper incisor show	At rest: 5 mm
	Smiling: 11 mm
Temporo-mandibular joint	Healthy with good range and co-ordination of movement

Intra-oral

Teeth present	654321/123456
	654321/123456
Dental health (restorations, caries)	Good
	No restorations or active caries
Oral hygiene	Good

Summary

A 12-year-old male presented with a class II division 1 incisor relationship on a moderate skeletal class II pattern with average vertical dimensions complicated by an increased overjet (11 mm) and overbite with well-aligned dental arches (Figure 4.7).

Summarize the occlusal features of this case

- Incisor relationship: Class II division 1
- Overjet is increased (11 mm)
- Overbite increased and complete
- Molar relationship: Class II bilaterally
- Canine relationship: Class II bilaterally
- Centre line discrepancy of 2 mm (⅓ tooth unit) (Upper dental centre line correct to facial midline, lower dental centre line deviated 2 mm to right)
- Lower arch:
  - Crowding: Mild
  - Incisor inclination: Average
  - Curve of Spee: Increased
- Upper arch:
  - Crowding: Mild
  - Incisor inclination: Proclined

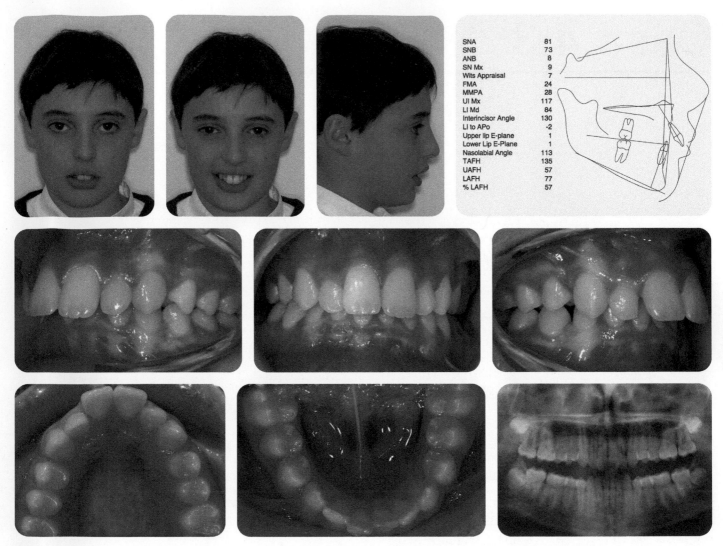

SNA	81
SNB	73
ANB	8
SN Mx	9
Wits Appraisal	7
FMA	24
MMPA	28
UI Mx	117
LI Md	84
Interincisor Angle	130
LI to APo	-2
Upper Lip E-plane	1
Lower Lip E-Plane	1
Nasolabial Angle	113
TAFH	135
UAFH	57
LAFH	77
% LAFH	57

Figure 4.7

Does the cephalometric analysis agree with the clinical appearance?

Yes. The cephalometric analysis is suggestive of a skeletal class II discrepancy (ANB = 8 degrees, Wits appraisal = 7 mm) with mandibular retrognathia (SNA = 81 degrees but SNB = 73 degrees); however, the vertical skeletal relationship is within the normal range (maxillary–mandibular planes angle [MMPA] = 28 degrees).

Treatment Plan

- Modified Twin Block functional appliance to reduce the overjet
- Upper and lower pre-adjusted edgewise appliances to align and co-ordinate the dental arches
- Long-term retention

Figure 4.8 shows the occlusion after 7 months of Twin Block therapy. What is characteristic about this appearance?

The overjet has reduced but bilateral lateral open bites are present. Overjet reduction usually takes place faster than correction of the vertical relationship. The appearance of bilateral lateral open bites is therefore commonly seen. Additional time will be required for these to close; however, overjet reduction will need to be maintained. Night-time wear of the appliance, occlusal trimming of the blocks on the Twin Block or the use of a simple removable appliance with an inclined anterior bite plane, which allows vertical development of the mandibular buccal dentition whilst maintaining the reduced overjet, can all be used.

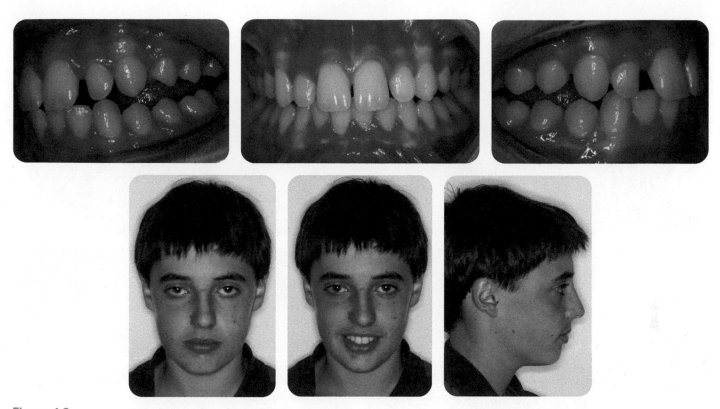

Figure 4.8

When is the best time to use a functional appliance?

Functional appliances are typically used in the late mixed dentition in growing patients. Prospective research has focused on the ability of functional appliances to modify mandibular growth in pre-pubertal children and overall, it seems that functional appliances are most efficient when used at this stage. Consequently, the functional phase can then be followed by fixed appliances to detail the occlusion in a single phase.

The chronological age corresponding to maximal pre-pubertal growth is variable, but generally treatment is commenced at 10–12 years of age in females and 11–14 years of age in males. This time period tends to coincide with establishment of the late mixed or early permanent dentition, permitting optimal retention of tooth-borne appliances.

Is there a greater risk of trauma with an increased overjet?

- An overjet exceeding 3 mm has an approximately two-fold increased risk of sustaining incisor trauma (Nguyen *et al.*, 1999).

- In children with an overjet exceeding 9 mm, up to 45% have sustained traumatic dental injury (Todd and Dodd, 1985).
- Risk of trauma is gender-specific, with excessive overjet more likely to be linked to trauma in females.

Has orthodontic treatment been shown to reduce the incidence of dental trauma?

A large prospective clinical study has failed to confirm the association between interceptive orthodontic treatment in 9–10-year olds with an overjet of 7 mm or more and prevention of trauma (Koroluk *et al.*, 2003). This finding may be related to the fact that traumatic injury often arises in the mixed dentition, before treatment would typically commence. Indeed, 29% had already been affected by trauma before participating in this research study. Therefore, from a public health viewpoint, initiating treatment in all children with excessive overjets at an early stage to prevent trauma would be inappropriate.

What soft tissue factor contributed to the increased overjet in this case?

A lower lip trap, with the lip acting palatal to the maxillary incisors, resulted in excessive proclination of

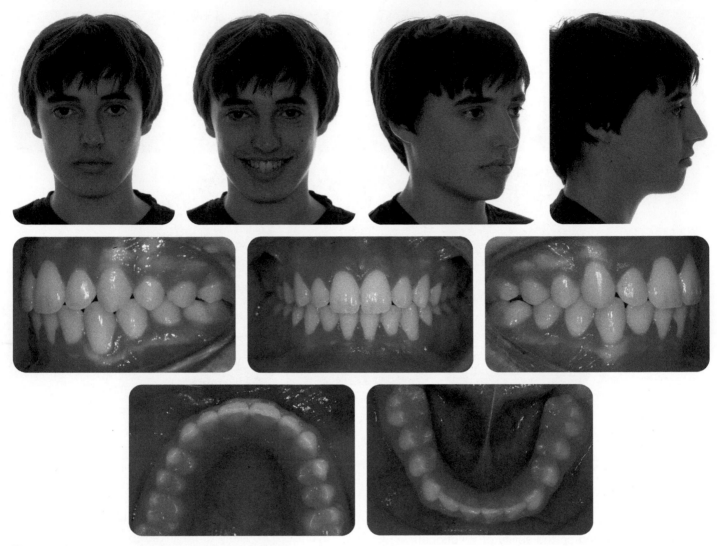

Figure 4.9

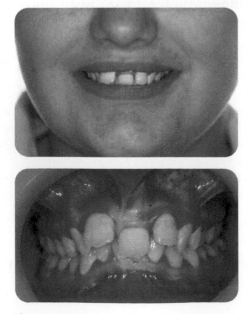

Figure 4.10

the central incisors. The lip trap may arise due to mandibular retrognathia; this in turn, increases maxillary incisor proclination with an additive effect on the overjet. The lip trap has been eliminated following treatment (Figure 4.9). Incompetent lips may also arise due to reduced tonicity, predisposing to proclination of the incisors. Asymmetric inclination changes can also occur due to resting lip position (Figure 4.10).

Case 4.4

This 18-year-old female was referred by her orthodontic specialist because she was concerned about the prominence of her upper front teeth. There was no relevant medical history.

Extra-oral

Skeletal relationship

Antero-posterior	Mild skeletal class II
Vertical	FMPA: Average
	Lower face height: Average
Transverse	Facial asymmetry: None
Soft tissues	Lip competence: Incompetent with lower lip acting behind the maxillary incisors
	Naso-labial angle: Average
Upper incisor show	At rest: 4 mm
	Smiling: 10 mm
Temporo-mandibular joint	Healthy with good range and co-ordination of movement

Intra-oral

Teeth present	7654321/1234567 7654321/1234567
Dental health (restorations, caries)	Good
Oral hygiene – periodontal	Good oral hygiene
Lower arch	Crowding: Mild
	Incisor inclination: Average
	Curve of Spee: Average
Upper arch	Crowding: Mild
	Incisor inclination: Proclined
	Canine position: Line of the arch
Occlusion	Incisor relationship: Class II division 1
	Overjet: Increased (10 mm)
	Overbite: Average and incomplete
	Molar relationship: Class II bilaterally
	Canine relationship: Class II bilaterally
	Centre lines: Maxillary centre line is 1 mm to the left side, the lower is coincident with the mid-facial axis
	Functional occlusion: Group function

Summary

An 18-year-old female presented with a class II division 1 malocclusion on a mild skeletal class II pattern with average vertical dimensions, an increased overjet of 10 mm and mild crowding of both dental arches (Figure 4.11).

Treatment Plan

- Upper and lower pre-adjusted edgewise appliances with extraction of maxillary first premolars bilaterally
- Temporary anchorage devices (TADs) between the maxillary second premolars and first molars (Figure 4.12)
- Long-term retention

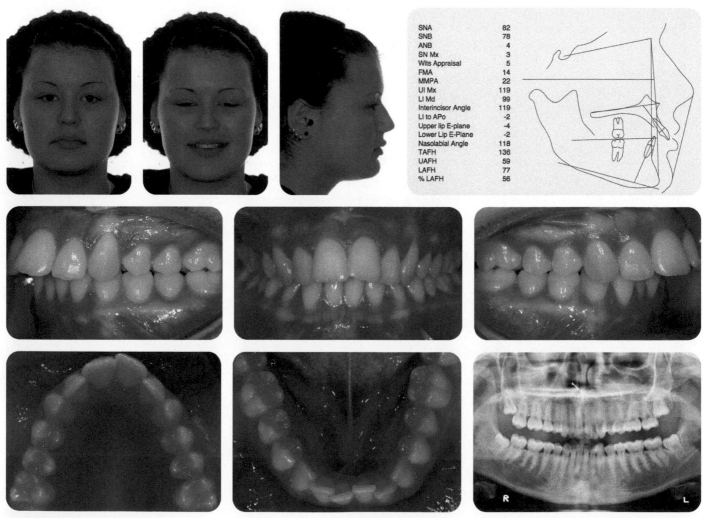

SNA	82
SNB	78
ANB	4
SN Mx	3
Wits Appraisal	5
FMA	14
MMPA	22
UI Mx	119
LI Md	99
Interincisor Angle	119
LI to APo	-2
Upper lip E-plane	-4
Lower Lip E-Plane	-2
Nasolabial Angle	118
TAFH	136
UAFH	59
LAFH	77
% LAFH	56

Figure 4.11

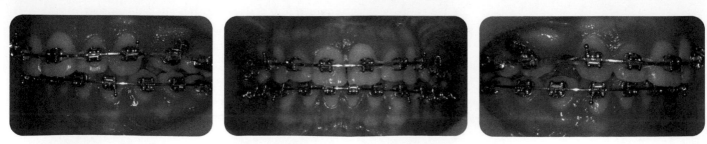

Figure 4.12

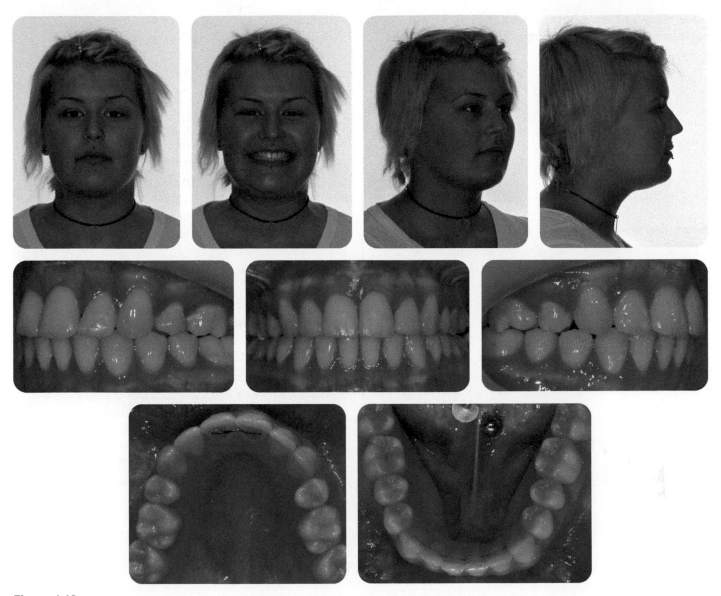

Figure 4.13

What is the primary aim of treatment in this case?

The primary aim of treatment was overjet reduction to camouflage the underlying skeletal class II discrepancy. The anchorage demand to facilitate overjet reduction was high because the pre-treatment molar relationship was a full unit class II bilaterally and the overjet was significantly increased. Consequently, maxillary first premolars were removed to maximize retraction of the upper labial segment. Some proclination of the mandibular incisors was also planned to reduce the maxillary arch anchorage requirement. In addition, TADs were placed mesial to the first permanent molars to prevent mesial migration of the maxillary buccal segments whilst retracting the maxillary incisors maximally. Consequently, the class II molar relationship was maintained and both the canine and incisor relationships were corrected to class I (Figure 4.13).

What is anchorage?

Anchorage is the resistance to unwanted tooth movement. In this case, anchorage was necessary to prevent mesial migration of the maxillary buccal segments during overjet reduction.

How may antero-posterior anchorage be supplemented to facilitate overjet reduction?

- **Intra-arch mechanics:**
  - Headgear
  - TADs
  - Nance palatal arch
  - Transpalatal arch
- **Inter-arch mechanics:**
  - Functional appliances
  - Class II elastics
  - Fixed class II correctors

What are the limitations of headgear?

- Patient compliance. Headgear wear of up to 14 hours per day may be required. The duration of wear is often less than half this time (Brandao *et al.*, 2006). Compliance is particularly poor in adults.
- Risk of injury. Reports of iatrogenic injury, including blindness, have been attributed to headgear injury, although this is extremely rare (Postlethwaite, 1989).
- For maximum effect, residual maxillary growth is required.
- Successful distal molar movement is difficult after maxillary second permanent molars have erupted.

How may compliance with headgear be improved?

- Encouragement and rewards
- Headgear charts (Cureton *et al.*, 1993)

- Headgear timers
- Patient should be actively growing

What are the risks of TAD use?

- Root damage
- Failure of the TAD

The risks of TADs would appear to be relatively minor, with evidence to suggest root damage relating to iatrogenic placement is transient. Nevertheless, it is suggested that patients are counselled on the advantages, disadvantages, risks and alternatives prior to TAD placement, and appropriately consented. A national audit is currently being undertaken by the British Orthodontic Society to investigate the relative merits of TAD use in the UK.

What are the problems associated with extracting premolar teeth in the maxillary arch only?

Space closure can be difficult, particularly if the lower incisor teeth are proclined during treatment. The main problem originates from the fact that a single maxillary premolar tooth width is often larger than a single tooth 'unit'. Therefore, with the overjet reduced, the molars in a full unit class II relationship and the canines class I, a small tooth size discrepancy can remain, which can result in a small amount of residual space. This can be completely closed by bringing the molars forward into a 'super' class II relationship or rotating the maxillary premolars slightly to increase their relative width.

Case 4.5

This 16-year-old female was referred by her orthodontic specialist because she was concerned with the gap between her teeth. She had a previous digit sucking habit.

Extra-oral

Skeletal relationship

Antero-posterior	Moderate skeletal class II
Vertical	FMPA: Reduced
	Lower face height: Reduced
Transverse	Facial asymmetry: None
Soft tissues	Lip competence: Incompetent with lower lip acting palatally to maxillary incisors
	Naso-labial angle: Average
Upper incisor show	At rest: 2mm
	Smiling: 5mm
Temporo-mandibular joint	Healthy with good range and co-ordination of movement

Intra-oral

Teeth present	7654321/1234567
	7654321/1234567
Dental health (restorations, caries)	Good
	No restorations or active caries
Oral hygiene – periodontal	Good
Lower arch	Crowding: Moderate
	Incisor inclination: Proclined
	Curve of Spee: Average
Upper arch	Crowding: Mild
	Incisor inclination: Proclined
	Canine position: Line of the arch
Occlusion	Incisor relationship: Class II division 1
	Overjet: 8mm to UR1
	Overbite: Reduced and incomplete
	Molar relationship: ½ unit class II bilaterally
	Canine relationship: ½ unit class II bilaterally
	Centre lines: Coincident
	Functional occlusion: Group function

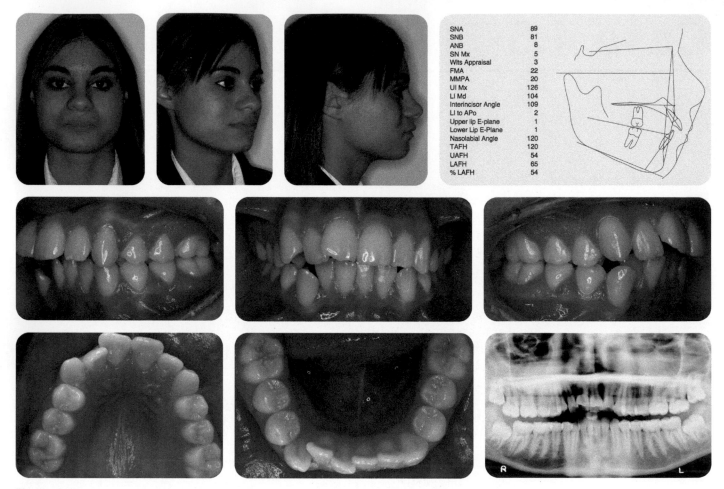

SNA	89
SNB	81
ANB	8
SN Mx	5
Wits Appraisal	3
FMA	22
MMPA	20
UI Mx	126
LI Md	104
Interincisor Angle	109
LI to APo	2
Upper lip E-plane	1
Lower Lip E-Plane	1
Nasolabial Angle	120
TAFH	120
UAFH	54
LAFH	65
% LAFH	54

Figure 4.14

Summary

A 16-year-old female presented with a class II division 1 malocclusion on a skeletal class II pattern with reduced vertical dimensions complicated by an increased overjet (8 mm), crowding of both dental arches and bi-maxillary proclination (Figure 4.14).

Treatment Plan

- Improve oral hygiene
- Upper and lower Tip Edge® appliances with extraction of maxillary first premolars and mandibular second premolars
- Long-term retention

What is orthodontic camouflage?

Orthodontic camouflage involves correcting the incisor relationship, whilst accepting the underlying skeletal discrepancy. Camouflage may be attempted to mask skeletal disproportions in all three spatial planes. Typically, mild or moderate skeletal class II discrepancies and mild skeletal class III discrepancies are amenable to orthodontic camouflage. More severe skeletal imbalances usually necessitate combined orthodontic–surgical treatment, addressing the underlying skeletal discrepancy, permitting stable correction of the incisor relationship and maximal improvement of facial aesthetics.

Why extract maxillary first premolars and mandibular second premolars in a class II case?

In class II malocclusions, extractions can be carried out in the maxillary arch in isolation or in both arches. When extracting in both arches in class II cases, it can be helpful to extract premolars further forward in the maxillary arch. Loss of upper first premolars facilitates overjet reduction by retraction of the upper labial segment. Mandibular second premolars may be removed to relieve crowding, while facilitating mesial movement of mandibular first molars to correct the

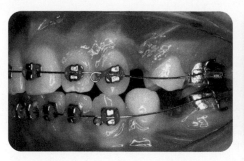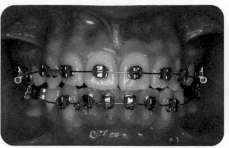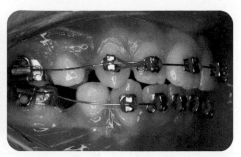

Figure 4.15

molar relationship and minimize retraction of the lower incisors. However, the ability to extract second premolars will depend upon the amount of crowding. If space requirements are high in the mandibular arch, first premolar extractions may be more suitable because they provide more space where it is usually required to relieve the crowding – in the labial segment.

What is the Tip Edge® appliance?

Tip Edge® is a fixed orthodontic appliance modelled on the Begg appliance (Kesling, 1989). The bracket design facilitates tipping of the teeth during the initial stages of treatment, which in combination with the use of rigid round stainless steel wires, anchor bends and class II elastics, allows rapid correction of the overjet and overbite during the first stage of treatment (Figure 4.15).

What are the three stages of Tip Edge® treatment?

Stage 1: Overjet and overbite reduction
Stage 2: Space closure
Stage 3: Angulation and torque correction

Why was the Tip Edge® appliance used in this case?

Tip Edge is a very effective appliance for class II camouflage. This case had a significant anchorage demand because of the increased overjet, class II molar relationship and presence of crowding. Tip Edge permits differential tooth movement with light class II traction from the outset, permitting distal tipping of the maxillary dentition and mesial tipping of the mandibular arch (Figure 4.16).

How is optimal inclination of the maxillary incisors maintained following loss of maxillary premolars?

With fixed orthodontic appliances, maxillary arch space closure can be performed with bodily control, permitting maintenance of adequate torque in the upper anterior region during overjet reduction. Torque may be enhanced by space closure on large dimension rectangular archwires, with use of supplementary palatal root torque and with the choice of bracket prescription. Torqueing auxiliaries are used with the Tip Edge® appliance to enhance maxillary incisor torque.

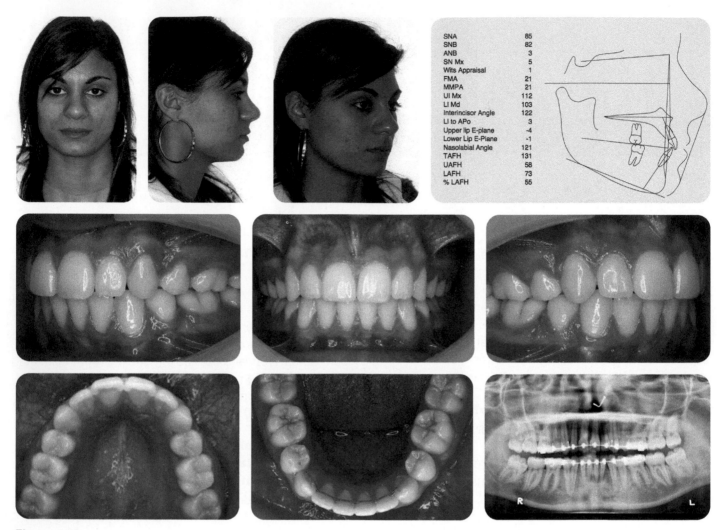

SNA	85
SNB	82
ANB	3
SN Mx	5
Wits Appraisal	1
FMA	21
MMPA	21
UI Mx	112
LI Md	103
Interincisor Angle	122
LI to APo	3
Upper lip E-plane	-4
Lower Lip E-Plane	-1
Nasolabial Angle	121
TAFH	131
UAFH	58
LAFH	73
% LAFH	55

Figure 4.16

Case 4.6

This 34-year-old female was referred by her orthodontic specialist because she was concerned by the crowding of her upper anterior teeth. She had previously undergone extraction-based orthodontic treatment as a teenager.

Extra-oral

Skeletal relationship
Antero-posterior	Mild skeletal class II
Vertical	FMPA: Average
	Lower face height: Average
Transverse	Facial asymmetry: None
Soft tissues	Lip competence: Competent
	Naso-labial angle: Average
Upper incisor show	At rest: 4mm
	Smiling: 9mm
Temporo-mandibular joint	Healthy with good range and co-ordination of movement

Intra-oral

Teeth present

$$\frac{765\ 321/123\ 5678}{7654321/1234567}$$

Dental health (restorations, caries)	Good
	Small occlusal restoration in LR6, no active caries
Oral hygiene – periodontal	Good oral hygiene, with generalized gingival recession
Lower arch	Crowding: Mild
	Incisor inclination: Average
	Curve of Spee: Average
Upper arch	Crowding: Mild
	Incisor inclination: Proclined
	Canine position: Line of the arch
Occlusion	Incisor relationship: Class II division 1
	Overjet: 9mm to UL1
	Overbite: Average and incomplete
	Molar relationship: Class II on right; 'super' class II on left
	Canine relationship: Class I on right; ½ unit class II on left
	Centre lines: Coincident (UL1 is a little to the right due to its crowded position)
	Functional occlusion: Group function

Summary

A 34-year-old female presented with a class II division 1 malocclusion on a mild skeletal class II pattern with average vertical dimensions, complicated by an increased overjet (of 9mm to the UL1), previous extraction of both upper first premolars and crowding of both dental arches (Figure 4.17).

Does the cephalometric analysis agree with the clinical findings in this case?

The ANB value is 3 degrees, which suggests a skeletal class I pattern; however, the Wits appraisal is 4mm, which indicates class II. The SNA value of 82 degrees is slightly high and as the SN-Mx plane value is within the normal range of 8 ± 5 degrees, this means that the position of Nasion is too high rather than Sella being too low. Application of the Eastman correction to the ANB value (subtract 0.5 from 3) leaves an ANB of 2.5

degrees, which is still indicative of a skeletal class I pattern in relation to the anterior cranial base. However, clinically there is a mild skeletal class II pattern.

Treatment Plan

- Upper and lower pre-adjusted edgewise appliances with extraction of UL6
- Long-term retention

The final occlusion is shown in Figure 4.18. How has overjet correction been achieved in this case?

The overjet has been reduced by some retroclination of the UL1 and more marked lower incisor proclination (from 98 to 111 degrees). There has been some gingival recession in the lower labial segment in association with this incisor proclination. The skeletal

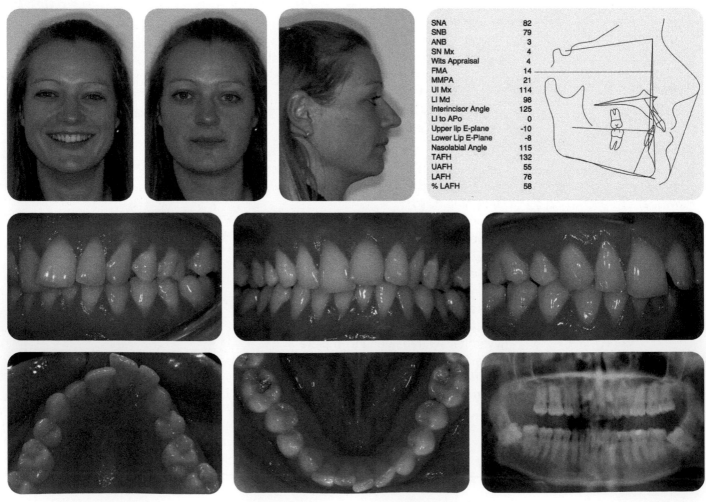

SNA	82
SNB	79
ANB	3
SN Mx	4
Wits Appraisal	4
FMA	14
MMPA	21
UI Mx	114
LI Md	98
Interincisor Angle	125
LI to APo	0
Upper lip E-plane	-10
Lower Lip E-Plane	-8
Nasolabial Angle	115
TAFH	132
UAFH	55
LAFH	76
% LAFH	58

Figure 4.17

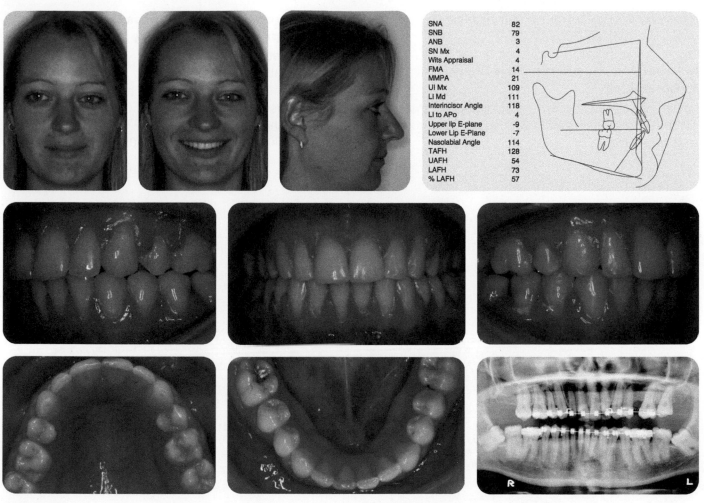

SNA	82
SNB	79
ANB	3
SN Mx	4
Wits Appraisal	4
FMA	14
MMPA	21
UI Mx	109
LI Md	111
Interincisor Angle	118
LI to APo	4
Upper lip E-plane	-9
Lower Lip E-Plane	-7
Nasolabial Angle	114
TAFH	128
UAFH	54
LAFH	73
% LAFH	57

Figure 4.18

relationship has remained the same, which would be expected in an adult.

Is there any association between occlusal para-function and orthodontic treatment?

This adult patient demonstrated significant occlusal wear. The association between orthodontic treatment, occlusal para-function and temporo-mandibular problems is unclear. A subset of patients experience worsening of their para-function during treatment; others show improvement. This is in keeping with the intermittent nature of para-functional habits. In relation to temporo-mandibular dysfunction, while some cross-sectional and longitudinal studies have noted a trend to improvement in symptoms with treatment, this change is unpredictable. Consequently, orthodontics is considered 'TMJ neutral' (Luther, 2007a,b). Nevertheless, it is advisable to carry out a thorough temporo-mandibular joint examination prior to treatment.

What are the risk factors for gingival recession during orthodontic treatment?

- Thin gingival biotype
- Pre-existing recession
- Gingival inflammation
- Poor oral hygiene (Melsen and Allais, 2005)

Is lower incisor proclination likely to exacerbate gingival recession?

Uncontrolled incisor proclination is inadvisable and risks further recession. However, the association between proclination and recession is weak and unpredictable. A retrospective study of 300 adult patients undergoing orthodontic treatment demonstrated an average increase in lower incisor recession of just 0.14 mm with incisor proclination (Allais and Melsen, 2003).

Is lower incisor proclination likely to be stable?

Lower incisor proclination is regarded as an unstable movement necessitating prolonged retention to limit relapse potential.

Are there any circumstances in which lower incisor proclination is likely to be stable?

- Pre-existing lip trap
- Digit habit
- Incisors held artificially upright by the occlusion (such as a class II division 2) (Mills, 1973)
- Following orthognathic surgery in class III malocclusion (Artun et al., 1990)

Case 4.7

This 9-year-old female was referred by her general dental practitioner, concerned about her upper front teeth; one tooth sticks out. There was no relevant medical history.

Extra-oral

Skeletal relationship

Antero-posterior	Moderate skeletal class II
Vertical	FMPA: Average
	Lower face height: Average
Transverse	Facial symmetry: None
Soft tissues	Lip competence: Incompetent with the lower lip resting behind the UL1
Upper incisor show	At rest: 3mm
	Smiling: 8mm
Temporo-mandibular joint	Healthy with good range and co-ordination of movement

Intra-oral

Teeth present	6EDC21/12CDE6
	6ED 21/12CDE6
Dental health (restorations, caries)	None present
Oral hygiene – periodontal	Good
Lower arch	Crowding: Mild
	Incisor inclination: Average
	Curve of Spee: Average
Upper arch	Crowding: Mild
	Incisor inclination: UL1 is proclined
Occlusion	Incisor relationship: Class II division 1
	Overjet: 9mm to UL1
	Overbite: Increased and complete
	Molar relationship: ½ unit class II bilaterally
	Centre lines: Coincident
	Functional occlusion: Group function

Summary

A 9-year-old female presented in the mixed dentition with a class II division 1 malocclusion on a skeletal class II pattern with average vertical facial proportions. She was concerned with the appearance of her maxillary teeth. The malocclusion was complicated by an increased overjet of 9 mm to the UL1 (Figure 4.19).

Treatment Plan

- Upper removable appliance for interceptive overjet reduction (Figure 4.20).
- Monitor further dental development

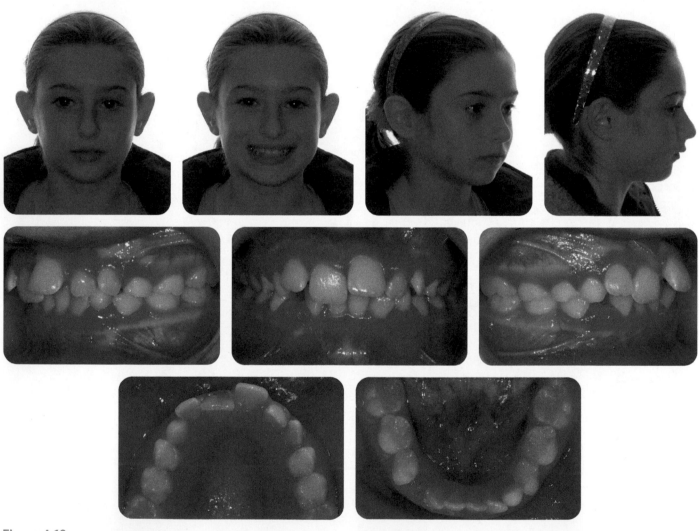

Figure 4.19

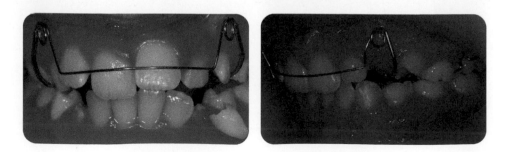

Figure 4.20

What are the indications for removable appliance therapy to reduce an increased overjet?

- Skeletal class I or mild class II pattern
- Proclined maxillary incisors
- Well-aligned arches

What are the limitations of removable appliance therapy

- Dependent on excellent co-operation
- Capable of tipping movements in isolation, but apical control is not feasible

Consequently, removable appliances are usually indicated as an adjunct or prelude to fixed appliances.

What type of removable appliance is being used and how is this constructed (Figure 4.20)?

This appliance incorporates a Robert's retractor, which is an active labial bow constructed from 0.5-mm stainless steel wire. This bow has increased flexibility because of the reduced diameter wire and increased length. However, it can be quite fragile and is easily distorted, so the buccal arms are sheathed laterally in stainless steel tubing to improve strength.

What were the indications for interceptive orthodontic treatment in this case?

Interceptive treatment was indicated for cosmetic reasons, to address psychosocial concerns in relation to teasing and to limit the risk of dental trauma.

How is overjet reduction achieved with removable appliances?

Overjet reduction is achieved by activation of the upper labial bow, which retracts the upper incisors by retroclination. Consequently, this form of treatment camouflages the underlying skeletal discrepancy.

What features would contra-indicate removable appliance therapy for overjet reduction?

- Poor co-operation
- Severe skeletal class II discrepancy with upright or retroclined maxillary incisors where tipping of the teeth would be inappropriate

Is overjet reduction likely to be stable in this case (Figure 4.21)?

Overjet reduction is likely to be stable if the upper incisors lie within the control of the upper lip following treatment. Further treatment, however, is likely to be required in the longer term to detail the occlusion and introduce optimal maxillary incisor torque.

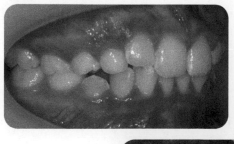
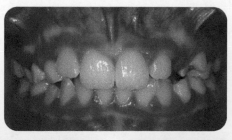
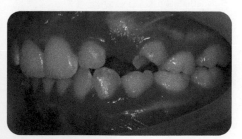
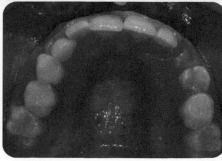
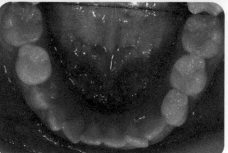

Figure 4.21

Case 4.8

This patient presented as a 12-year-old class II division 1 malocclusion. She was concerned about the prominence of her upper front teeth and had previously avulsed the UR1. The overjet on the UL1 was 9mm.

Summarize her malocclusion (Figure 4.22)

This is a class II division 1 on a moderate skeletal class II base with reduced anterior lower face height. The overjet is increased and the overbite is increased and complete. The buccal segments are ½ unit class II bilaterally and the centre lines are coincident. The

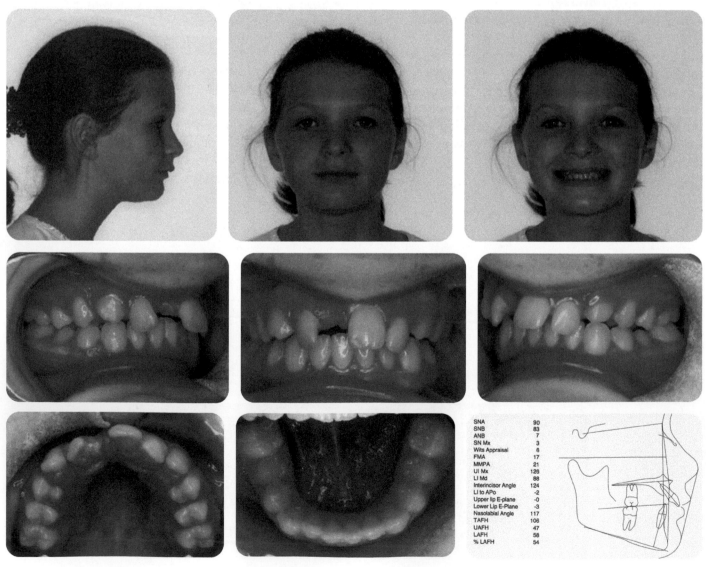

SNA	90
SNB	83
ANB	7
SN Mx	3
Wits Appraisal	6
FMA	17
MMPA	21
UI Mx	126
LI Md	88
Interincisor Angle	124
LI to APo	-2
Upper lip E-plane	-0
Lower Lip E-Plane	-3
Nasolabial Angle	117
TAFH	106
UAFH	47
LAFH	58
% LAFH	54

Figure 4.22

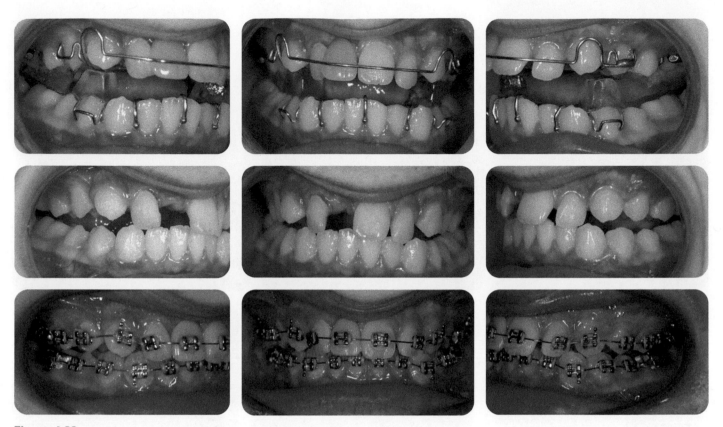

Figure 4.23

lower arch is well aligned and there is mild crowding in the upper arch. The UR1 has been previously lost but there is adequate space available for prosthetic replacement of this tooth.

Comment on the pre-treatment cephalometric analysis (Figure 4.22)

Moderate skeletal class II (ANB = 7 degrees; Wits = +6 mm; although an Eastman correction can be applied to the ANB value due to the position of Nasion [SN-Mx plane is just within the normal range], which gives a corrected value of 2.5 degrees for ANB). There is maxillary prominence (SNA = 90 degrees) and a reduced MMPA (21 degrees). The upper incisors are proclined and the lower incisors are upright.

What treatment has been carried out (Figure 4.23)?

A Twin Block functional appliance has been used (in combination with cervical headgear), followed by pre-adjusted edgewise fixed appliances.

Comment on the design of the Twin Block

This modified Twin Block incorporates a prosthetic UR1 to maintain space for this tooth and improve aesthetics. Headgear tubes have been placed on the Adams cribs on the maxillary first molars. The lower first permanent molars have not been cribbed to aid in bite opening.

How has this malocclusion been corrected (Figure 4.24)?

There has been some restraint of maxillary growth and forward movement of the mandible (SNA has reduced, SNB has increased and ANB has reduced). The MMPA has increased slightly. The upper incisors have been retroclined and the lower incisors have proclined.

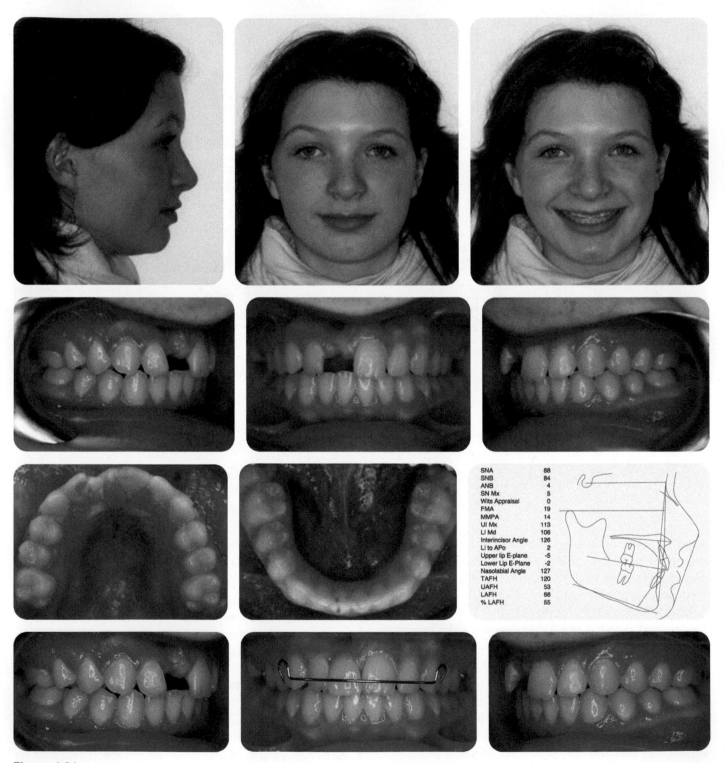

SNA	88
SNB	84
ANB	4
SN Mx	5
Wits Appraisal	0
FMA	19
MMPA	14
UI Mx	113
LI Md	106
Interincisor Angle	126
LI to APo	2
Upper lip E-plane	-5
Lower Lip E-Plane	-2
Nasolabial Angle	127
TAFH	120
UAFH	53
LAFH	66
% LAFH	55

Figure 4.24

Case 4.9

This 10-year-old boy was referred by his general dental practitioner who was concerned about the prominence of his upper front teeth. He is medically fit and well. The overjet is increased to 14 mm and both maxillary permanent canines are palpable buccally. The general dental practitioner has sent a dental panoramic radiograph that was taken 6 months previously.

Summarize the main features of this malocclusion (Figure 4.25)

- Class II division 1 case on a skeletal class II base with reduced vertical proportions
- Mixed dentition and poor oral hygiene
- Overjet is increased to 14 mm, the overbite is increased and complete, and the buccal segments are a full unit class II
- Centre lines are coincident
- Mild crowding in the mandibular arch but the maxillary arch is reasonably well aligned

Describe the stage of development of the dentition (Figure 4.25)

This child is in the late mixed dentition. In the mandibular arch, all permanent teeth are present and erupted, with the exception of the second and third molars. In the maxillary arch, the primary canines are still present as well as the URE, which is carious. The ULE has recently been exfoliated and the UL5 is erupting.

Why does this boy have an increased overjet?

The increased overjet is due to the presence of a significant skeletal class II discrepancy, which is caused primarily by mandibular retrognathia. As a result of the retrognathic mandible and reduced vertical facial proportions, there is a lip trap, with the lower lip lying habitually behind the upper incisors. This has caused proclination of the upper incisors and retroclination of the lowers, which together further increases the overjet caused by the retrognathic mandible.

This boy was fitted with a Twin Block functional appliance, which he wore on a full-time basis for 7 months (Figure 4.26, upper panel). His dental appearance at this stage is shown in Figure 4.26 (lower panel).

Describe the features of his malocclusion at this stage

This boy is now in the early permanent dentition, with dental development more advanced in the mandibular arch. In the maxillary arch, the UL3, UR3, UR4, and UR5 are all partially erupted. The overjet and overbite have been reduced. The maxillary arch has been expanded with the functional appliance. There are marked lateral open bites. The oral hygiene is poor.

Are there any contraindications to a phase of fixed appliance treatment following the successful use of a functional appliance?

- Poor oral hygiene
- Mixed dentition
- History of poor compliance
- Well aligned class I occlusion with no open bites

What will need to be addressed in the management of this malocclusion?

The lateral open bites need to close and the overjet reduction needs to be maintained. Once this has been achieved, a decision needs to be made regarding progression to fixed appliances.

A common problem associated with the transition from a Twin Block functional appliance to a fixed appliance is relapse. How does this usually manifest?

- Increase in the overjet
- Molar and canine relationships becomes more class II

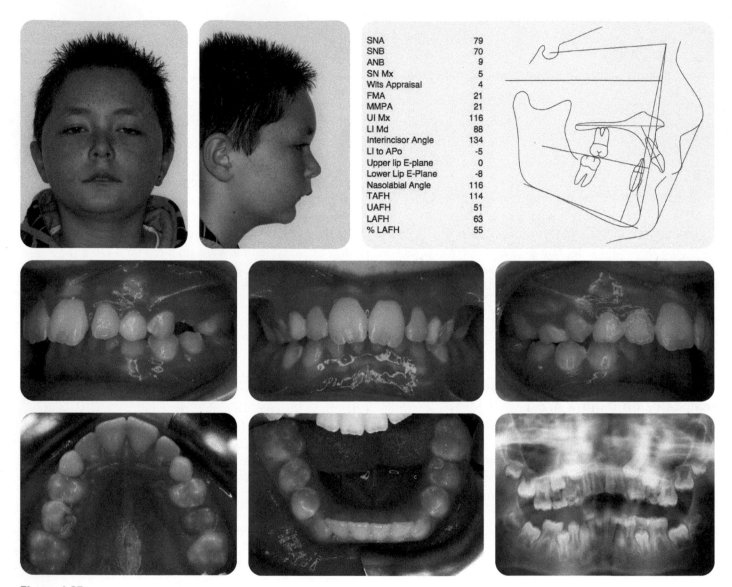

SNA	79
SNB	70
ANB	9
SN Mx	5
Wits Appraisal	4
FMA	21
MMPA	21
UI Mx	116
LI Md	88
Interincisor Angle	134
LI to APo	-5
Upper lip E-plane	0
Lower Lip E-Plane	-8
Nasolabial Angle	116
TAFH	114
UAFH	51
LAFH	63
% LAFH	55

Figure 4.25

How can these problems be avoided?

- Achieving overcorrection in both the incisor and molar relationship
- Completing the functional appliance phase in the permanent dentition
- If posterior open bites are present, continued wear of the functional appliance whilst they close (nocturnal and then progressive reduction in wear of the functional appliance; or full time wear and occlusal trimming of the bite blocks or wear of an upper removable appliance with a 'steep and deep' inclined anterior bite plane)
- Headgear during the early phase of fixed appliance treatment
- Class II elastics early on in the fixed phase

This boy continued to wear his Twin Block appliance at night for a period of 6 months. The lateral open bites have closed down and he is now in the permanent dentition (Figure 4.27). There has been a small increase in the overjet to 4 mm.

Summarize the changes that have enabled overjet reduction to occur during this period of functional appliance treatment

- The antero-posterior skeletal pattern has improved, the maxilla has been restrained, the mandible has come forward and the ANB angle has reduced.
- The lower facial profile has improved markedly and the lip trap has been eliminated.

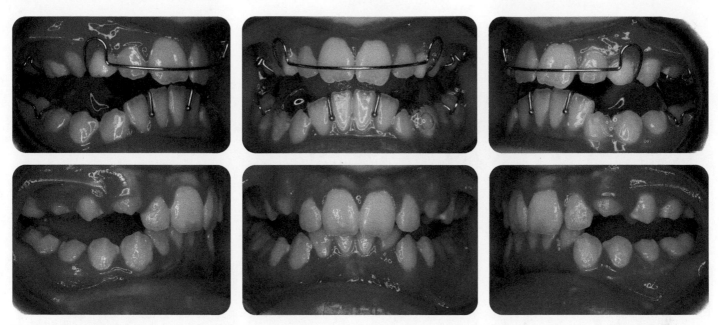

Figure 4.26

- The upper incisors have been retroclined and the lower incisors proclined.
- The maxillary buccal dentition has been restrained, whilst the mandibular buccal dentition has moved mesially.
- There has been an increase in the MMPA.

What further options are there for treatment?

A further option is a course of fixed appliance treatment to detail the occlusion (Figure 4.28). This will be carried out on a non-extraction basis and the reasons for this are primarily because:

- There is only mild crowding
- Although the lower incisors have moved forward during the functional appliance phase of treatment, they were originally quite retroclined (due to the lower lip position)
- Currently the lower incisors are behind the A-Pog line.

Because of the small increase in overjet that has occurred, some headgear support would also be useful during the early stages of fixed appliance treatment.

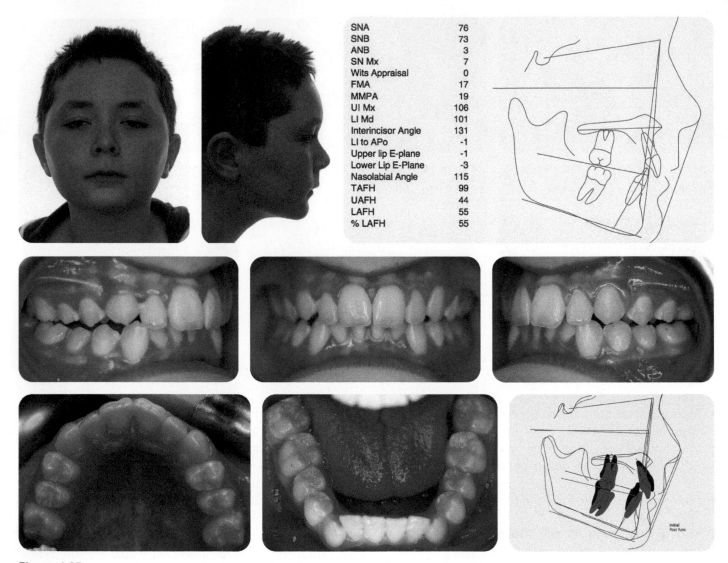

SNA	76
SNB	73
ANB	3
SN Mx	7
Wits Appraisal	0
FMA	17
MMPA	19
UI Mx	106
LI Md	101
Interincisor Angle	131
LI to APo	-1
Upper lip E-plane	-1
Lower Lip E-Plane	-3
Nasolabial Angle	115
TAFH	99
UAFH	44
LAFH	55
% LAFH	55

Figure 4.27

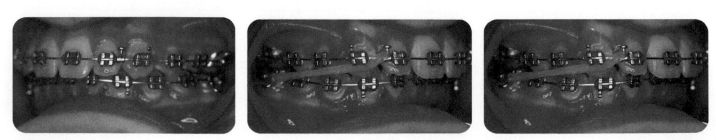

Figure 4.28

Case 4.10

This 12-year-old female was referred by her general dentist in relation to her prominent upper front teeth. There was no relevant medical history.

Extra-oral

Skeletal relationship

    Antero-posterior   Moderate skeletal class II base

    Vertical   Average FMPA

                                        Average lower face height

    Transverse   No facial asymmetry

Soft tissues   Lips appear incompetent with a lower lip trap at rest

                                        Naso-labial angle is normal

                                      Upper incisor show at rest and smiling is within the normal range

Intra-oral

Late mixed dentition

Teeth present

$$\frac{\text{6E4321/123456}}{\text{76E4321/1234E67}}$$

Dental health (restorations, caries)   UL6 is carious on the panoramic radiograph but this has been restored

                                      Generalized marginal gingivitis

Lower arch   Crowding: Moderate

                                        Incisor inclination: Average

                                        Canines: Erupted and mesially angulated

                                        Curve of Spee: Average

Upper arch   Crowding: Mild

                                        Incisor inclination: Proclined

                                        Canine position: Erupted and mesially angulated

Occlusion   Incisor relationship: Class II division 1

                                        Overjet: Increased (to 9 mm)

                                        Overbite: Average and complete

                                        Molar relationship: Full unit class II bilaterally

                                        Canine relationship: ½ unit class II bilaterally

                                        Centre lines: Coincident

Summary

A 12-year-old female presented with a class II division 1 incisor relationship on a skeletal class II pattern with average vertical dimensions and mild crowding in both arches (Figure 4.29) complicated by:

- Increased overjet (10 mm)
- Palatally-displaced UR2 and UL2
- Missing LL5
- Infra-occluded LLE.

What are the treatment options in this case?

- Combined orthodontic–surgical treatment with upper and lower fixed appliances and mandibular advancement surgery
- Orthodontic camouflage with removal of both maxillary first premolars, upper and lower fixed appliances and anchorage support

As the patient had no concerns in relation to her facial appearance and has a full soft tissue profile, a decision was made to camouflage her overjet (Figure 4.30).

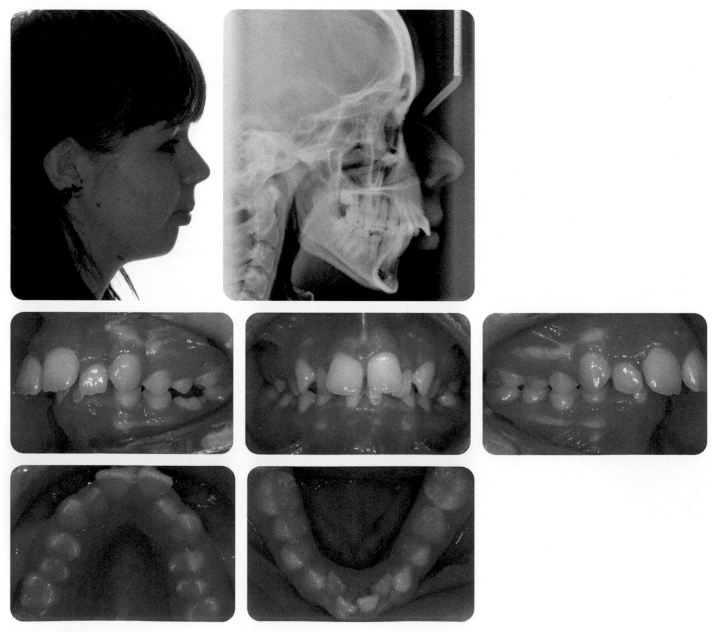

Figure 4.29

What are the options to conserve anchorage and facilitate overjet reduction?

Anchorage is required to facilitate overjet reduction. Intra-arch auxiliaries that could be considered include headgear, a Nance palatal arch or temporary anchorage devices. Headgear tends to be poorly tolerated in adult patients. Palatal arches can be problematic during orthodontic space closure and overjet reduction, and are traditionally dispensed with prior to this treatment stage. In addition, there is some evidence that palatal arches may be of little real value for antero-posterior anchorage (Stivaros et al., 2010). Consequently, temporary anchorage devices were used to facilitate overjet reduction. Other options that could have been considered include use of differential tooth movement, e.g. Tip Edge® appliance and inter-arch mechanics, including elastics or fixed class II correctors.

How can temporary anchorage devices be used to effect overjet reduction?

Temporary anchorage devices can be used directly or indirectly. Direct use involves placement of the active

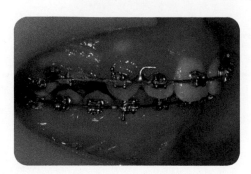

Figure 4.31

mechanics directly between the fixed anchorage unit and the active unit (Figure 4.31). The advantage of this technique is that forces can be directed along the occlusal plane, limiting unwanted vertical reactionary forces. Indirect anchorage involves ligation of the reactive or anchorage unit.

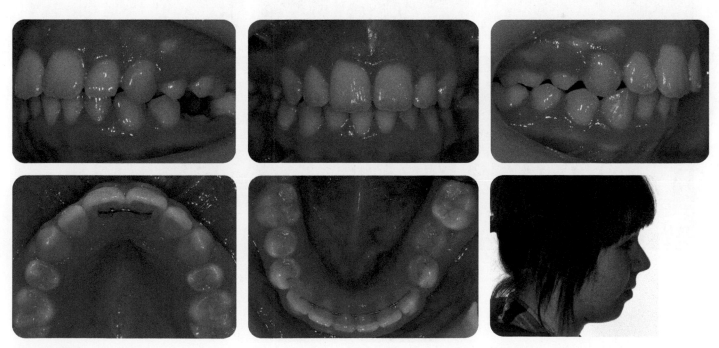

Figure 4.30

Case 4.11

This 12-year-old girl presented following referral by her general dental practitioner (Figure 4.32).

Summary

A 12-year-old female presented with a class II division 1 incisor relationship on a moderate skeletal class II pattern with average vertical dimensions complicated by:

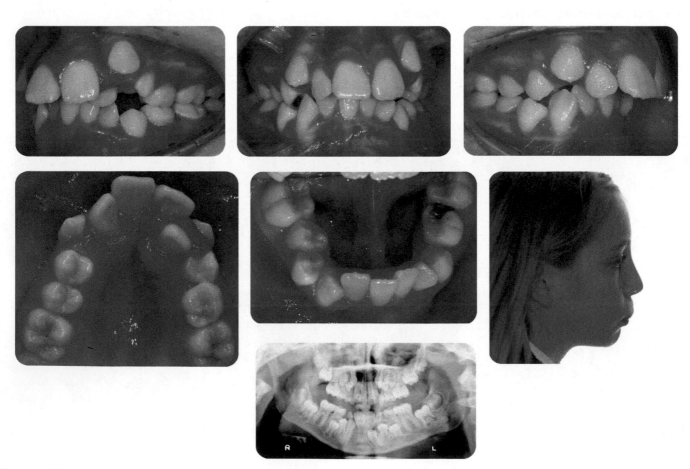

Figure 4.32

- Increased overjet (11 mm)
- Ectopic LL3
- Severe upper and lower arch crowding
- Upper centre line shift
- Palatally displaced UL2
- Possible occlusal caries in the UL6.

What treatment plan would you suggest in this case?

The panoramic radiograph does not show clear evidence of caries in the UL6; however, given the clinical appearance, bite-wing radiographs should be taken to obtain a definitive diagnosis. In this case, there proved to be no caries in this tooth.

As this is a growing patient, growth modification could be utilized to facilitate overjet reduction. In addition, the crowding and centre line deviation could be addressed with extraction of four premolar units. Given the degree of displacement of the LL3, its loss could be considered in conjunction with the removal of four first premolars.

In this case, a functional appliance was used first to reduce the overjet and correct the buccal segment relationship. The functional appliance therapy progressed well, and all four first premolars and the LL3 were then removed prior to a treatment phase involving fixed appliances (Figure 4.33).

What do you notice in Figure 4.34? What mechanics could be considered to achieve an ideal buccal segment relationship?

The canine relationship has been corrected to class I; there is 4 mm of extraction space remaining in the

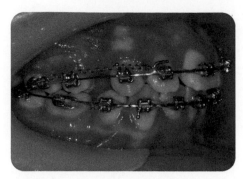

Figure 4.34

upper right quadrant. Therefore, to achieve an ideal result, space closure will need to occur by mesial movement of the buccal segment rather than retraction of the anterior teeth or reciprocal space closure. As the initial malocclusion involved a large overjet, this situation is acceptable. However, to promote space closure from behind, additional torque may be added to the maxillary incisors; the archwire could be rounded and reduced in dimension in the buccal segment to reduce frictional resistance locally; the UR5 and UR6 could be protracted individually; and class III inter-arch traction could be considered.

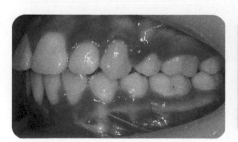
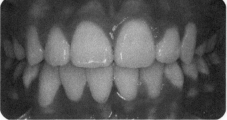
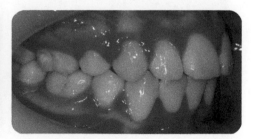

Figure 4.33

Case 4.12

This 13-year-old boy was referred by his general dental practitioner, complaining of prominent upper front teeth (Figure 4.35).

Summary

A 13-year-old male presented with a class II division 1 incisor relationship on a mild skeletal class II pattern with average vertical dimensions complicated by:

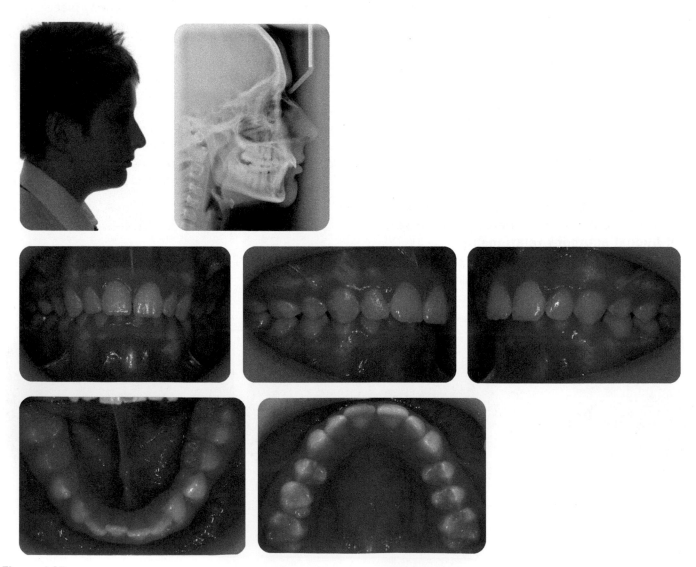

Figure 4.35

- Increased overjet (9mm)
- Mild mandibular arch crowding.

What treatment options would you consider in this case?

As this is a growing patient, growth modification should be considered. Options include either headgear followed by fixed appliances or a functional appliance followed by fixed appliances, both on a non-extraction basis. The latter option was chosen in this case (Figure 4.36).

What are the likely effects of functional appliance therapy in this case?

In the short-term, skeletal and dento-alveolar changes are likely. Skeletal effects are likely to include restraint of maxillary growth, temporary acceleration and redirection of mandibular growth, and an increase in lower facial height. The majority of the changes are likely to be dento-alveolar, including retroclination of the maxillary incisors, distal tipping of the maxillary buccal segments and proclination of the mandibular incisors.

What bracket prescription would you suggest following the functional phase?

A prescription with increased palatal root torque in the maxillary incisors and labial root torque in the mandibular incisors would be beneficial to counteract excessive dento-alveolar change during the functional phase. Furthermore, if maxillary expansion was undertaken during the functional phase, buccal root torque would be helpful to counteract unwanted buccal flaring of the maxillary buccal segments (Fleming et al., 2007).

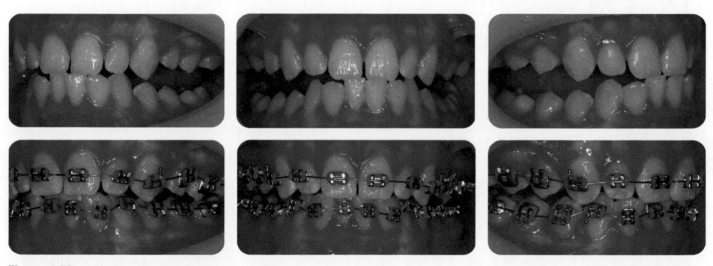

Figure 4.36

Case 4.13

This 14-year-old girl, who is fit and well, has been referred complaining about the appearance of her upper front teeth. She has no previous history of orthodontic treatment and is quite happy to undertake orthodontic treatment (Figure 4.37).

Summary

A 14-year-old female presented with a class II division 1 malocclusion on a moderate skeletal class II base with reduced vertical proportions. There is an increased overjet, an increased and complete overbite, and severe crowding in both dental arches. The molar

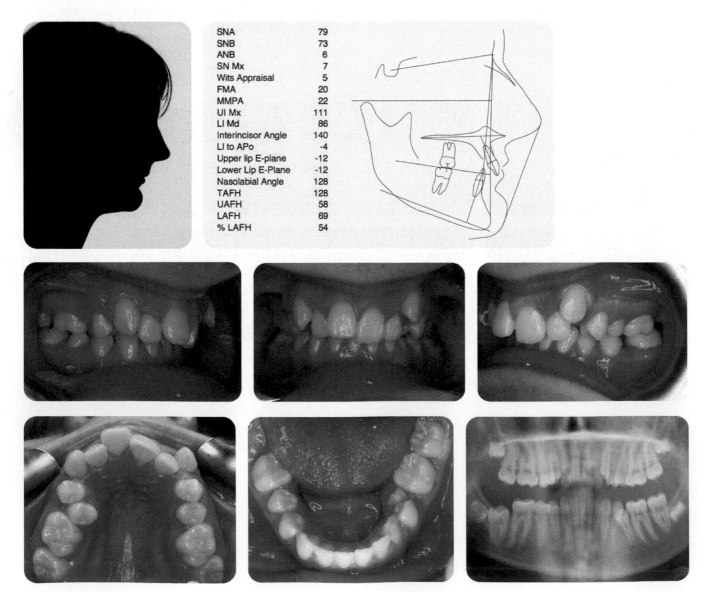

SNA	79
SNB	73
ANB	6
SN Mx	7
Wits Appraisal	5
FMA	20
MMPA	22
UI Mx	111
LI Md	86
Interincisor Angle	140
LI to APo	-4
Upper lip E-plane	-12
Lower Lip E-Plane	-12
Nasolabial Angle	128
TAFH	128
UAFH	58
LAFH	69
% LAFH	54

Figure 4.37

relationship is class II bilaterally and there is a centre line discrepancy.

Describe the extra-oral features

- Skeletal class II discrepancy
- Retruded facial profile with a prominent chin button
- Reduced vertical proportions

Describe the intra-oral features

- Oral hygiene is good
- No evidence of caries or previous restorative work
- Teeth present: $\dfrac{7654321/1234567}{654321/1234567}$
- LL5 is crowded and only partially erupted

Describe the occlusion

- Severe crowding in the lower arch, with the LL5 partially erupted. The LR7 is unerupted
- Lower incisors are retroclined and both canines distally angulated
- Severe crowding in the upper arch, with the UR5 palatally excluded and both upper canines crowded buccally
- UR1 is proclined with a 9mm overjet but the UL1 is retroclined
- Upper canines are mesially angulated
- Incisor relationship is class II division 1 with an increased overjet on the UR1
- Molar relationship is class II bilaterally
- Lower centre line is over to the left of the face and the upper is over to the right, almost certainly due to the dental crowding

What additional information does the panoramic radiographic examination provide?

The panoramic radiograph confirms the absence of caries and shows all four third molars developing. The LR7 is distally angulated and unerupted. There is some evidence of over-eruption of the UR7, although clinically this tooth occludes with the LR6 as there is a class II molar relationship.

What information does the cephalometric examination give regarding the skeletal pattern?

The lateral skull radiograph has been digitized and confirms a skeletal class II pattern (ANB = 6 degrees; Wits = +5mm) with reduced vertical proportions (MMPA 22 degrees). In addition, the lip relationship to Rickett's E-line (both lips −12mm) suggests a retrusive profile.

What information does it provide about the incisor position?

The lower incisors are retroclined, both in relation to the mandibular plane (86 degrees) and to the A-Pog line (−4mm). The position of these teeth might be expected to be upright because of the reduced MMPA. A guide to the expected lower incisor inclination to the mandibular plane can be achieved by subtracting the MMPA from 120, which in this case would give an ideal value of 98 degrees; therefore, they are retroclined at 88 degrees.

The most prominent upper incisor is proclined at 111 degrees, although this is within the normal range.

What is the main problem list for this patient?

- Skeletal class II pattern with reduced vertical proportions
- Retrognathic profile
- Increased overjet and overbite
- Severe crowding
- Centre line discrepancy
- Class II buccal segment relationship

What are the main options for treatment?

As with any case that has a class II skeletal discrepancy and an increased overjet, the main options are between:
- Orthodontic camouflage
- Growth modification
- Combined orthodontics and orthognathic surgery.

If this patient declined to wear a functional appliance and refused jaw surgery, how would you achieve orthodontic camouflage?

Orthodontic camouflage could be achieved using fixed orthodontic appliances.

Although there is severe crowding in the lower arch, this only affects the partially erupted/impacted LL5. Given that there is an increased overbite and some retroclination of the lower incisors, one option would be to treat the lower arch on a non-extraction basis, creating space by expansion to align the LL5.

A further factor to consider is accommodating the unerupted LR7. This tooth requires exposure and extrusive mechanics to bring it into occlusion. However, this will be time-consuming, technically difficult and complicated by lack of space, particularly if a non-extraction approach is taken in the lower arch.

Alternatively, second premolar extractions could be carried out in the lower arch. This would have the advantage of providing some space at the back of the arch for the LR7 and also some anchorage to facilitate overjet reduction via the use of some inter-arch class II traction.

In the upper arch, anchorage requirements are high. There is severe crowding, an increased overjet and a buccal segment relationship that is class II. The extraction of first premolars alone will not provide enough space. In order to generate further space, headgear could be used; however, compliance will need to be very good in order to achieve distal movement of the first molars, particularly as most facial growth will be complete in a 14-year-old girl.

Headgear wear could be supplemented with a removable appliance with finger springs mesial to the upper first molar (Ten Hoeve, ACCO or nudger appliance), which could also incorporate a bite plane to aid overbite reduction (see Figure 4.4). Alternatively, a non-compliance technique could be applied using temporary anchorage devices to aid molar distalization.

This patient was successfully treated with a functional appliance followed by fixed appliances in conjunction with the extraction of UR4, UL4, LL5, exposure of the LR7 and headgear support (Figure 4.38).

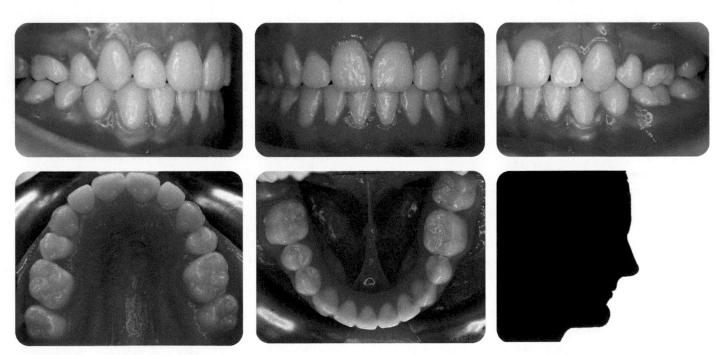

Figure 4.38

Case 4.14

This 12-year-old patient is fit and well and was referred with an increased overjet of 9 mm (Figure 4.39).

What are the main features of the malocclusion?

- Skeletal class II pattern
- Some increase in the vertical proportions

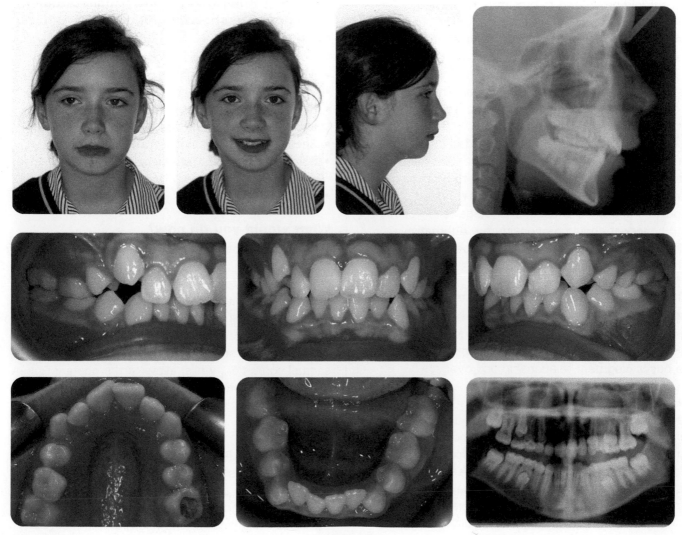

Figure 4.39

- Late mixed dentition
- Mild crowding in both dental arches
- Increased overjet of 9mm
- Buccal segments ½ unit class 2
- Centre line discrepancy (the lower deviated to the left)
- Occlusal caries in the UL6 (present on OPG but restored in the clinical records)

A Twin Block functional appliance was prescribed to reduce the overjet, which was to be followed by a review of the need for extractions and fixed appliances to align and co-ordinate the dental arches. Can you suggest two alternative treatment plans?

There is mild crowding in the lower dental arch, with both second primary molars (Es) present. A lingual arch could be fitted and following loss (or extraction) of the Es and eruption of the 5s, the E space could be utilized to provide space to align the lower arch with a fixed appliance. In the upper arch, space is required to correct the buccal segment relationship, reduce the overjet and align the teeth. This could be provided by distalization of the upper first permanent molars using headgear. The presence of an URE gives this distalization process a head-start in the upper right quadrant.

Alternatively, space could be provided by the extraction of upper first premolars and lower second premolars, and fixed appliances used to produce a well-aligned class I occlusion. If a pre-adjusted edgewise appliance is used, anchorage reinforcement with headgear should be considered. Alternatively a light-wire Tip Edge® appliance could be used in combination with class II traction.

What are the main advantages and disadvantages of these approaches?

The non-extraction approach is dependent upon good compliance and favourable growth to correct the buccal segment relationship and overjet. Space requirements in the lower arch will mean that some proclination of the lower incisors is almost inevitable with this treatment plan and this might not be stable in the long-term. The extraction of permanent teeth is required for the second approach and some headgear wear. Both of these strategies are likely to be quicker than a functional/fixed approach. However, the open naso-labial angle and upper lip trap combined with mandibular retrognathia

make retraction of the upper labial segment less desirable in this case due to the risk of further deterioration of the soft tissue profile. The use of a Twin Block is a very effective way to correct the buccal segment relationship and overjet in a manner that, whilst dependent upon good compliance, is generally very achievable in most growing adolescent children.

What are the space requirements in the lower arch?

Space is required primarily to relieve mild crowding, but there is also an increased curve of Spee and the lower canines are upright, which is anchorage-demanding to correct. In addition, the lower second permanent molars are erupting and the lower incisor crowding can increase when this takes place.

The occlusion and cephalometric changes following 8 months of functional appliance treatment are shown in Figure 4.40. What has been achieved?

- Overjet has been reduced
- Buccal segment relationship has been corrected
- Centre line has been corrected
- Remaining second deciduous molars have been lost and the second premolars have erupted
- Second permanent molars have erupted
- Some upper incisor retroclination and lower incisor proclination
- Profile remains class II

What would you do now?

The posterior open bites need to be closed down. The patient should now wear the functional appliance at night-time only for a month, then on alternate nights until the open bites have gone. Alternatively, the acrylic can be trimmed on the blocks of the Twin Block to facilitate guidance of eruption in the buccal segments. The goal of this phase is to maintain the sagittal correction, whilst allowing the posterior open bites to close, prior to moving into a fixed appliance phase of treatment.

What decision needs to be made prior to placing fixed appliances?

A key decision is the need for extractions. The fixed appliances are primarily concerned with levelling and aligning the arches and maintaining the class I relationship. The need for extractions,

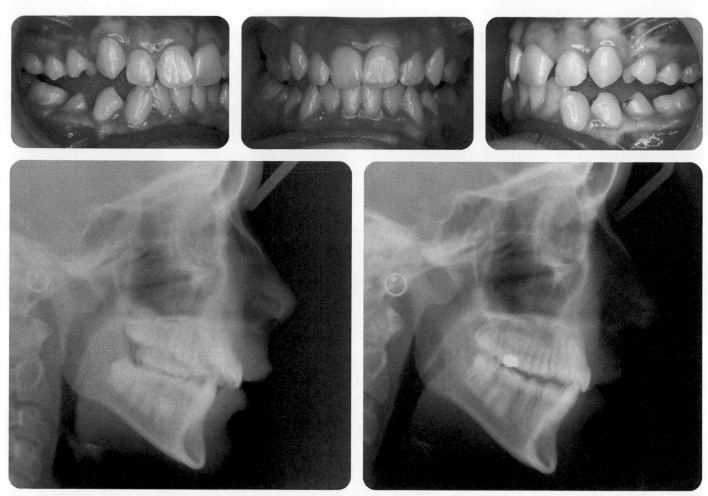

Figure 4.40

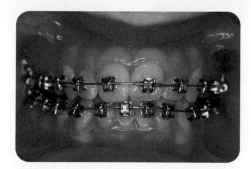

Figure 4.41

and which teeth should be extracted, is influenced by:

- Space requirements in the arches for levelling and aligning
- The existing inclinations of the labial segments.

As the space requirements were low in the lower arch, the lower incisors had not been proclined excessively and the overjet remained reduced, a decision was made to progress into fixed appliances on a non-extraction basis. A self-ligating Damon bracket system was used (Figure 4.41).

The clinical records after removal of the fixed appliances are shown in Figure 4.42. Treatment with the fixed appliances took approximately 18 months and with the Twin Block 12 months, giving an overall treatment time of 30 months.

Comment on the facial profile changes (compare Figure 4.39 with Figure 4.42)

The skeletal pattern remains class II but the chin point has improved following treatment. There has been some further lower incisor proclination during the fixed appliance phase.

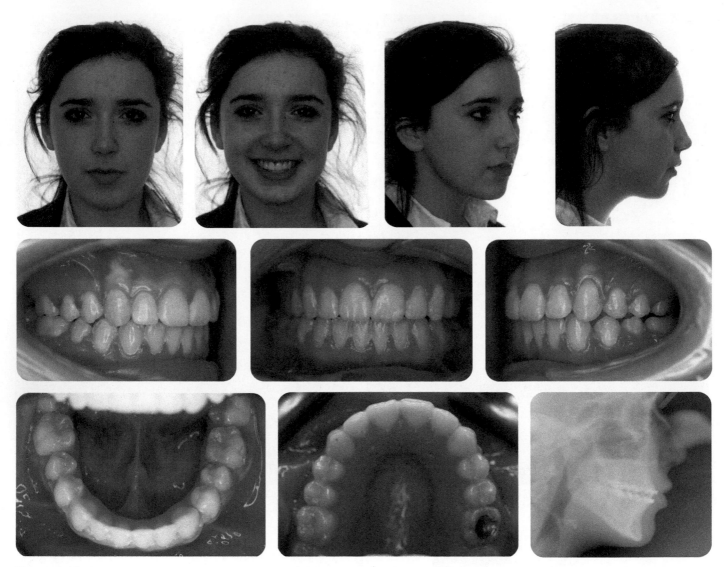

Figure 4.42

Case 4.15

Give a brief summary of this malocclusion

The patient presents with a class II division 1 malocclusion on a skeletal class II base with a prominent soft tissue pogonion. The lower anterior face height and FMPA are average. The malocclusion

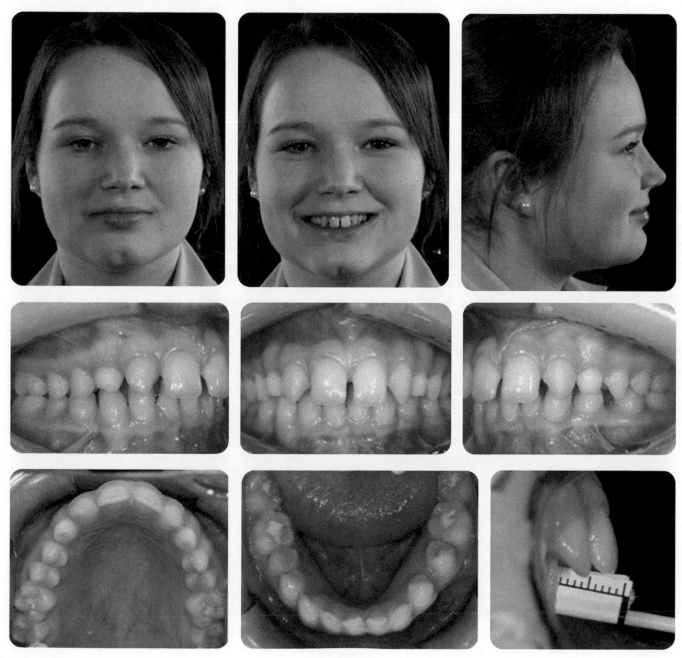

Figure 4.43

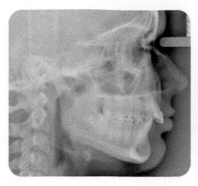
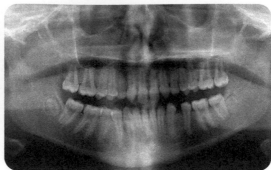

Figure 4.44

is in the late mixed dentition and both the upper and lower arches are reasonably well aligned. The malocclusion is complicated by:

- Congenital absence of the upper lateral incisors and one lower incisor
- Increased overjet (8 mm)
- Slightly increased overbite
- Buccal segment relationship that is ½ unit class 2 bilaterally.

What essential approaches should be considered when planning treatment to reduce an increased overjet?

- Potential growth modification with a functional appliance or headgear
- Orthodontic camouflage
- Orthognathic surgery

What would be the most appropriate approach in this case?

As the patient is still growing, treatment with a functional appliance to reduce the overjet or orthodontic camouflage with fixed appliances are both possible. Both approaches require decisions to be made regarding management of the missing lateral incisors.

Discuss the following two treatment options
Option 1

- Removal of retained upper primary canines
- Headgear to distalize the maxillary molars to class I
- Upper and lower fixed appliances to distalize the maxillary canines into a class I relationship and create space for future prosthetic replacement of the upper lateral incisors
- Closure of all the lower arch space

Option 2

- Removal of the maxillary primary canines
- Upper and lower fixed appliances to achieve space closure in the upper arch, accepting the maxillary canines in the position of the upper lateral incisors, with a view to camouflaging the canines with composite resin on completion of the orthodontic treatment
- Closure of all the lower arch space

Option 1 is anchorage demanding as space is required to reduce the overjet in addition to creating space for prosthetic replacement of the upper lateral incisors. Headgear is required to distalize the upper buccal segments and this relies on patient compliance.

This option has the aesthetic advantage of enabling prosthetic replacement of the maxillary lateral incisors; however, this does commit the patient to long-term maintenance and replacement of the restorative work.

Option 2 is less anchorage demanding than option 1, although anchorage support will be required for reduction of the overjet. Space for overjet reduction will be provided by removal of the retained maxillary primary canines. Both permanent maxillary canines will require restorative masking with composite resin on completion of the orthodontics. The colour match between maxillary canines and central incisors is good.

For both options, consideration will need to be given to the developmental absence of one lower incisor, which will result in a tooth-size discrepancy. As a result, for both options, if the upper centre line is coincident with the coronal midpoint of a single incisor positioned in the midline, there will be a slightly increased overjet and overbite at the end of treatment.

Alternatively, a lower canine tooth (given the starting position, almost certainly the LR3) could be used as the LR2 and a normal centre line relationship achieved. In this case the right buccal segment relationship would be class III for option 1 or class I for option 2. However, there would still be a tooth-size discrepancy, as a canine is bigger than a lateral incisor, so these relationships would be imperfect. They could be predicted in advance using a Kesling set-up.

Case 4.16

A 19-year-old male was referred in relation to crowding and an increased overjet (Figure 4.45). He is unhappy with the appearance of his teeth and is anxious to have orthodontic correction. A simple cephalometric analysis was carried out and provided the following data:

SNA	80°
SNB	75°
ANB	5°
Wits	1 mm
MMPA	31°
LAFH proportion	57%
UI-Mx	112°
LI-Mn	90°

Comment on the facial profile (Figure 4.45)

The skeletal profile appears to be mild class II with a slightly increased lower anterior face height (LAFH). The mandibular symphysis is flat with poor chin projection; this is in keeping with a backward mandibular growth rotation, which usually results in increased vertical proportions. The lower facial profile is convex, reflecting mandibular retrognathia. The soft tissues are retrusive to Rickett's E-line, indicating that the lips are thin. The naso-labial angle is within normal limits. The upper lip hangs vertically with acceptable upper lip curl.

What is the relevance of these findings?

The fact that the skeletal discrepancy is mild suggests that it is acceptable. Consequently, unless facial

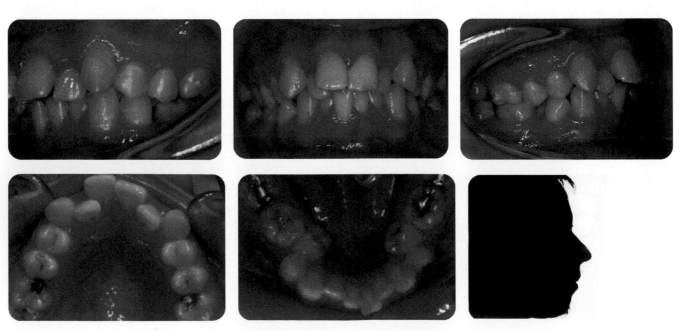

Figure 4.45

change is requested or orthodontics risks compromising the facial profile, orthodontic camouflage is a viable option.

As the soft tissues are relatively thin and retrusive, it would be unwise to retract the dentition excessively, as this would risk prematurely ageing the soft tissue profile. However, as the mandibular arch is severely crowded, in this case excessive retraction of the dentition is unlikely.

Comment on the inter-arch relationships

- Incisor relationship: Class II division 1, with an increased overjet
- Canine relationships: Also class II bilaterally, indicating that there is a significant anchorage demand to achieve a class I relationship
- Molar relationships: Class I

Are you surprised to note that the molar relationships are class I?

Given the skeletal class II discrepancy, it would be intuitive to think that the first molars would also tend toward a class II relationship. In addition, the increased overjet would also suggest that the molar relationships would also be class II. However, it is likely that the mandibular first molars have migrated mesially secondary to premature loss of mandibular second primary molars. There is also severe lower arch crowding, with lingual displacement of the second premolars. Therefore, it appears that the class I molar relationships are somewhat artificial and mask an underlying anchorage demand.

Summarize the presenting malocclusion

A 19-year-old male with a class II division 1 incisor relationship on a mild skeletal class II base with increased FMPA complicated by:

- Increased overjet
- Crowding of both arches
- Class II canine relationships
- Lingual displacement of both mandibular second premolars.

What are the likely aetiological factors underlying the malocclusion?

- Skeletal class II relationship: contributing to increased overjet and class II canines
- Increased LAFH: leading to a slightly reduced overbite

- Dento-alveolar disproportion: tooth-arch size mismatch has led to crowding of both arches. The mandibular arch is severely crowded
- Premature loss of primary teeth: early loss of the mandibular second primary molars resulted in mesial migration of the first permanent molars inducing crowding; which in turn resulted in lingual displacement of the second premolars
- Bolton tooth-size discrepancy: the lower second premolars are macrodont, exacerbating the lower arch crowding
- Soft tissues: incompetent lips may be exacerbating the increased proclination of the maxillary incisors and keeping the mandibular incisors upright

How would you treat this malocclusion?

In view of the mild skeletal discrepancy, orthodontic camouflage is indicated. Treatment will therefore involve upper and lower pre-adjusted edgewise appliances. Extractions will be necessary to alleviate the crowding and to facilitate overjet reduction.

Discuss the relative merits of extraction of mandibular first or second premolars in this case

Extraction of first premolars would favour relief of anterior crowding as they are more mesially placed. It would generate sufficient space to relieve crowding without advancement of the mandibular incisors. However, the lingually-displaced second premolars would require alignment. The second premolars are also enlarged mesio-distally; consequently, by maintaining them, the final occlusion may be compromised by an inter-arch tooth-size discrepancy.

Extraction of second premolars involves a slightly greater challenge for the dentist. However, as these teeth are macrodont and lingually-displaced, second premolar extraction would be sensible. In addition, a differential extraction pattern of maxillary first premolars and mandibular second premolars would promote overjet reduction and correction of the class II canine relationships to class I.

What form of anchorage support could be considered to reduce the overjet and address the malocclusion fully?

Palatal arches or headgear could be considered to maintain the position of the maxillary first molars. Headgear is often poorly tolerated in adults. Palatal arches offer little benefit in terms of antero-posterior anchorage and Nance palatal arches should be discarded prior to space closure as they may become imbedded in the palatal vault. Class II elastics may be used to guide space closure; however, extrusion of both lower molars and upper anterior teeth would be unhelpful here in view of the reduced overbite, increased LAFH and increased maxillary incisor display at rest. Therefore, temporary anchorage devices in the form of micro-implants or screws could be considered during space closure. They could be positioned in a variety of areas, including distal to the maxillary first permanent molars to effect overjet reduction providing either direct or indirect anchorage.

Anchorage may also be preserved by using light forces, including maxillary second molars in the appliance during space closure, and by individual retraction of maxillary first molars prior to *en masse* space closure.

Would you suggest any local bracket variations in this case?

Local bracket variations are not essential to addressing this malocclusion. However, as the UR2 is palatally displaced, both the crown and root must be moved labially to achieve a stable and aesthetic result. Use of an inverted bracket on this tooth could therefore be considered to promote additional buccal root torque as the crown is moved buccally.

As there is a significant anchorage demand, use of maxillary canine brackets with little mesial crown tip (angulation) would be wise to reduce anchorage demands and allow the roots of the maxillary canines to move distally.

This case was treated with the removal of all four second premolars. The treated occlusal result is shown in Figure 4.46.

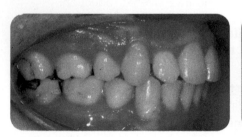 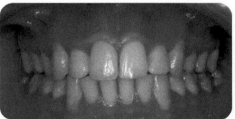 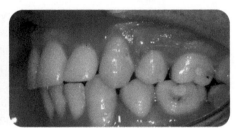

Figure 4.46

Case 4.17

A 13-year-old male was referred in relation to crowding and an unerupted UL3 (Figure 4.47). He was unhappy with the appearance of his teeth. Cephalometry indicated that the skeletal pattern was mild class II with average vertical skeletal proportions. The maxillary incisors were also slightly proclined (119 degrees) with the mandibular incisors of average inclination. The panoramic view confirmed the presence of all teeth, including the third molars. Root length and morphology were favourable with no evidence of pathology. The UL3 is impacted but situated buccally and in a favourable position for eruption following space creation.

Summarize the malocclusion

A 13-year-old male with a Class I malocclusion on a mild skeletal class II pattern complicated by:
- Impacted UL3 and LL5
- Crowding of both arches.

The centre lines are mutually coincident but both are not aligned with the facial midline. Which side do you think the centre lines have deviated to?

In view of the asymmetric crowding, the centre lines are likely to have deviated to the left side. In particular, the UL3 is impacted with associated space loss; there is also more crowding in the lower left quadrant than the lower right side, being concentrated in the LL2 and LL5 regions.

Describe the aetiology of this malocclusion

- Mild skeletal class II: contributing to the increased overjet on the UR1
- Dento-alveolar disproportion: tooth-arch size mismatch producing crowding of both arches. The maxillary arch is severely crowded (>8 mm) and the mandibular arch moderately crowded (4–8 mm)
- Premature loss of primary teeth: Early loss of the LLE has resulted in mesial movement of the LL6, leading to localized crowding and impeded eruption of the LL5

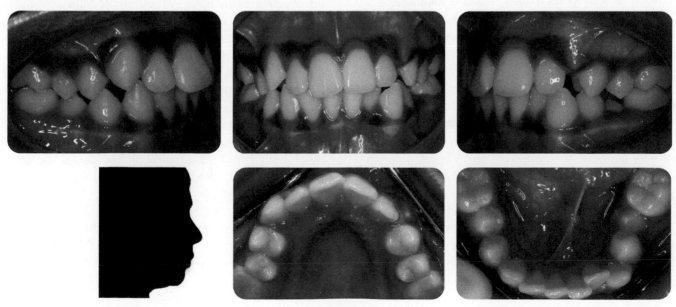

Figure 4.47

• Soft tissues: A lower lip trap on the UR1 may have resulted in excessive proclination of this tooth with a resultant increase in overjet

What extraction pattern would you consider in this case?

The lower arch is moderately crowded and the upper severely crowded; hence premolar extractions are warranted to alleviate the crowding and facilitate arch alignment and levelling. Maxillary first premolars could be extracted to facilitate eruption of the UL3. Alternatively, maxillary second premolars could be removed and space created using push mechanics between the UL2 and UL4 to encourage eruption of the UL3 and simultaneously promote centre line correction. If maxillary second premolars are extracted, removal of both mandibular premolars would also be sensible to avoid introducing an antero-posterior anchorage problem. If both maxillary first premolars were removed, either mandibular first or second premolars could be extracted to alleviate mandibular arch crowding. Loss of second premolars may be preferable as alignment of LL5 may be time-consuming. This extraction pattern would also facilitate overjet reduction and maintenance of class I buccal segment relationships.

Is centre line correction likely to be problematic in this case?

The centre line discrepancy is mild (2 mm). It also has an obvious cause: asymmetric crowding in both arches. The crowding will be corrected simply by arch alignment as part of treatment. There is also no skeletal component to the problem. Consequently, centre line correction will be relatively straightforward and would not necessitate an asymmetric extraction pattern.

Why did the impacted UL3 lie buccal to the arch and the impacted LL5 lingual?

The maxillary canine has a long and tortuous eruption path, moving over 20 mm from 5 to 15 years. Prior to eruption the canine becomes palpable buccally. If adequate space exists, the tooth will finally move palatally and inferiorly to assume a position in the dental arch. If inadequate space is present, the tooth is deflected from its normal course and remains buccally excluded from the dental arch. Similarly, the mandibular second premolar develops lingual to the arch. Premature loss of the second primary molar often results in mesial displacement of the first permanent molar. Consequently, there is insufficient space for the second premolar to erupt in its normal position. It therefore follows a path of least resistance and erupts lingual to its normal position.

If this patient declined treatment, what would the likely result be?

There is unlikely to be a significant change in the skeletal pattern. In relation to the occlusion, inter-arch relationships are also likely to be largely preserved. Sinclair and Little (1983) evaluated the dental casts of 65 untreated normal occlusions to determine the nature and extent of maturational changes on the normal dentition from 9 to 20 years. Decreases arose in arch length and inter-canine width with minimal overall changes in inter-molar width, overjet and overbite, and increases in lower incisor irregularity. More marked changes occurred in females, with the individual changes being variable and unpredictable.

In this case it is likely that both the UL3 and LL5 will erupt, in a buccal and lingual position, respectively. The imbrication in the lower anterior region will deteriorate. Oral hygiene may also become problematic locally.

What compromise approach might be considered? What are the likely results of this?

Interceptive extractions without immediate orthodontics could be considered. Depending on the patient's likely compliance, consideration may be given to extraction of four first premolars. In the medium-term this is likely to facilitate eruption of UL3 and LL5, eliminating plaque stagnation areas. The crowding in the LL2 region is likely to improve due to natural drift. In the longer-term, further space closure is likely to occur (Persson et al., 1989). Space closure is likely to result both from bodily migration and dental tipping, especially in the mandibular arch; nevertheless periodontal consequences are unlikely (Persson et al., 1989). Typically, natural space closure is more likely to result from movement of posterior teeth than distal tipping and migration of anterior teeth (Yoshihara et al., 2002).

Case 4.18

This patient presented unhappy with the appearance of his teeth (Figures 4.48 and 4.49).

What is the key problem list?

- Mild skeletal class II pattern
- Increased vertical proportions

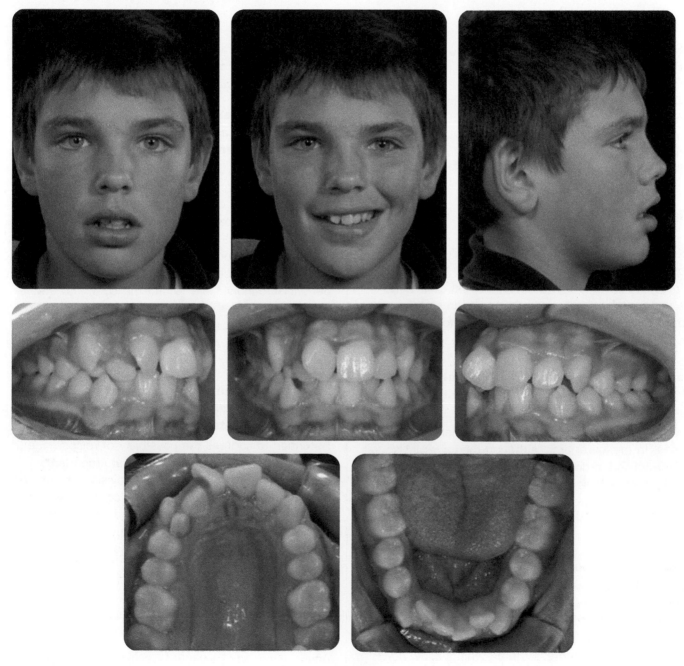

Figure 4.48

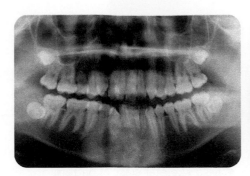 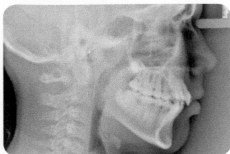

Figure 4.49

- Severe upper and lower arch crowding
- Rotated UR1
- Retained URC
- Centre line discrepancy (both centre lines off to the right)
- Increased overjet (to the UR1 – due to rotation of the tooth as a result of the crowding)
- Reduced overbite

What are the space requirements in this case?

Space is required in the lower arch to alleviate the crowding, maintain the inclination of the lower incisors to preserve the overbite, and correct the centreline. In the upper arch, space is required to address the crowding, in particular to provide space to de-rotate the UR1 and to correct the upper centre line.

Does this case require the removal of teeth to treat?

An extraction approach is appropriate in this case in view of the crowding present in the upper and lower arches. In the lower arch, although the lower incisors are retroclined, proclination of the lower incisors will not produce sufficient space to address the crowding or correct the centre line. In addition, a non-extraction approach by proclination of the lower incisors will reduce the already reduced overbite.

Which teeth would you extract in this case?

Extraction of the lower first premolars would address the crowding and would enable maintenance of lower incisor inclination. In the upper arch, extraction of the upper first premolars and the retained URC will provide sufficient space to address the crowding, allow de-rotation of the UR1 and correct the upper centre line.

Alternatively, extraction of first premolars on the right and second premolars on the left would help with centre line correction.

Discuss the treatment mechanics in the upper arch to allow alignment of the rotated upper central incisor

Alignment of the upper arch can be completed with a nickel–titanium archwire with partial ligation of the UR1. Full ligation of this tooth can only be carried out once sufficient space has been created for alignment. Space will be created following some initial alignment on a nickel–titanium archwire and then a round stainless steel archwire. In the first instance it will be beneficial to individually retract the UR3, into the space created by the removal of the UR4 and URC. Individual retraction of the UL3 will help provide additional space, whilst also enabling correction of the upper centre line.

What are the long-term considerations required for maintenance of the alignment of a severely rotated tooth?

Retention to address the possibility of relapse due to recoil of the supra-crestal fibres is an important consideration. In addition to the provision of removable retainers, it would be important to consider additional retention in the form of a bonded retainer to maintain the UR1 in its new position, or even a supra-gingival circumferential fibreotomy or pericision.

References

Allais D, Melsen B (2003) Does labial movement of lower incisors influence the level of the gingival margin? A case-control study of adult orthodontic patients. *Eur J Orthod* 25:343–352.

Artun J, Krogstad O, Little RM (1990) Stability of mandibular incisors following excessive proclination: a study in adults with surgically treated mandibular prognathism. *Angle Orthod* 60:99–106.

Bass NM, Bass A (2003) The Dynamax system: a new orthopedic appliance. *J Clin Orthod* 37:268–277.

Brandao M, Pinho HS, Urias D (2006) Clinical and quantitative assessment of headgear compliance: a pilot study. *Am J Orthod Dentofacial Orthop* 129:239–244.

Cureton SL, Regennitter FJ, Yancey JM (1993) The role of the headgear calendar in headgear compliance. *Am J Orthod Dentofacial Orthop* 104:387–394.

Fleming PS, Scott P, DiBiase AT (2007) Managing the transition from functional to fixed appliances. *J Orthod* 34:252–259.

Foster TD, Day AJW (1974) A survey of malocclusion and need for orthodontic treatment in a Shropshire school population. *Br J Orthod* 1:723–778.

Helm S (1968) Malocclusion in Danish children with adolescent dentition: an epidemiological study. *Am J Orthod* 54:352–368.

Johal A, Cheung MY, Marcene W (2007) The impact of two different malocclusion traits on quality of life. *Br Dent J* 202:E2.

Kesling PC (1989) Dynamics of the Tip-edge bracket. *Am J Orthod Dentofacial Orthop* 96:16–25.

Koroluk LD, Tulloch JF, Phillips C (2003) Incisor trauma and early treatment for Class II Division 1 malocclusion. *Am J Orthod Dentofacial Orthop* 123:117–125; discussion 125–126.

Luther F (2007a) TMD and occlusion part I. Damned if we do? Occlusion: the interface of dentistry and orthodontics. *Br Dent J* 202:E2; discussion 38–39.

Luther F (2007b) TMD and occlusion part II. Damned if we don't? Functional occlusal problems: TMD epidemiology in a wider context. *Br Dent J* 202:E3; discussion 38–39.

Marques LS, Filogonio CA, Filogonio CB, *et al.* (2009) Aesthetic impact of malocclusion in the daily living of Brazilian adolescents. *J Orthod* 36:152–159.

McNamara JA Jr (1981) Components of Class II malocclusion in children 8–10 years of age. *Angle Orthod* 51:177–202.

Melsen B, Allais D (2005) Factors of importance for the development of dehiscences during labial movement of mandibular incisors: a retrospective study of adult orthodontic patients. *Am J Orthod Dentofacial Orthop* 127:552–561; quiz 625.

Mills JR (1973) The problem of overbite in Class II, division 2 malocclusion. *Br J Orthod* 1:34–48.

Nguyen QV, Bezemer PD, Habets L, Prahl-Andersen B (1999) A systematic review of the relationship between overjet size and traumatic dental injuries. *Eur J Orthod* 21:503–515.

O'Brien K, Wright J, Conboy F, *et al.* (2003) Effectiveness of treatment for Class II malocclusion with the Herbst or twin-block appliances: a randomized, controlled trial. *Am J Orthod Dentofacial Orthop* 124:128–137.

O'Brien K, Wright J, Conboy F, *et al.* (2009) Early treatment for Class II Division 1 malocclusion with the Twin-block appliance: a multi-center, randomized, controlled trial. *Am J Orthod Dentofacial Orthop* 135:573–579.

Pancherz H (1991) The nature of Class II relapse after Herbst appliance treatment: a cephalometric long-term investigation. *Am J Orthod Dentofac Orthop* 100:220–233.

Persson M, Persson EC, Skagius S (1989) Long-term spontaneous changes following removal of all first premolars in Class I cases with crowding. *Eur J Orthod* 11:271–282.

Postlethwaite K (1989) The range and effectiveness of safety headgear products. *Eur J Orthod* 11:228–234.

Proffit WR, Fields Jr HW, Moray LJ (1998) Prevalence of malocclusion and orthodontic treatment need in the United States: estimates from the NHANES III survey. *Int J Adult Orthod Orthog Surg* 13:97–106.

Shaw WC, Meek SC, Jones DS (1980) Nicknames, teasing, harassment and the salience of dental features among school children. *Br J Orthod* 7:75–80.

Sinclair PM, Little RM (1983) Maturation of untreated normal occlusions. *Am J Orthod* 83:114–123.

Stivaros N, Lowe C, Dandy N, Doherty B, Mandall NA (2010) A randomized clinical trial to compare the Goshgarian and Nance palatal arch. *Eur J Orthod* 32:171–176.

Thiruvenkatachari B, Sandler J, Murray A, Walsh T, O'Brien K (2010) Comparison of Twin-block and Dynamax appliances for the treatment of Class II malocclusion in adolescents: a randomized controlled trial. *Am J Orthod Dentofacial Orthop* 138:144 e1–9; discussion 144–145.

Todd JE, Dodd T (1985) Children's dental health in the United Kingdom. *Her Majestey's Stationary Office*.

Yoshihara T, Matsumoto Y, Suzuki J, Ogura T (2002) Effect of serial extraction alone on crowding: relationship between closure of residual extraction space and changes in dentition. *J Clin Pediatr Dent* 26:147–153.

5

Class II Division 2 Malocclusion

Introduction

A class II division 2 malocclusion is a subdivision of the Angle class II classification and is defined by a class II division 2 incisor relationship, with the incisal edges of the mandibular incisors occluding posterior to the cingulum plateau of the maxillary central incisors, which are retroclined.

Typically, there is an increased and complete overbite stemming from both dento-alveolar and skeletal factors, namely the retroclined labial segments, and reduced Frankfort–mandibular planes angle and lower anterior face height. A traumatic overbite to the gingivae of the lower labial segment labially or the upper incisors palatally is occasionally seen, which in the presence of poor oral hygiene can result in stripping of the gingival attachment.

Skeletally the antero-posterior relationship can range from class I or even a mild class III to severe class II, although the latter is rare and usually associated with a class II division 1 malocclusion. Typically the skeletal pattern is mild class II with a reduced maxillary–mandibular planes angle and a hypo-divergent or brachy-facial form.

The dental arches tend to be short and broad with retroclination of the maxillary central incisors. The lateral incisors are often proclined and rotated mesio-buccally as they escape the control of the lower lip. The lower labial segment can also be retroclined, particularly if the skeletal base relationship is class I or mild skeletal class II, as the lower incisors become trapped behind a retroclined upper labial segment

(Mills, 1973). This can result in posterior positioning of B-point compared to pogonion (Fischer-Brandies, 1985). The buccal segment relationship can range from class I to a full unit II, again depending on the severity of the underlying skeletal relationship. Transversely, maxillary buccal crossbites or scissor bites affecting the premolars are common, particularly in more severe low angle skeletal class II cases.

The lips are typically competent, with a high lower lip line, which may rest on the cervical one-third of the maxillary central incisors. The lower lip also covers a greater surface of the upper central incisors as they erupt, leading to retroclination. If, however, the lower lip rests below the lateral incisors, these tend to be proclined. The position of the lower lip is believed to have a significant role in the development of a class II division 2 incisor relationship. If both labial segments are retroclined, there may be little support for the lips in relation to Rickett's E-line, resulting in a retrusive soft tissue profile. The position of the lower lip in combination with reduced lower face height can also result in a deep labio-mental fold and relative prominence of the chin button.

Class II division 2 malocclusions occur in approximately 10% of Caucasian populations. Classically, hyperactive or hypertonic lips have been implicated in the aetiology of the class II division 2 incisor relationship (Karlsen, 1994). In reality, however, a combination of a reduced lower face height, an increased overbite, a mild skeletal class II base and specific lip position and morphology are usually central to the class II division 2 incisor relationship (McIntyre and Millett, 2006). Indeed, in view of the recognized association of skeletal, dental and soft tissue features, the phrase 'class II division 2 syndrome' has been coined. This concept is borne out by the high heritability of class II division 2 malocclusion, complete penetrance being reported in familial studies of monozygotic twins (Markovic, 1992). A reduced crown–root angle has also been reported for the upper incisors in class II division 2 malocclusions, which can contribute to their characteristic inclination (McIntyre and Millett, 2003).

To correct a class II division 2 incisor relationship, overbite reduction is often critical. To promote stability, the inter-incisal angle requires correction by placing the incisal edge of the mandibular incisors anterior to the midpoint or centroid of the upper incisor roots (Houston, 1989). To achieve this, the use of fixed appliances is invariably required to apply torque to the upper labial segment. Space will be required in the upper arch if proclination of the upper incisors is to be prevented during torque delivery. This space can be created by mid-arch extractions or distal movement of the buccal segments.

In a growing patient, the overbite can be reduced effectively using removable appliances with a flat anterior bite plane. Alternatively, in the presence of a skeletal class II pattern, a functional appliance may also be helpful to reduce the overbite. Both of these treatment modalities can allow unimpeded eruption of the molars and premolars. Consequently, the lower face height increases and compensatory growth and adaptation at the condyles stabilizes overbite reduction.

In non-growing patients overbite reduction is more problematic, because without active growth, it is solely reliant on tooth movement. There is usually some scope for proclination of the mandibular incisors, particularly if they are retroclined, which aids overbite reduction and correction of the inter-incisor angle (Mills, 1973; Selwyn-Barnett, 1991). Otherwise, intrusion of the anterior dentition is required to reduce the overbite. True intrusion is mechanically difficult and in severe cases, typically with markedly reduced lower face height, overbite reduction may only be achievable with a combination of fixed appliances and orthognathic surgery.

Case 5.1

This 13-year-old female was referred by her general dental practitioner regarding impacted upper second premolars and buccally placed LR3. There was no relevant medical history.

Extra-oral

Skeletal relationship

Antero-posterior	Skeletal class II
Vertical	FMPA reduced, lower anterior face height reduced
Transverse	No facial asymmetry
Soft tissues	Retrusive profile
	Incompetent lips
	Nasio-labial angle: Average
	Labio-mental fold: Pronounced
Incisor show	At rest: 2mm
	Smiling: 5mm
Temporo-mandibular joint	Healthy with good range and co-ordination of movement

Intra-oral

Teeth present	76 4321/1234 67
	7654321/1234 67
Dental health (restorations/caries)	UL6 and LL6 heavily restored
	Occlusal caries LR7
Lower arch	Severe crowding with retroclined mandibular incisors
	Both mandibular canines are disto-angular
	LR4 is excluded buccally and the LL5 excluded lingually
Upper arch	Severe crowding with retroclined maxillary incisors
	Both canines are excluded buccally and distally angulated
Occlusion	Class II division 2 incisor relationship
	Overjet: 1mm
	Overbite: Increased and complete
	Molar relationship:
	½ unit class II on the right and class I on the left
	Unilateral posterior mandibular buccal crossbite on right side with displacement of the mandible to the right on closure from centric relation (CR) to centric occlusion (CO)
	Centre lines: Lower centre line is to the right

Summary

A 13-year-old female presented with a class II division 2 malocclusion on a mild skeletal class II base with reduced vertical dimensions (Figure 5.1). There is severe crowding in both arches, heavily restored first permanent molars on the left hand side and caries in the LR7.

Treatment Plan

- Extraction of the impacted UR5, the UL6, LR4 and LL6
- Upper and lower pre-adjusted edgewise fixed appliances with anchorage re-inforcement
- Retention

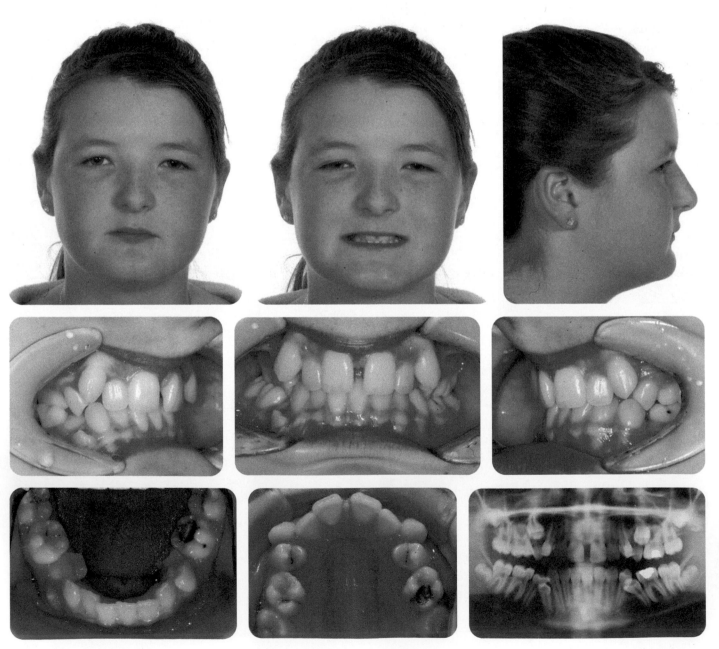

Figure 5.1

What should be done before commencing orthodontic treatment?

The LR7 should first be restored by the general dental practitioner.

This is a case with high anchorage demand. What factors contribute to this?

- **Severe crowding:**
  - There is severe crowding in the lower arch with impeded eruption of both the LL5 and LR4 due to space deficiency.
  - In the maxillary arch the upper buccal segments are severely crowded with both upper second premolars impacted palatally. The upper labial segment is moderately crowded with both canines buccally positioned.
- **Canine angulations:** All canines are distally angulated. This is especially marked in the upper arch, which will increase the anchorage demands during alignment of the upper labial segment.
- **Inclination of the upper labial segment:** The upper labial segment is retroclined; this will require torque application to improve the inclination of the teeth.
- Centre line correction is required in both arches.

What is the rationale for the extraction pattern in this case?

The LR4 was extracted due to severe crowding and an ectopic position.

The decision to extract the UL6 and the LL6 was based on dental health concerns as both teeth were restored. Removal of these teeth would provide sufficient space to relieve crowding in the buccal segments.

In the maxillary arch, the ectopic unerupted UR5 was extracted due to its unfavourable position.

How do you think anchorage might have been reinforced in this case?

In the upper arch, anchorage reinforcement was provided by use of a Nance palatal arch. This was placed to prevent mesial movement of the upper buccal segments. Alternatively, headgear could have been used; given the increased overbite and reduced vertical dimensions, cervical pull headgear would have been the best option.

In the lower arch, anchorage was reinforced by the use of a lingual arch. This facilitated correction of the lower centre line.

Discuss the mechanics for centre line correction in this case

Placement of the lingual arch facilitated lower centre line correction. At the time of appliance placement, a laceback was tied in the lower left quadrant to prevent tip from being expressed in the LL3 bracket. Once in a round 0.018-inch stainless steel archwire centre line, correction was continued by distalizing the LL5 initially, followed by individual retraction of teeth to the left side. The final result is shown in Figure 5.2.

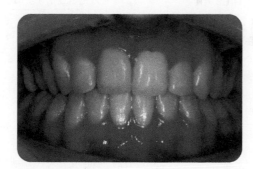

Figure 5.2

Case 5.2

This 14-year-old female was referred by her orthodontic specialist due to palatal displacement of the UR3. The patient did not like her crooked front teeth. There was no relevant medical history.

Extra-oral

Skeletal relationship

Antero-posterior	Mild skeletal class II
Vertical	FMPA: Reduced
	Lower face height: Reduced
Transverse	Facial symmetry: None
Soft tissues	Lip competence: Competent and retrusive to Rickett's E-line
	Naso-labial angle: Obtuse and open
Upper incisor show	At rest: 4 mm
	Smiling: 11 mm
Temporo-mandibular joint	Healthy with good range and co-ordination of movement

Intra-oral

Teeth present

7654C21/1234567

7654321/1234567

Dental health (restorations, caries)	Good
	No active caries and good oral hygiene
Lower arch	Mild crowding
	Incisor inclination: Retroclined
Upper arch	Mild crowding
	Incisor inclination: Retroclined
	Canine position: Left buccal
	Right unerupted and not palpable buccally
Occlusion	Incisor relationship: Class II division 2
	Overjet: 4 mm to UR2
	Overbite: Increased and complete
	Molar relationship: ½ unit II bilaterally
Radiographic examination	UR3 was unerupted and ectopic; this tooth was confirmed to be in a palatal position using vertical parallax
	All third molars present
Cephalometric examination	Confirms the clinical impression of a mild skeletal class II base relationship with reduced FMPA and retroclined upper labial segment (Figure 5.3)

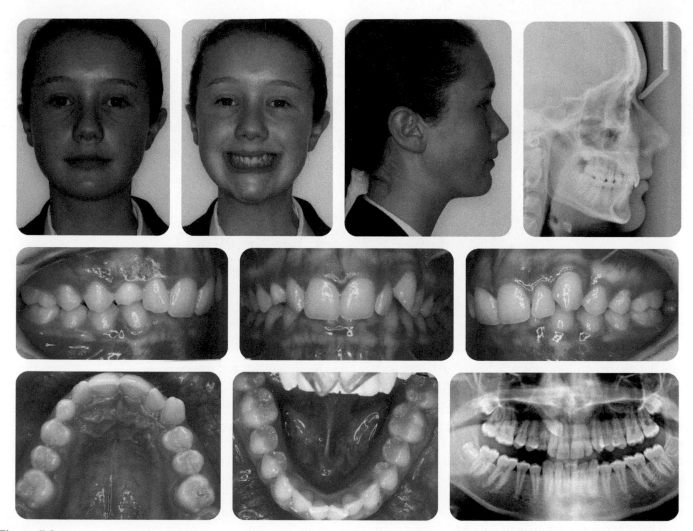

Figure 5.3

Summary

A 14-year-old Caucasian female presented with a class II division 2 incisor relationship on a mild skeletal class II base with reduced vertical proportions. The malocclusion was complicated by a palatally impacted UR3, mild crowding of the upper and lower arches, an increased overbite and decreased overjet, and ½ unit class II molar relationship bilaterally (Figure 5.3).

Treatment Plan

- Use of headgear and removable appliance to correct the buccal segment relationship to class I while commencing overbite reduction
- Upper and lower pre-adjusted edgewise fixed appliances to level and align arches and correct the incisor relationship
- Exposure and bonding of the UR3 to allow mechanical traction to align UR3
- Long-term retention

What treatment is being carried out in Figure 5.4?

To correct the incisor relationship, the overbite should first be reduced. An effective way of doing this in a growing patient is the use of an anterior bite plane. A removable appliance incorporating a flat anterior bite plane was therefore placed initially.

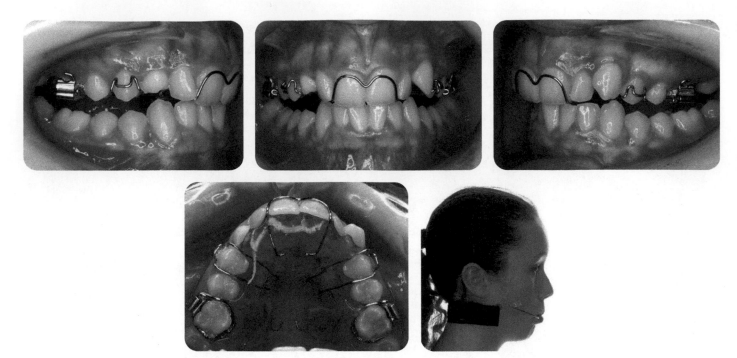

Figure 5.4

In addition, space is required in the maxillary arch to correct the buccal segment relationship, torque the upper labial segment and achieve a class I incisor relationship. The removable appliance was supplemented with cervical pull extra-oral traction, directly to bands on the maxillary first molars. The patient was instructed to wear this for 14 hours daily with a 400-g force applied bilaterally. The direction of pull of the headgear creates an extrusive force on the maxillary molars, which aids overbite reduction.

What are the principles of providing a patient with headgear?

As well as direction of pull, the other important principles when using headgear are duration of wear, level of force and safety.

For anchorage support when no movement of the molars is desirable, the patient should be instructed to wear the headgear for 10–12 hours a day with a force of between 250 and 350 g applied bilaterally.

To distalize upper molars, as in this case, or to restrict maxillary growth, the force should be increased above 400 g and the headgear worn for at least 14 hours a day. As such, the main limitation of headgear is compliance, as success is reliant on a highly co-operative patient.

There have been a few cases reported in the literature of headgear facebows becoming disengaged from the molar tubes and causing soft tissue injury. The most serious of these is ocular damage with the inner part of the bow penetrating the eye and resulting in infection and blindness. Fortunately, these types of injuries are extremely rare, but given the serious consequences, action should be taken to prevent them. Therefore, at least two safety features should be incorporated in headgear design:

- A locking facebow preventing detachment of the inner bow at night is advocated
- Use of snap-away headgear modules that disengage when excessive force is applied is sensible to prevent catapult injuries.

What other features are apparent in the design of the upper removable appliance in Figure 5.4?

The removable appliance also had palatal finger springs placed mesial to the maxillary first molars to aid in their distalization. A Southend clasp on the upper central incisors was also added for retention. The design is a modification of the Acrylic Cervical-Occipital (ACCO) appliance popularized by Cetlin and Ten Hoeve (1983).

What are the principles of overbite reduction in class II division 2 malocclusions?

Class II division 2 malocclusions require a reduction of the inter-incisal angle, to achieve a class I incisor relationship and stable overbite reduction. A key element in this is the relationship between the lower incisor tip and what is known as the centroid of the upper incisor root (a constructed point half-way along the root). If the lower incisor tip is placed anteriorly to the centroid of the upper incisor, it should lead to greater stability of overbite reduction (Houston, 1989). To achieve this, the maxillary incisor roots require palatal root torque, necessitating fixed appliances and space as retroclined teeth result in a shorter arch length than teeth with appropriate torque. In this case, space was created with headgear and distal movement of the maxillary buccal segments.

What mechanics are being used in Figure 5.4 to reduce the increased overbite?

There are essentially three ways in which an increased overbite can be reduced:
- Intrusion of the incisors
- Extrusion of the buccal segments
- Proclination of the labial segments.

In this case, the overbite is being reduced initially by extrusion of the buccal segments. This extrusion is achieved primarily using of an upper removable appliance with a flat anterior bite plane. By discluding the posterior teeth, they are free to erupt, giving the effect of extrusion. In a growing patient, this is

relatively stable as the resulting increase in lower face height is compensated by vertical growth at the condyle. In an adult, significant growth potential is lacking and these mechanics are more likely to result in a downward and backward rotation of the mandible, which is usually undesirable when there is an underlying skeletal class II relationship. In addition, without vertical condylar growth, significant increases in the vertical dimension are prone to relapse. The use of cervical pull headgear will also cause some extrusion of the maxillary molars and aid overbite reduction.

What is happening in Figure 5.5?

Considerable maxillary first molar distalization has been achieved. A pre-adjusted edgewise fixed appliance has been placed in the lower arch to commence arch levelling and aligning on a non-extraction basis.

What is the next stage of treatment?

Having corrected the buccal segment relationship, created space in the upper arch and begun aligning and levelling in the lower arch, an upper fixed appliance was placed and the UR3 exposed surgically. The maxillary arch was aligned and space consolidated to accommodate the UR3 using open nickel–titanium coil spring. Once space was available, mechanical

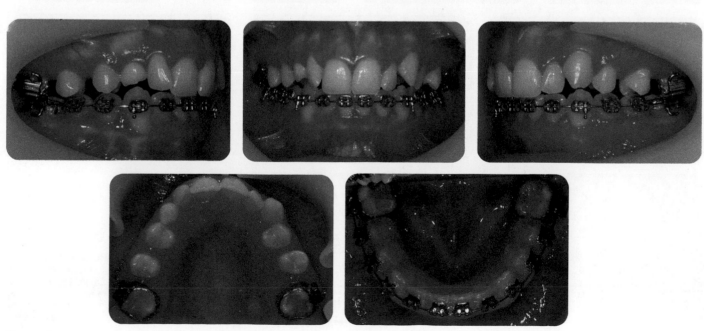

Figure 5.5

traction was applied to the tooth initially using elastomeric thread and followed by a nickel–titanium piggy-back archwire. Once the tooth had been erupted mechanically, it was fully aligned using rectangular nickel–titanium and then stainless steel archwires.

Why was this case treated on a non-extraction basis?

In the lower arch, extractions were avoided because there was minimal crowding. In addition, during space closure following extractions, invariably some retraction of the lower incisors will occur, which can complicate overbite reduction – another reason to avoid extractions in this case. This non-extraction approach has to be considered in the knowledge that some space will be required to align the mildly

crowded incisor teeth and reduce the increased curve of Spee in the lower arch.

Depending upon how much space is needed in the upper arch, this can either be created by mid-arch extractions or distalization of the buccal dentition. In this case, the ½ unit class II molar relationship and underlying growth potential favoured an attempt at distal movement using headgear. An additional anchorage burden was presented by the impacted UR3, but co-operation with headgear was good and a successful result obtained (Figure 5.6).

Following active treatment, a lower bonded retainer was placed as some proclination of the lower incisors took place during treatment. This was supplemented with night-time wear of removable retainers (Figure 5.6). The duration of active treatment was 26 months.

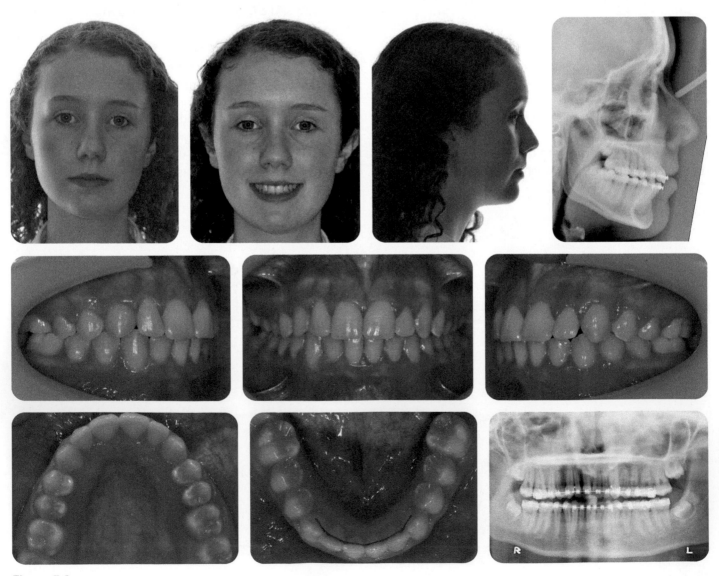

Figure 5.6

Case 5.3

This 13-year-old female was referred by her general dental practitioner because she did not like the position of her maxillary lateral incisors. There was no relevant medical history.

Extra-oral

Skeletal relationship	
Antero-posterior	Moderate skeletal class II
Vertical	FMPA: Increased
	Lower face height: Increased
Transverse	Facial symmetry: None
Soft tissues	Lip competence: Competent and retrusive to Rickett's E-line
	Naso-labial angle: Obtuse and open
Upper incisor show	At rest: 6 mm
	Smiling: 11 mm
Temporo-mandibular joint	Healthy with good range and co-ordination of movement

Intra-oral

Teeth present	7654C21/1234567
	654321/1234567
Dental health (restorations, caries)	Good
	No active caries and good oral hygiene
Lower arch	Mild crowding
	Incisor inclination: Upright
Upper arch	Mild crowding
	Incisor inclination: Retroclined
	Canine position: Left line of the arch
	Right unerupted and palpable buccally
Occlusion	Incisor relationship: Class II division 2
	Overjet: 7 mm to UR2
	Overbite: Increased and complete
	Molar relationship: Full unit class 2 bilaterally
Radiographic examination	All third molars and LR7 present
	UR3 also present and in line of the arch
Cephalometric examination	Moderate skeletal class II base relationship with increased MMPA and retroclined upper labial segment

Summary

A 13-year-old Caucasian female presented with a class II division 2 incisor relationship on a moderate skeletal class II base and slightly increased lower facial height. The malocclusion was complicated by mild crowding in the upper and lower arches, with an increased overbite, decreased overjet and bilateral full unit class II molar relationship (Figure 5.7).

Treatment Plan

- Sagittal correction with a functional appliance combined with a sectional fixed appliance to decompensate the upper labial segment
- Pre-adjusted edgewise fixed appliances to level and align the arches and detail the occlusion
- Long-term retention

What treatment has been carried out in Figure 5.8?

In growing individuals, class II division 2 malocclusions with mild-to-moderate skeletal class II base relationships and a class II buccal segment relationship can be successfully treated with a combination of functional and fixed appliances. The main problem with this approach in a class II division 2 incisor relationship is that the retroclined upper labial segment will not

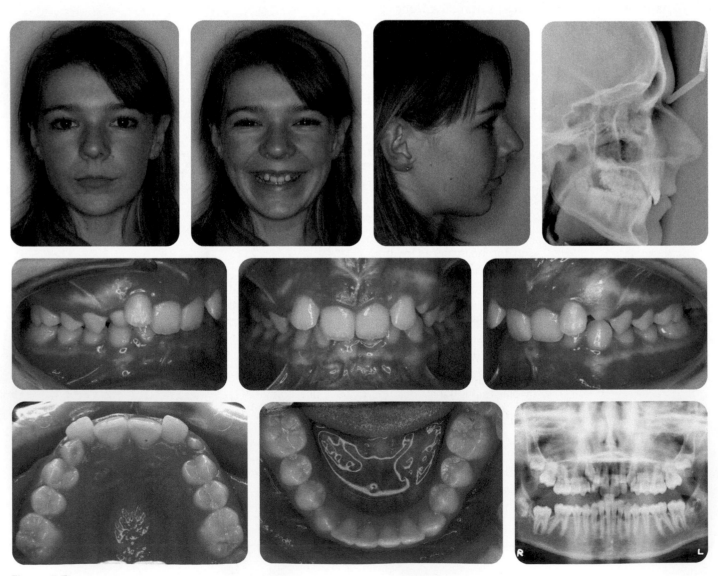

Figure 5.7

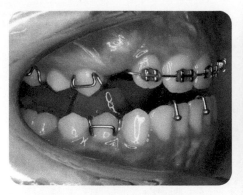
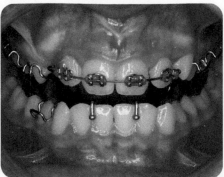
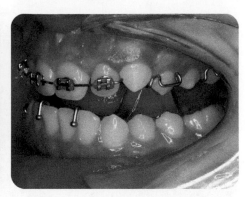

Figure 5.8

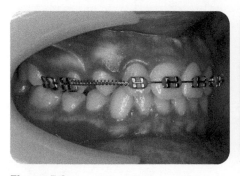
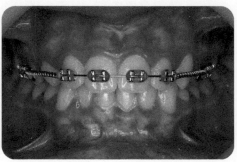
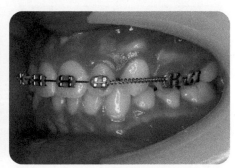

Figure 5.9

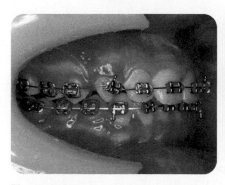
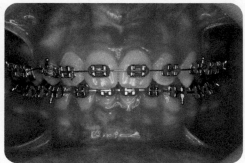
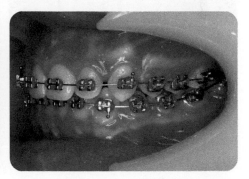

Figure 5.10

permit full antero-posterior posture with the functional appliance. In order to achieve this, proclination or decompensation of the maxillary incisors is required prior to or during the functional phase of treatment.

In this case, a sectional upper fixed appliance was initially placed on the upper incisors to procline the upper labial segment. To then reduce the resulting increased overjet, a modified Clark Twin Block appliance was fitted at the second visit. The patient was instructed to wear this on a near full-time basis.

Compliance was very good and the overjet was fully reduced in 9 months, at which point, the patient was instructed to wear the appliance for a further 3 months at night only to permit settling of the buccal occlusion (Figure 5.9).

Complete pre-adjusted edgewise appliances were subsequently placed in both arches, with initial nickel–titanium wires for alignment (Figure 5.10). Subsequent rectangular nickel–titanium wires were used for full alignment and then rectangular stainless steel

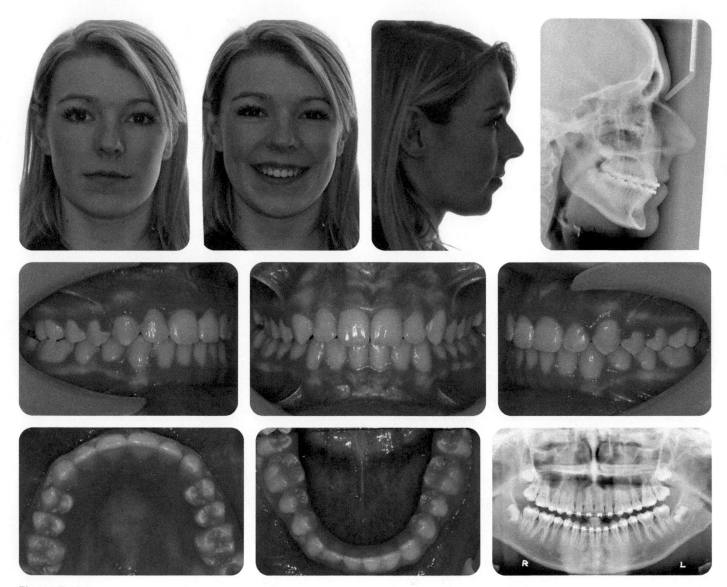

Figure 5.11

archwires for complete overbite and overjet control. Final occlusal settling was achieved using a braided stainless steel rectangular archwire in the mandibular arch. Following removal of the appliances, the patient was given upper and lower removable vacuum-type retainers to wear at night (Figure 5.11).

Are there any other ways of decompensating the upper labial segment prior to the use of a functional appliance?

Whilst the case described utilized a fixed appliance prior to use of a functional appliance, removable appliances can be used to the same effect. Expansion and Labial Segment Alignment Appliances (ELSAAs),

which incorporate springs to procline the maxillary incisors, are very useful for this (Figure 5.12). The appliances can also incorporate midline expansion screws to expand the maxillary arch, which is beneficial if using a monobloc-type functional appliance that does not incorporate a midline expansion screw. Further, the ELSAA appliance can also incorporate an anterior bite plane to start the process of overbite reduction.

Undertaking an initial course of treatment prior to the functional phase risks extending treatment time unnecessarily. Given that most of these cases will progress to a final phase of treatment with upper and lower fixed appliances, this can place an unacceptable strain on compliance. Therefore, attempts have been

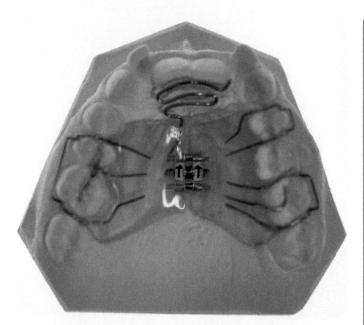

Figure 5.12

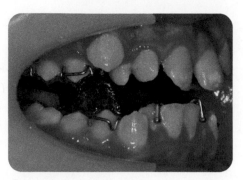

Figure 5.13

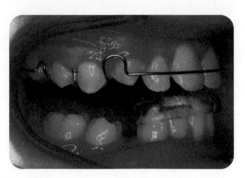

Figure 5.14

made to integrate an upper sectional appliance with the functional appliance itself to reduce the overall treatment time. In addition, modifications to the Twin Block appliance have been described, with springs or screws to procline the maxillary incisors while allowing simultaneous antero-posterior correction (Dyer *et al.*, 2001). A potential problem with these appliances is excessive bite opening, which can make them more difficult to tolerate (Clark, 2010).

Are there any disadvantages associated with the Twin Block appliance?

The Twin Block is just one of a plethora of functional appliances in common use. Whilst primarily designed to correct an antero-posterior discrepancy, functional appliances are also effective at reducing overbites, especially if they are designed to allow unimpeded eruption of the buccal segments. A disadvantage of Twin Block use in cases with an increased overbite and increased curve of Spee is that occlusal coverage in the buccal segments does not allow free eruption of the posterior teeth and hence levelling of the curve of Spee. This often results in lateral open bites as the overjet is reduced much more rapidly than the overbite. To address this, the appliance can either be worn on a part-time basis, the blocks selectively

trimmed or cribbing the lower first molars can be avoided to allow buccal segment eruption, whilst still maintaining a postural element (Figure 5.13). Alternative functional appliances allowing differential eruption of the posterior dentition, such as a Median Opening Activator (Figure 5.14), can be used.

Are there any alternative ways to treat this patient?

This patient presented with a moderate skeletal class II base relationship. This was complicated by a retrusive soft tissue pattern, the naso-labial angle being obtuse or open. Any treatment should avoid opening this further. Indeed, treatment should aim to enhance support for the upper lip. Therefore, orthodontic camouflage involving loss of upper premolars and retraction of the upper incisors would be inappropriate. An alternative approach would be to decompensate and co-ordinate the dental arches prior to mandibular advancement surgery to address the mandibular retrognathia.

Case 5.4

This 14-year-old female was referred by her general dental practitioner because she did not like her crooked front teeth. There was no relevant medical history.

Extra-oral

Skeletal relationship	
Antero-posterior	Severe skeletal class II
Vertical	FMPA: Reduced
	Lower face height: Reduced
Transverse	Facial symmetry: None
Soft tissues	Lip competence: Competent with normal protrusion relative to Rickett's E-line
	Naso-labial angle: Average
Upper incisor show	At rest: 4mm
	Smiling: 7mm
Temporo-mandibular joint	Healthy with good range and co-ordination of movement

Intra-oral

Teeth present	7654321/1234567
	7654321/1234567
Dental health (restorations, caries)	Heavily restored upper first molars
Lower arch	Mild crowding
	Incisor inclination: Upright
Upper arch	Mild crowding
	Incisor inclination: Retroclined
	Canine position: Both in the line of the arch
Occlusion	Incisor relationship: Class II division 2
	Overjet: 5mm to upper right lateral incisor
	Overbite: Increased and complete
	Molar relationship: ½ unit on the right; class I left
Radiographic examination	All third molars are present
	UR6 is heavily restored
Cephalometric examination	Severe skeletal class II base relationship with average MMPA and retroclined maxillary incisors

Summary

A 14-year-old Caucasian female presented with a class II division 2 incisor relationship on a severe skeletal class II base with reduced vertical proportions, mandibular retrognathia and mild crowding in both upper and lower labial segments complicated by heavily restored maxillary first molars (Figure 5.15).

Treatment Plan

- Extraction of upper first molars
- Tip Edge® fixed appliance to level and align the arches and correct the incisor and buccal segment relationship
- Long-term retention

How else could this patient have been treated?

Ideally, to achieve an optimum outcome from a facial perspective, the mandibular retrognathia would be addressed using a combination of fixed appliances to decompensate and co-ordinate the dental arches prior to a mandibular advancement osteotomy.

However, the patient declined the surgical option and therefore it was decided to treat her with orthodontics alone to achieve a class I occlusion and accept the skeletal base relationship. The rationale for this was that whilst there was significant mandibular retrognathia, the lip form and protrusion were acceptable and, if these were maintained during

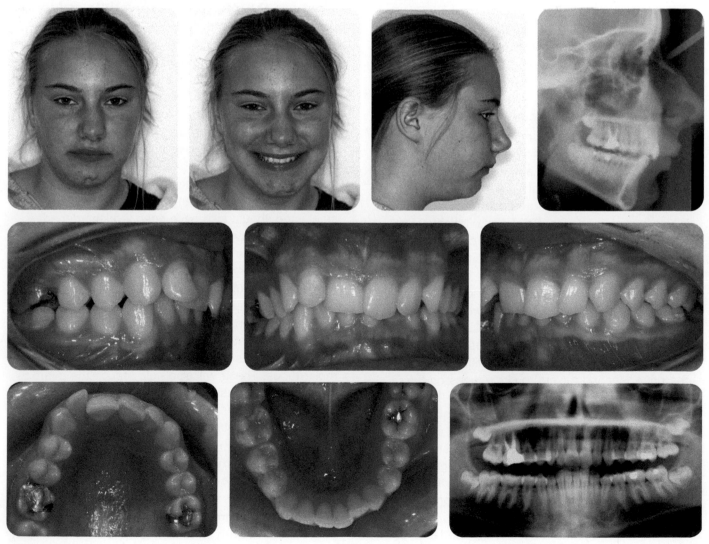

Figure 5.15

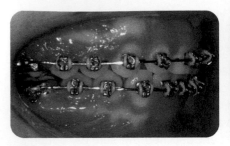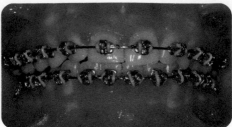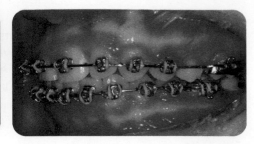

Figure 5.16

treatment, an acceptable compromise could be achieved. Treatment, therefore, involved the loss of upper first molars, which were heavily restored, and placement of upper and lower fixed appliances to level and align the arches and correct the incisor relationship. Due to a high anchorage demand in the maxillary arch, a Tip Edge® appliance was used.

What are the stages of treatment using the Tip Edge® appliance for this patient?

- **Stage 1** of treatment involves overbite and overjet correction and correction of the molar relationship. Initially, an appliance is placed on the upper labial segment only and a nickel–titanium archwire placed to align the teeth, increasing the overjet as a result. Following this, appliances are placed on the lower labial segment and upper and lower 016-inch stainless steel by-pass arches are placed with tip-back bends mesial to the upper second and lower first molar bands. Light class II elastics are worn on a full-time basis, which in combination with the tip-back bends, facilitates overbite and overjet reduction.
- **Stage 2** involves space closure. Once the overbite and overjet are fully reduced, the premolar attachments and upper and lower 020-inch stainless steel wires are placed. Space is closed in the maxillary arch using intra-arch elastics running from the upper second molars to circle loops on the archwire, again supported by light class II traction.
- **Stage 3** involves second- (angulation) and third- (torque) order correction. Once space is closed, upper and lower 21 × 25-inch stainless steel archwires are placed with auxiliary springs inserted into the vertical bracket slots to express the correct angulation and torque for each bracket prescription (Figure 5.16).

Finally the lower second molars were bonded and settling elastics were run to a lower braided rectangular steel archwire. Following removal of the appliances, a lower bonded retainer was placed and the patient was provided with removable vacuum-type retainers to wear at night.

In this case, active treatment time was 22 months (Figure 5.17).

What are the principles of overbite reduction with the Tip Edge® appliance?

In edgewise mechanics overbite reduction takes place following the initial alignment stage, generally using heavy rectangular stainless steel archwires. With the Tip Edge® appliance, the reduction of overbite and overjet is an aim of stage 1 of treatment. To achieve this, only the labial segments (including the canines and first molars) are initially included in the appliance. The first archwires in stage 1 are usually 016-inch stainless steel, which, because they bypass the premolars, have a long range action. The stainless steel used should also have been work-hardened, making it stiff and resilient. Light class II elastics are worn and, as the brackets permit free tipping of the teeth, this is very effective at reducing the overjet by retroclining the upper labial segment. The elastics also extrude the lower molars, helping to reduce the overbite. The tendency for the lower molars to roll forwards is resisted by the use of tip-back or anchorage bends placed just in front of the lower molar tubes. These will also help reduce the overbite by placing an intrusive force on the lower incisors. Similar tip-back bends are used in the upper arch, which also help maintain anchorage.

What types of bypass arches can be used with pre-adjusted edgewise appliances?

Bypass arches can be used with edgewise brackets, particularly if true intrusion of the labial segments is desired. The Rickett's intrusion arch is inserted directly into the incisor brackets (Ricketts, 1976) (Figure 5.18),

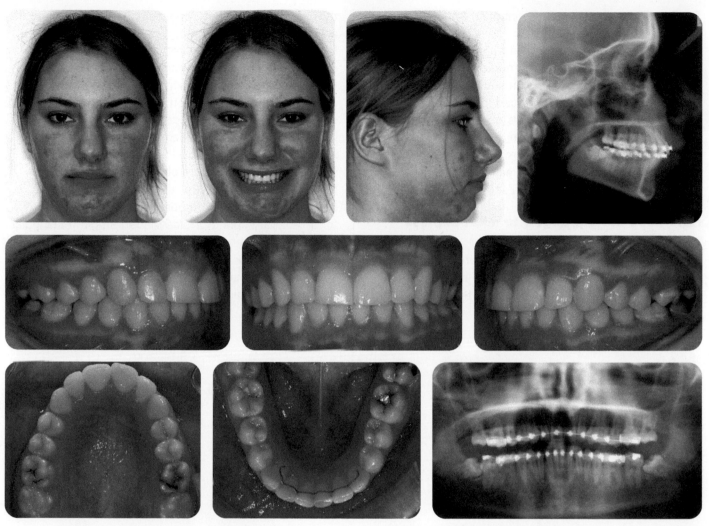

Figure 5.17

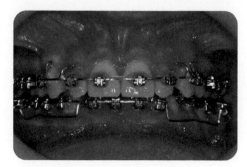

Figure 5.18

whilst the Burstone-type arch is tied above a sectional archwire (Burstone, 1977). The principle behind this is to control the rotational effects of the intrusion arch in relation to the centre of resistance of the teeth by varying the point at which the intrusion arch is ligated to the archwire.

Why is the Tip Edge® appliance theoretically less demanding on anchorage than an edgewise fixed appliance?

With the edgewise slot, the angulation or second-order movement in the bracket is expressed as the teeth are initially aligned and therefore any antero-posterior movement of the teeth will occur in a bodily fashion. This means that with edgewise mechanics, a premium is placed on anchorage for antero-posterior correction. The design of the Tip Edge® bracket allows initial tipping of the teeth in the direction of the desired tooth movement, which requires less initial force and hence less anchorage (Lotzof *et al.*, 1996). This is the concept of differential tooth movement, whereby the tipping of the active unit is pitted against the bodily movement of the reactive or anchorage unit (Kesling, 1989). The roots of the teeth are then uprighted during the final stage of

Tip Edge® treatment, using uprighting springs known as sidewinders.

The Tip Edge® appliance can be particularly efficient in terms of antero-posterior correction. It was chosen in this case because of the high anchorage demand in the maxillary arch due to enforced loss of the first molars. Second maxillary molars offer little anchorage value due to the size and shape of their roots and the use of headgear directly to them is not recommended for similar reasons; in addition, palatal arches are of questionable anchorage value (Zablocki et al., 2008).

How does the Tip Edge® bracket express torque?

The Tip Edge® appliance expresses torque using full dimension stainless steel archwires in stage 3 of treatment. The principle underscoring this is that as the Tip Edge® bracket uprights under the influence of an auxiliary uprighting spring (or sidewinder) (Figure 5.16), the slot of the bracket closes down and fully engages the rectangular archwire (Parkhouse, 1998). Therefore, the torque prescription of the bracket slot becomes expressed, as is the case with a pre-adjusted edgewise bracket on engagement of a rectangular wire. More recently, a horizontal slot has been introduced in the Tip Edge-PLUS® bracket, which is situated deep to the main bracket slot. By placing a flexible superelastic nickel–titanium archwire in this slot, the brackets can be uprighted without the need for an auxiliary spring or sidewinder; a rigid rectangular archwire is present in the main bracket slot, permitting torque expression (Parkhouse, 2007). Overall, this innovation has made stage 3 a little less complicated for the orthodontist.

Case 5.5

This 21-year-old female was referred by her general dental practitioner concerned with the appearance of her upper front teeth. There was no relevant medical history.

Extra-oral

Skeletal relationship

Antero-posterior	Skeletal class II
Vertical	FMPA: Reduced
	Lower face height: Reduced
Transverse	Facial symmetry: None
Soft tissues	Lip competence: Competent with high lower lip retroclining the maxillary central incisors
	Naso-labial angle: Normal
Upper incisor show	At rest: 4 mm
	Smiling: 8 mm
Temporo-mandibular joint	Healthy with good range and co-ordination of movement

Intra-oral (initial consultation is represented by the panoramic radiograph in Figure 5.19)

Teeth present	7654321/1234567
	7654321/1234567
Dental health (restorations, caries)	Large restoration UR6
Oral hygiene	Good
Occlusion	Incisor relationship: Class II division 2
	Overjet: 1 mm
	Overbite: Increased and complete
	Molar relationship: ½ unit class II on right; essentially class I on left
	Canine relationship: Class I on left; ½ unit class II on right
	Centre lines: Upper slightly to the left
	Functional occlusion: Canine guidance
Lower arch	Crowding: Mild
	Incisor inclination: Average
Upper arch	Crowding: Moderate
	Incisor inclination: Retroclined
	Canine position: Line of arch (UL3 upright)

Summary

A 21-year-old female presented with a class II division 2 malocclusion on a skeletal class II base with reduced vertical dimensions complicated by an increased overbite, crowding of both dental arches and a heavily restored UR6 (Figure 5.19).

Describe the main features of the panoramic radiograph in Figure 5.19

- All teeth are present, including the third molars, which are all unerupted
- No caries (although clinically there is occlusal staining on the LL6)
- UR6 has a large coronal restoration and is root canal treated

- Abnormal calcified structure in the region of the UR6 and UR7; either an unusual root form associated with the UR7 or possibly a supernumerary tooth

Further investigation of the UR6–UR7 region was required and a cone beam computed tomographic scan (CBCT) of this region was ordered (Figure 5.19) What is the likely diagnosis based upon this scan?

The UR7 has an unusual enamel-covered odontome-like structure that extends between the roots of the UR6.

Although there was a skeletal class II pattern and a retrusive facial profile, the facial appearance was not

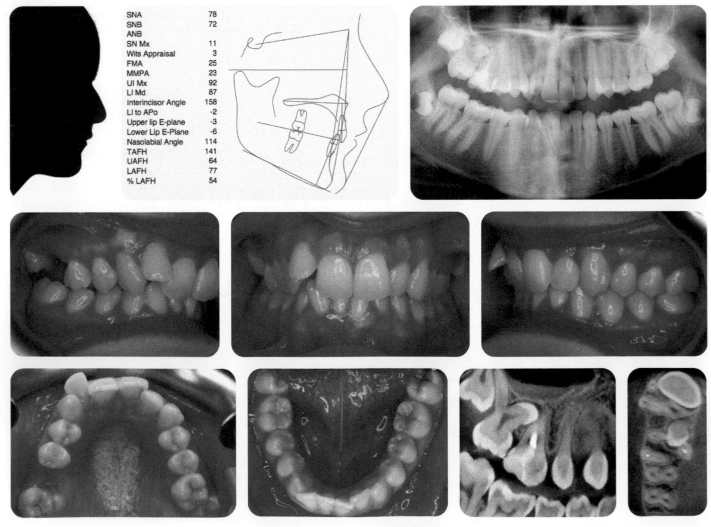

SNA	78
SNB	72
ANB	
SN Mx	11
Wits Appraisal	3
FMA	25
MMPA	23
UI Mx	92
LI Md	87
Interincisor Angle	158
LI to APo	-2
Upper lip E-plane	-3
Lower Lip E-Plane	-6
Nasolabial Angle	114
TAFH	141
UAFH	64
LAFH	77
% LAFH	54

Figure 5.19

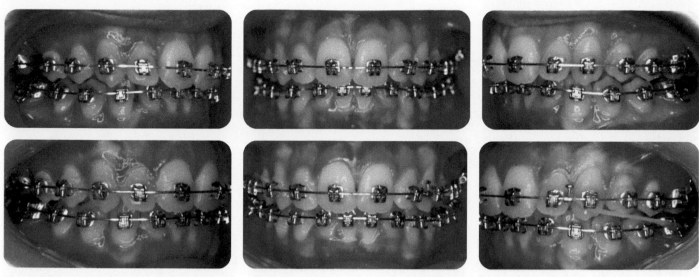

Figure 5.20

felt to be unattractive and the patient was anxious to avoid extractions or surgery. A decision was made to treat this patient with pre-adjusted edgewise self-ligated appliances on a non-extraction basis. However, prior to starting treatment the patient began experiencing pain in the UR6, and after consultation with the general dental practitioner this tooth was extracted (Figure 5.19).

Why were class II elastics required on the left side at the end of treatment (Figure 5.20)?

The maxillary centre line was displaced to the left at the start of treatment, reflected in a canine relationship that was ½ class II on the right and essentially class I on the left. However, during treatment, significant intra-arch traction was required in the upper right quadrant to close space following extraction of the UR6. This led to the maxillary centre line becoming displaced to the right. This was corrected at the end of treatment with unilateral class II inter-arch traction on the left side.

How has this malocclusion been corrected (Figure 5.21)?

The incisor relationship, overbite and buccal segment relationships have been corrected using arch expansion and class II elastic traction. Space closure in the upper right quadrant was achieved with intra-arch traction. A major contributor to overbite reduction and

sagittal correction has been proclination of the lower incisors.

Comment on the lower incisor proclination that has taken place during treatment

Orthodontic teaching in the UK has historically discouraged anterior movement of the lower incisors during treatment because of evidence that this is likely to relapse (Mills, 1966; 1968). However, in many class II division 2 malocclusions the lower incisors are retroclined and essentially trapped behind the upper incisors. For this reason, it has been suggested that in some cases space can be created to relieve lower arch crowding and reduce the overbite by allowing proclination of the lower incisor teeth. Indeed, where the lower incisors are retroclined and behind the uppers in a class II division 2 malocclusion, proclination may be justified if the lower incisors are not moved beyond the original sagittal position of the upper incisors. In this case, the relative position of the anterior dentition will not change in relation to the lips (Selwyn-Barnett, 1991).

There is little evidence that lower incisor proclination is any more stable when carried out during the treatment of a class II division 2 malocclusion compared to any other. In this case, the post-treatment lower incisor position should be regarded as unstable and the patient should be informed of this. Long-term retention is recommended.

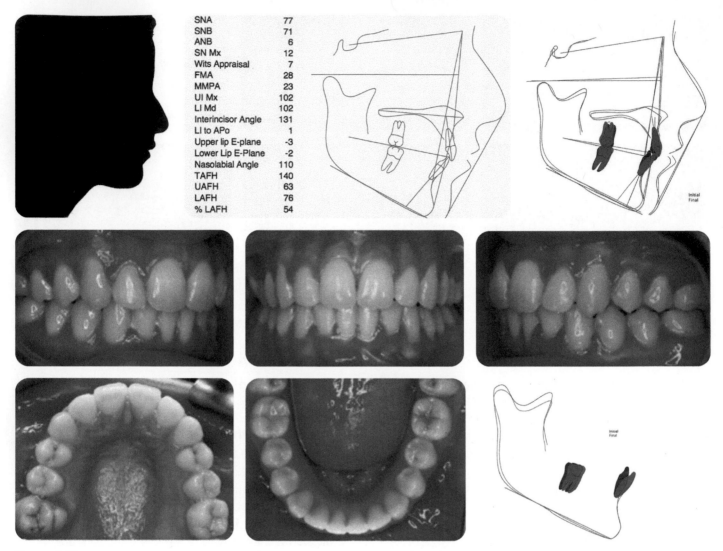

SNA	77
SNB	71
ANB	6
SN Mx	12
Wits Appraisal	7
FMA	28
MMPA	23
UI Mx	102
LI Md	102
Interincisor Angle	131
LI to APo	1
Upper lip E-plane	-3
Lower Lip E-Plane	-2
Nasolabial Angle	110
TAFH	140
UAFH	63
LAFH	76
% LAFH	54

Figure 5.21

Case 5.6

This 13-year-old female was referred by her paediatric dentist following the extraction of all four hypoplastic first permanent molars.

Summarize the clinical examination (Figure 5.22)

- A 13-year-old class II division 2 case on a skeletal class II base with average vertical proportions Lips are competent and there is good soft tissue morphology
- Late mixed dentition with the following teeth present:

  7 E4C21/1234E 7
  7   4321/1234 7

- Some alteration in the enamel of the UL1, possibly due to previous trauma or infection associated with the ULA. Alternatively, this may be a manifestation of molar–incisor hypomineralization (MIH)
- Upper Es have overerupted
- Retained URC
- A class II division 2 incisor relationship with an increased and incomplete overbite
- Upper centre line is displaced to the right, with the left canine relationship ½ class II and the right class I (to the URC)
- Both labial segments are well aligned but there is spacing in the buccal segments, particularly the lower

What information does the radiographic examination provide (Figure 5.23)?

The cephalometric radiograph confirms the clinical findings. It demonstrates that the mandibular incisors are at a normal inclination and the maxillary incisors are retroclined.

The panoramic radiograph shows that all four third molars, all four second premolars and the UR3 are present. The lower second premolars are unerupted and distally angulated. The UR3 is ectopic, high and horizontal in orientation.

Vertical parallax with the panoramic and anterior occlusal radiographs demonstrates that the UR3 is palatal. It also has an enlarged follicle and is closely associated with the apex of the UR1; however, the outline of this apex is identifiable and intact.

What is the problem list associated with this case?

- Class II division 2 incisor relationship
- Palatal impacted and horizontal UR3
- Centre line discrepancy
- Asymmetric buccal segment relationship
- Retained URC, upper Es
- Unerupted distally angulated LL5 and LR5
- Previous loss all first molars with excess space in the lower arch

Why are the LL5 and LR5 distally angulated?

The lower first molars were almost certainly lost early, which has resulted in distal movement of the second premolar crowns and an ectopic position of these teeth. However, the position of the erupted second molars at some distance from the first premolars does suggest that the first molars were extracted late!

What treatment options should be considered?

Assuming the patient is prepared to undergo fixed appliance treatment, accommodating the UR3 in the maxillary arch following surgical exposure of this tooth and extraction of the URC is the best option.

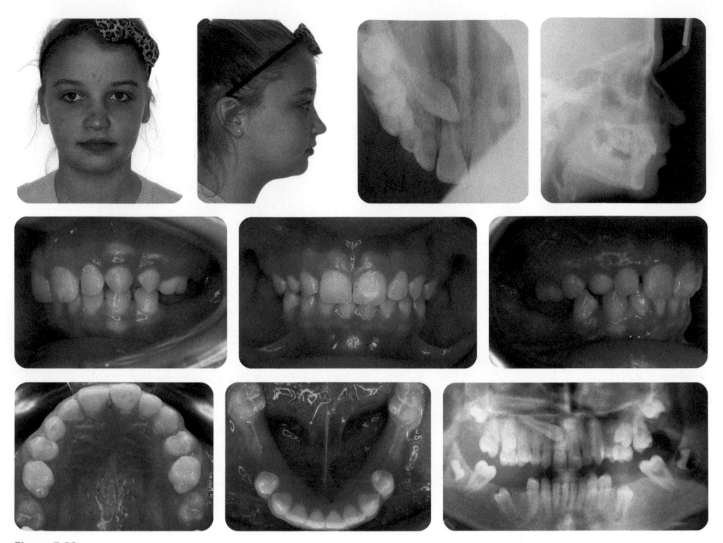

Figure 5.22

Anchorage requirements are quite high in the maxillary arch given the position of the UR3 and the mesial eruption of the second molars. In the lower arch, consideration could be given to exposure of the second premolars at the same time as the UR3 to allow traction to be placed early in treatment, although these teeth will probably erupt independently eventually. There is significant lower arch spacing, which will allow for unilateral (left-sided) class II traction to be used during centre line and buccal segment correction. However, complete space closure will be difficult in the lower arch, particularly as there

is necking of the alveolar ridge and a significant amount of space to be closed. Prolonged space closure will also complicate correction of the incisor relationship.

If the patient declines orthodontic treatment, consideration should be given to extraction of the UR3; the URC has a good root and has a good medium-term prognosis. The lower second premolars would be expected to erupt eventually. However, this would result in a compromised occlusion and residual space in the lower buccal segments.

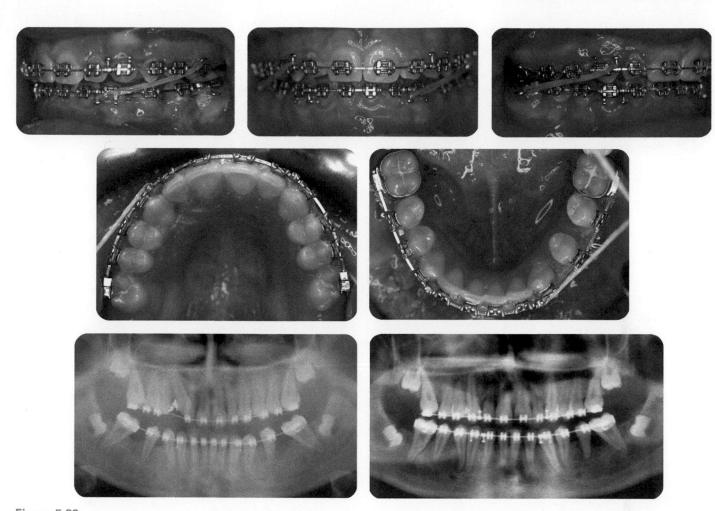

Figure 5.23

References

Burstone CR (1977) Deep overbite correction by intrusion. *Am J Orthod* 72:1–22.

Cetlin NM, Ten Hoeve A (1983) Nonextraction treatment. *J Clin Orthod* 17:396–413.

Clark W (2010) Design and management of Twin Blocks: reflections after 30 years of clinical use. *J Orthod* 37:209–216.

Dyer FM, McKeown HF, Sandler PJ (2001) The modified twin block appliance in the treatment of Class II division 2 malocclusions. *J Orthod* 28:271–280.

Fischer-Brandies H, Fischer-Brandies E, König A (1985) A cephalometric comparison between Angle Class II, division 2 malocclusion and normal occlusion in adults. *Br J Orthod* 12:158–162.

Houston WJ (1989) Incisor edge-centroid relationships and overbite depth. *Eur J Orthod* 11:139–143.

Karlsen AT (1994) Craniofacial morphology in children with Angle Class II div. 2 malocclusion combined with extreme deep bite. *Angle Orthod* 64:123–130.

Kesling PC (1989) Dynamics of the Tip-edge bracket. *Am J Orthod Dentofacial Orthop* 96:16–25.

Lotzof LP, Fine HA, Cisneros GJ (1996) Canine retraction: a comparison of two preadjusted bracket systems. *Am J Orthod Dentofacial Orthop* 110:191–196.

Markovic MD (1992) At the cross-roads of orofacial genetics. *Eur J Orthod* 14:469–481.

McIntyre GT, Millett DT (2003) Crown-root shape of permanent maxillary incisors. *Angle Orthod* 73:710–715.

McIntyre GT, Millett DT (2006) Lip shape and position in Class II division 2 malocclusion. *Angle Orthod* 76:739–744.

Mills JR (1966) The long-term results of the proclination of lower incisors. *Br Dent J* 120:355–363.

Mills JR (1968) The stability of the lower labial segment. A cephalometric survey. *Dent Pract Dent Rec* 18:293–306.

Mills JR (1973) The problem of overbite in Class II, division 2 malocclusion. *Br J Orthod* 1:34–48.

Parkhouse RC (1998) Rectangular wire and third-order torque: a new perspective. *Am J Orthod Dentofacial Orthop* 113:421–430.

Parkhouse RC (2007) Current products and practice: Tip-Edge Plus. *J Orthod* 34:59–68.

Ricketts RM (1976) Bioprogressive therapy as an answer to orthodontic needs. Part II. *Am J Orthod* 70:359–397.

Selwyn-Barnett BJ (1991) Rationale of treatment for Class II division 2 malocclusion. *Br J Orthod* 18:173–181.

Zablocki HL, McNamara JA Jr, Franchi L, Baccetti T (2008) Effect of the transpalatal arch during extraction treatment. *Am J Orthod Dentofacial Orthop* 133:852–860.

6

Class III Malocclusion

Introduction

A class III malocclusion is defined by the presence of a class III incisor relationship, which may range from a reduced overjet or edge-to-edge incisor relationship to a frank reversed overjet, the severity typically reflecting the underlying skeletal pattern. However, in some cases, considerable dento-alveolar compensation can be seen masking the skeletal discrepancy. The maxilla is often deficient in all three spatial planes, which may lead to significant crowding and the presence of posterior crossbites, which are often bilateral and exacerbated by an antero-posterior skeletal discrepancy. A full range of overbite depth may also occur and can be associated with an anterior displacement on closure from the retruded contact position (RCP) to inter-cuspal position (ICP), making the skeletal class III pattern appear more severe than it actually is. The term 'pseudo-class III' has been coined for this situation where an anterior displacement disguises what is in fact an underlying skeletal class I base relationship.

However, the skeletal pattern is usually class III, and unlike most skeletal class II patterns, which are primarily due to mandibular deficiency, skeletal class III discrepancies can be related to maxillary retrusion, mandibular prognathism or a combination of these two features with a large range of individual variation (Guyer et al., 1986; Battagel, 1993). The extent of the antero-posterior skeletal discrepancy is usually the defining feature of the malocclusion. In the vertical dimension, variation is common, with patients presenting with a full range of vertical growth patterns from hypo- to hyper-divergent facial types. Skeletal asymmetries, particularly in conjunction with mandibular prognathism, are also relatively common in class III malocclusions (Severt and Proffit, 1997).

The prevalence of class III malocclusion is generally low in Western societies, being reported at 3–5%. There is a higher prevalence in Oriental populations. The aetiology is multifactorial, although there certainly appears to be a familial tendency, particularly in relation to mandibular prognathism (Xue et al., 2010). Patients with a history of a repaired cleft lip and palate exhibit a higher incidence of class III malocclusion, which is thought often to be iatrogenic in nature and related to scarring from the primary surgical repair in infancy.

Treatment planning in class III cases is notoriously difficult and influenced primarily by the skeletal discrepancy, size of the reverse overjet, extent of crowding, degree of existing dento-alveolar compensation and the likelihood of future growth. However, as with other types of malocclusion, there are really three main approaches to the correction of a class III malocclusion:

- **Growth modification:** Class III malocclusions usually present in the early mixed dentition following eruption of the permanent incisors. A decision is required at this stage as to whether correction of the incisor relationship and the underlying skeletal discrepancy should be attempted with interceptive treatment. This treatment can be aimed at modifying growth, either with reverse-pull headgear (with or without maxillary expansion) or a functional appliance. Success of this treatment will depend on establishing a positive overjet and overbite, and the

Clinical Cases in Orthodontics, First Edition. Martyn T. Cobourne, Padhraig S. Fleming, Andrew T. DiBiase, and Sofia Ahmad.
© 2012 Martyn T. Cobourne, Padhraig S. Fleming, Andrew T. DiBiase, and Sofia Ahmad. Published 2012 by Blackwell Publishing Ltd.

nature and direction of future growth. An alternative strategy is to attempt mandibular growth suppression; however, long-term mandibular growth restraint using chin caps has met with little success (Sugawara *et al.*, 1990).

- **Orthodontic camouflage:** Definitive treatment can be carried out in the permanent dentition if the skeletal discrepancy is mild and facility for dento-alveolar compensation still exists. While removable appliances and sectional fixed appliances are useful to camouflage the incisor relationship as an interceptive measure in the mixed dentition, comprehensive correction in the permanent dentition typically involves the use of fixed appliances with class III inter-arch elastic traction. Extractions are often required in the upper arch of class III cases because of crowding; however, when attempting camouflage, lower arch extractions are also commonly required to create space for retraction of the lower labial segment. Mid-arch extractions are usually undertaken in both arches, although in adult patients a single lower incisor extraction can be considered. The prolonged success of treatment depends on establishing a positive overjet and overbite, and the pattern and magnitude of further growth.

  Orthodontic camouflage is not appropriate in the presence of a severe skeletal class III relationship with compensated incisors (i.e. proclined maxillary incisors and retroclined mandibular incisors). Further growth is also an important consideration as mandibular prognathism tends to deteriorate during the adolescent growth period and beyond (Battagel, 1993). If orthodontic camouflage is attempted in a case who subsequently grows unfavourably and requires surgery to definitively correct the class III relationship, lower incisor decompensation will subsequently be required as part of the pre-surgical set-up. This is difficult to achieve if teeth have been previously extracted in the lower arch without re-opening space. Several studies have attempted to provide cephalometric guidelines to distinguish cases who will be suitable for camouflage, but it is sensible in significant class III cases to delay final treatment planning until near the end of adolescent growth (Kerr *et al.*, 1992; Burns *et al.*, 2010).

- **Surgery:** For those cases with a significant antero-posterior or vertical skeletal component to their malocclusion, combined orthodontic–surgical treatment is required for definitive correction. Surgery should ideally be deferred until growth is complete; otherwise continued mandibular growth will result in skeletal relapse. Therefore, monitoring mandibular growth during adolescence prior to committing to a surgical plan is considered best practice. Superimposition of serial cephalograms to confirm that active growth has reduced to acceptable levels has been advocated prior to instituting treatment (Fudalej *et al.*, 2007).

Case 6.1

This 9-year-old female was referred by her orthodontic specialist concerned about a "back to front" bite.

Extra-oral

Skeletal relationship

Antero-posterior — Skeletal class I

Vertical — FMPA: Average

Lower face height: Average

Transverse — Facial symmetry: None

Soft tissues — Lip competence: Competent with protrusive lower lip

Naso-labial angle: Normal

Upper incisor show — At rest: 2 mm

Smiling: 5 mm

Temporo-mandibular joint — Healthy, with good range and co-ordination of movement

Intra-oral

Teeth present

6E4C21/123456
6EDC21/123DE6

Dental health — Good

(restorations, caries) — No active caries and good oral hygiene

Occlusion — Incisor relationship: Class III

Overjet: −2 mm

Overbite: Average and incomplete

Molar relationship: Class I bilaterally

Anterior displacement on closure from RCP to ICP

Centre line: Mandibular to the right by 2 mm

Lower arch — Crowding: Aligned

Incisor inclination: Proclined

Upper arch — Crowding: Mild crowding

Incisor inclination: Upright

Canine position: Palpable buccally

Summary

A 9-year-old female presented in the mixed dentition with a class III malocclusion on a skeletal class I base with an average lower face height, mild crowding and an anterior crossbite (Figure 6.1).

Treatment Plan (Figure 6.2)

The aims of treatment were to correct the anterior crossbite and eliminate the displacement.

A pre-adjusted edgewise appliance was placed on the upper incisors, primary canines and first permanent molars. The initial aligning archwire was a 014-inch heat-activated nickel–titanium fully engaged into the brackets on the maxillary incisors. The wire was supported in the buccal segments with 0.8 mm steel tubing to prevent distortion.

At the second visit, the initial archwire was re-activated. At the third visit a 0.020 × 0.020-inch heat-activated nickel–titanium archwire was placed and the glass ionomer bite plane removed. Thereafter, a 019 × 025-inch beta titanium archwire was placed with a vertical offset to extrude the upper central incisors and establish a positive overbite. The appliance was then removed (Figure 6.3).

Why was treatment carried out in the mixed dentition?

An anterior crossbite with an associated displacement is an indication for early orthodontic interception, particularly if the displacement is greater than 2 mm. An anterior crossbite can result in occlusal wear and gingival recession in the presence of an associated displacement.

Why was glass ionomer cement placed on the occlusal surface of the posterior dentition?

This was placed to eliminate potential occlusal interferences to tooth movement.

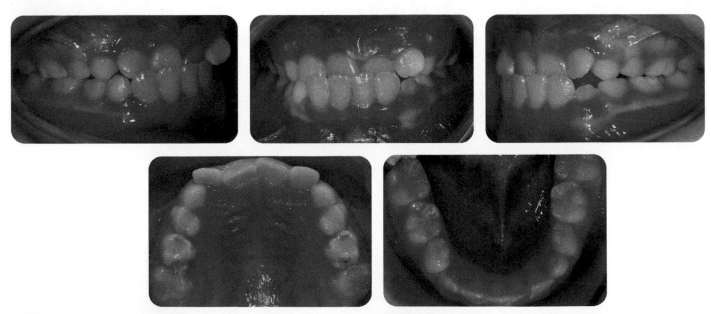

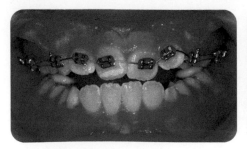

Figure 6.1

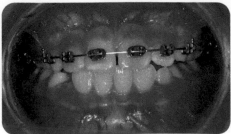

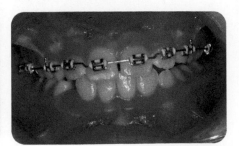

Figure 6.2

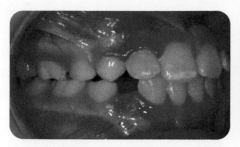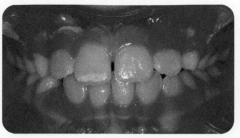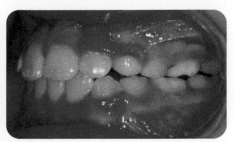

Figure 6.3

What retention regime should be used?

In this case, no retention was prescribed, as a positive overbite and overjet was established which should maintain the new incisor position (Figure 6.3).

What were the advantages of using a fixed appliance in this case?

In the mixed dentition, a fixed appliance can result in the rapid correction of a crossbite, is well tolerated and is less dependent on compliance than a removable appliance (McKeown and Sandler, 2001). Fixed appliances also offer three-dimensional control, including vertical repositioning, which is key to creating a positive overbite at the end of treatment (Skeggs and Sandler, 2002). Another advantage of a fixed appliance is that it can allow for space creation if necessary. In this case, the maxillary central incisors were actively extruded to create a positive overbite at the end of treatment to improve long-term stability.

What other methods are available to correct an anterior crossbite?

Removable appliances can also be used, although these are reliant on good retention and compliance, and are only capable of tipping teeth. As such, removable appliances are most effective with only one or two teeth in crossbite, with space available to procline them. Alternatively, a functional appliance, such as a Functional Regulator or reverse Twin Block, can be used, although these also depend on good co-operation.

Case 6.2

This 10-year-old male was referred by his orthodontic specialist as he did not like the position of his maxillary canines and bite. There was no relevant medical history.

Extra-oral

Skeletal relationship
Antero-posterior	Moderate skeletal class III
Vertical	FMPA: Average
	Lower face height: Average
Transverse	Facial symmetry: None
Soft tissues	Lip competence: Competent with protrusive lower lip
	Naso-labial angle: Normal
Upper incisor show	At rest: 2 mm
	Smiling: 5 mm
Temporo-mandibular joint	Healthy with good range and co-ordination of movement

Intra-oral

Teeth present

654321/1234 6
6E4 21/1234E6

Dental health	Good
(restorations, caries)	No active caries and good oral hygiene
Lower arch	Aligned
	Incisor inclination: Upright
Upper arch	Severely crowded. UL5 impacted palatally
	Incisor inclination: Proclined
	Canine position: Palpable buccally

Summarize the occlusal findings

- Incisor relationship: Class III
- Overjet: −3 mm
- Overbite: Average and incomplete
- Molar relationship: ¼ unit class III bilaterally
- No anterior displacement on closing from RCP to ICP

Summary

A 10-year-old male presented with a class III malocclusion on a moderate skeletal class III pattern with average lower face height, severe crowding, an impacted UL5 with an anterior crossbite without displacement in the late mixed dentition (Figure 6.4).

Treatment Plan

A bonded rapid maxillary expansion device with a HYRAX screw was initially placed and the patient asked to activate the screw once daily for 10 consecutive days. Thereafter, protraction headgear was fitted and an anterior force applied to the maxilla via elastics between hooks on the bonded appliance

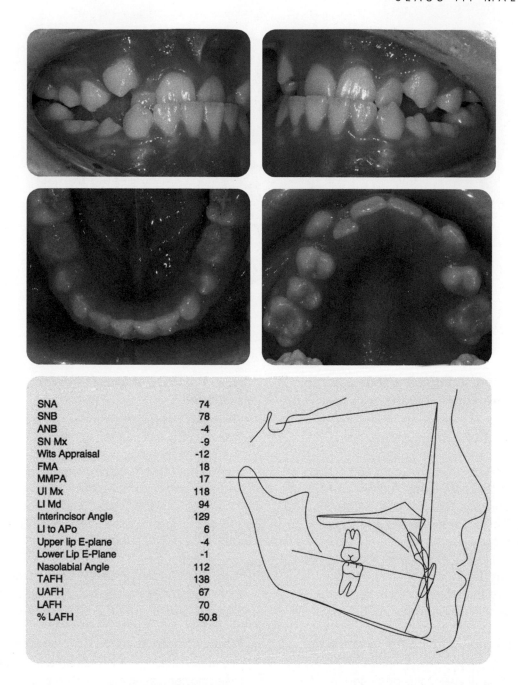

SNA	74
SNB	78
ANB	-4
SN Mx	-9
Wits Appraisal	-12
FMA	18
MMPA	17
UI Mx	118
LI Md	94
Interincisor Angle	129
LI to APo	6
Upper lip E-plane	-4
Lower Lip E-Plane	-1
Nasolabial Angle	112
TAFH	138
UAFH	67
LAFH	70
% LAFH	50.8

Figure 6.4

and the facemask of the protraction headgear. The force was increased incrementally over a period of 8 weeks to 400 g bilaterally and the position of the bar on the facemask adjusted to direct the force parallel to the occlusal plane, limiting rotational effects on the maxilla. The patient was instructed to wear the facemask for a minimum of 16 hours daily (Figure 6.5).

Comment on the principles and design of protraction headgear

Protraction headgear is not a new innovation in orthodontics, having been originally described over a century ago. However, it was re-introduced and popularized by Delaire in the early 1970s. The principles are straightforward and involve applying a force to an appliance bonded or banded to the maxilla via a frame or facemask that is primarily supported on the forehead and chin. The facemask either consists of a frame that sits lateral to the cheeks, as originally described by Delaire, or a single midline rod based on a design by Petit. With either of these appliances, the principle is the same – a force of around 400 g is applied bilaterally using heavy elastics.

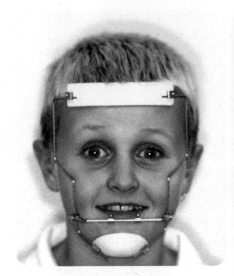

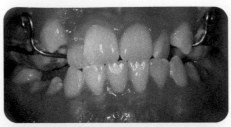

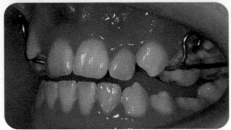

Figure 6.5

Why is protraction headgear often used in combination with rapid maxillary expansion?

Protraction headgear is often preceded by rapid maxillary expansion (RME) because in many class III malocclusions the maxilla is also narrow in the transverse plane, resulting in crowding and a posterior crossbite. Theoretically, the combined use of RME will also loosen or disengage the circum-maxillary sutures, which in theory facilitates downward and forward movement of the maxillary complex under the force of the headgear (Haas, 1973). However, current evidence would suggest that this combination does not necessarily improve maxillary advancement with protraction headgear (Vaughn et al., 2005).

What is the rationale for using protraction headgear?

The majority of class III malocclusions seen in juveniles and adolescents who have an underlying skeletal component will demonstrate some maxillary hypoplasia (Guyer et al., 1986). Ideally, treatment in these cases should be aimed at redirecting and stimulating maxillary antero-posterior growth. One way of achieving this is with the use of extra-oral force in the form of protraction headgear. This is designed to give an 'orthopaedic' effect, achieving skeletal change in addition to dento-alveolar movement. The facemask is worn for as close to 24 hours per day as possible, until a positive overjet has been achieved. In this case, the overjet was corrected in 9 months, at which stage it was +4 mm (Figure 6.6).

How has this occlusal correction been achieved?

There has been some forward movement of the maxilla (SNA has increased from 74 to 79 degrees) and this has been accompanied by a clockwise rotation of the maxilla (SN-Mx plane has changed from −9 to +5 degrees) and mandible. Interestingly, maxillary incisor inclination has remained essentially the same (UI-Mx, 118 degrees at the start versus 117 degrees at the end).

The bonded expansion appliance was removed and the patient underwent a course of fixed appliance therapy in the maxillary arch to create space for and align the UL5 (Figure 6.7 and Figure 6.8).

When should protraction headgear be used?

Protraction headgear is indicated in class III malocclusion associated with maxillary hypoplasia. Use of this appliance appears to be more effective in pre-adolescent (under the age of 10 years) patients than adolescents (Suda et al., 2000).

Are any class III patients unsuitable for protraction headgear?

Patients who present with frank mandibular prognathism are not suitable for protraction headgear therapy. Various other treatment techniques have been described for these patients, including the use of chin caps in an attempt to control mandibular growth. However, even with prolonged treatment, in the long-term this has little effect on the

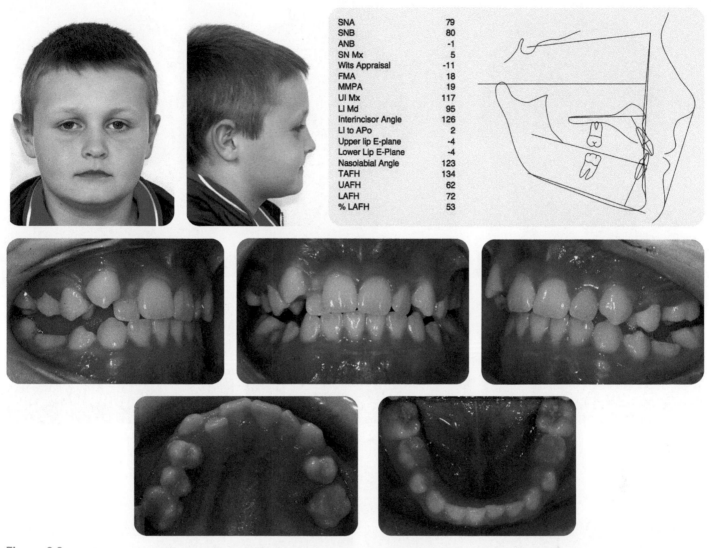

SNA	79
SNB	80
ANB	-1
SN Mx	5
Wits Appraisal	-11
FMA	18
MMPA	19
UI Mx	117
LI Md	95
Interincisor Angle	126
LI to APo	2
Upper lip E-plane	-4
Lower Lip E-Plane	-4
Nasolabial Angle	123
TAFH	134
UAFH	62
LAFH	72
% LAFH	53

Figure 6.6

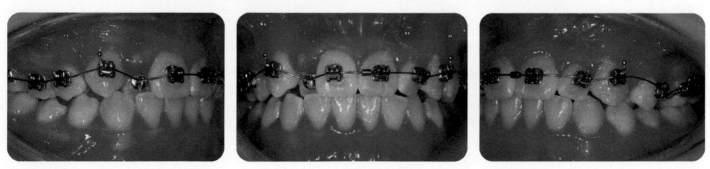

Figure 6.7

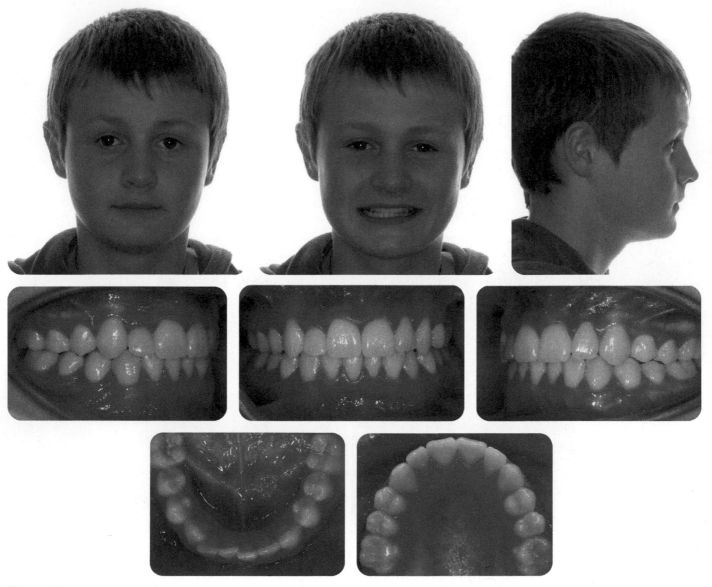

Figure 6.8

underlying prognathic growth pattern (Sugawara et al., 1990).

What are the main effects of protraction headgear?

Protraction headgear therapy will usually result in forward displacement of the maxillary complex of 1–3 mm and a downwards and backwards rotation of the mandible (Kim et al., 1999; Ngan et al., 1998). This will result in an increase in the SNA angle, a decrease in SNB and an increase in ANB. Treatment will also produce dento-alveoler compensation, with proclination of maxillary incisors and some retroclination of the mandibular incisors.

One problem with many of the studies that have been carried out to investigate the effects of protraction headgear has been the lack of an appropriate control group or the use of historical class I or class III controls from longitudinal cephalometric growth studies. Some investigations have tried to overcome this by having each subject act as his or her own control, using the pre-treatment period to measure growth (Ngan et al., 1998), although this is not ideal.

How stable is this treatment?

Following treatment, a class III growth pattern will tend to re-impose itself (Baccetti et al., 2000) with

25–30% of patients exhibiting some relapse following successful protraction headgear therapy. Relapse appears to be primarily related to mandibular growth (Hagg *et al.*, 2003; Wells *et al.*, 2006). Unfavourable long-term outcomes are also associated with patients who exhibit an increased vertical growth pattern and in those starting treatment after the age of 10 years (Baccetti *et al.*, 2004; Hagg *et al.*, 2003).

Case 6.3

This 11-year-old male was referred by Orthodontic specialist. Concerned about "back to front" bite. There was no relevant medical history.

Extra-oral

Skeletal relationship
   Antero-posterior   Mild skeletal class III
   Vertical   FMPA: Average
                               Lower face height: Average
   Transverse   Facial symmetry: None
Soft tissues   Lip competence: Competent with protrusive lower lip
                               Naso-labial angle: Normal
Upper incisor show   At rest: 2 mm
                               Smiling: 5 mm
Temporo-mandibular joint   Healthy with good range and co-ordination of movement

Intra-oral

Teeth present   6E4C21/123456
                         6EDC21/123 E6

Dental health   Good
(restorations, caries)   No active caries and good oral hygiene
Occlusion   Incisor relationship: Class III
                               Overjet: −3 mm
                               Overbite: Average and incomplete
                               Molar relationship: Class I bilaterally
                               Anterior displacement on closing from RCP to ICP
Lower arch   Crowding: Aligned
                               Incisor inclination: Proclined
Upper arch   Crowding: Aligned
                               Incisor inclination: Upright
                               Canine position: Palpable buccally

Summary

An 11–year-old male presented with a class III malocclusion on mild skeletal class III base with average lower face height, well aligned arches and an anterior crossbite with a displacement, in the late mixed dentition (Figure 6.9).

Treatment Plan

The aims of treatment were correction of the anterior crossbite and elimination of the displacement.

The patient was successfully treated with a modified Twin Block functional appliance for approximately 6 months (Figure 6.10). The design included cantilever springs behind the upper incisors, a midline expansion screw, a lower labial bow and intersecting blocks at 70 degrees with a vertical height of 7 mm. The patient was instructed to wear the appliance on a full-time basis initially, activating the midline expansion screw twice a week. On the second visit the cantilever

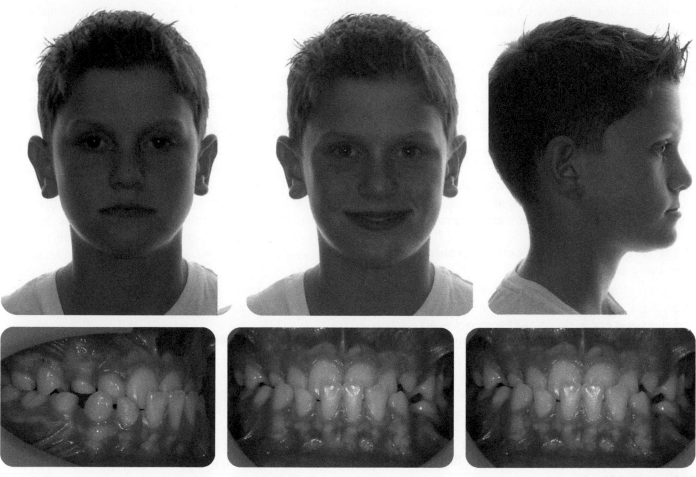

Figure 6.9

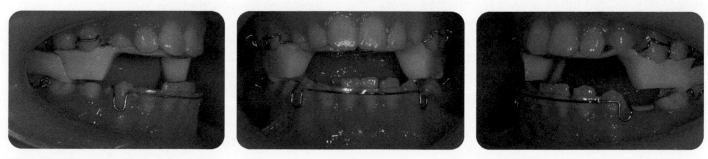

Figure 6.10

springs were activated to procline the upper labial segment.

Why are functional appliances not routinely used in the treatment of class III malocclusions?

Functional appliances are routinely used for the correction of class II malocclusions. However, whilst numerous appliances have been described for the treatment of class III malocclusions, none is in routine use. This is partly because the majority of class II malocclusions present with some degree of mandibular retrognathia. Advocates of functional appliances would argue that they stimulate mandibular growth and thereby make a significant contribution to correction of this type of malocclusion. However, class

III malocclusions are more disparate, presenting with maxillary hypoplasia, mandibular prognathism or a combination of these (Guyer et al., 1986). While it is possible to advance the maxilla using extra-oral force, control of mandibular prognathism is more difficult. Prolonged chin cap therapy has been shown to have a positive short- term effect on growth. However, following treatment, catch-up mandibular growth has been observed as the original growth pattern is re-established (Sugawara et al., 1990). Nevertheless, some patients with class III malocclusion are amenable to treatment using a functional appliance, and with careful case selection can be treated successfully.

What were the main effects of treatment in this case (Figure 6.11)?

The main effects of treatment were proclination of the upper labial segment, retroclination of the lower labial segment and some downward and backward rotation of the mandible. Following correction of the anterior crossbite, the appliance was discontinued to allow closure of the lateral open bites as the positive overbite and overjet that were achieved were judged to be self-retaining.

What factors determine whether interceptive treatment is attempted in class III malocclusions?

The decision to treat a growing class III malocclusion is a difficult one and depends on the underlying aetiology, predicted future growth and the degree of dento-alveolar compensation present, which in turn indicates how much further compensation is possible. Indicators that early correction is possible include the presence of:
• Anterior mandibular displacement
• Average or increased overbite
• Average or reduced lower face height
• Upright or proclined lower incisors
• Upright or retroclined upper incisors.
The present case had these features; such a malocclusion has been described as a 'pseudo-class III', implying that it is essentially is skeletal class I but appears to be skeletal class III due to the anterior displacement. Several studies have tried to establish pre-treatment predictors for those class III malocclusions that will be treatable orthodontically as opposed to surgically (Kerr et al., 1992; Schuster et al., 2003). However, the main determinant is future growth, particularly in the vertical dimension.

How do functional appliances work in the treatment of class III malocclusions?

The mode of action of functional appliances for class III correction has been subject to some limited retrospective investigation. This has shown that correction is achieved primarily by dental movement (Kidner et al., 2003; Loh and Kerr, 1985; Ulgen and Firatli, 1994). There is no sustained effect on growth of either the maxilla or mandible, although there is a reduction in SNB and an increase in ANB due to the backwards and downwards rotation of the mandible and an increase in lower face height. Therefore, this type of treatment is inappropriate for high angle cases with an already increased FMPA.

Are there any alternative methods of treatment?

Accepting that the effects of this type of treatment are dento-alveolar, other treatment modalities include:
• **Removable appliances with palatal springs:** The problem with using an upper removable appliance is retention; on activation of the palatal springs, the appliance is displaced vertically. With the reverse Twin Block, by occluding with the lower component of the appliance, the upper plate is re-seated and activated. Therefore, simple upper removable appliances are only effective with one or two teeth in crossbite.
• **Fixed appliances:** Use of a fixed appliance to correct a class III incisor relationship with a displacement can be effective and avoids the problems of compliance associated with removable appliances.

How stable is this treatment?

The determinant for initial stability will be a positive overbite and overjet at the end of treatment following elimination of the anterior displacement. In the long-term, stability is reliant on the magnitude and direction of mandibular growth. With correct case selection, avoiding treatment in class III malocclusions with an overtly skeletal aetiology, stability is more predictable.

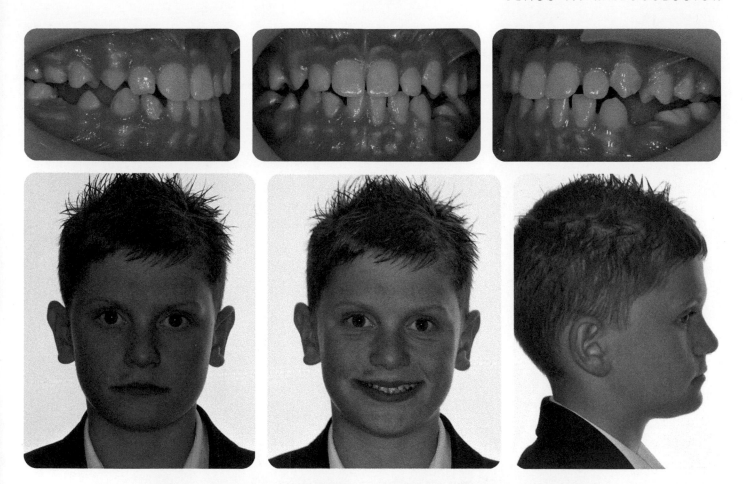

Pre-Twin block Post-Twin block

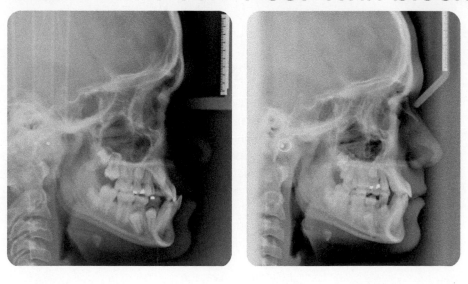

Figure 6.11

Case 6.4

This 13-year-old female was referred by her dental practitioner as she was concerned about the prominence of her upper canine teeth.

Extra-oral

Skeletal relationship

Antero-posterior	Mild skeletal class III
Vertical	FMPA: Increased
	Lower face height: Increased
Transverse	Facial symmetry: None
Soft tissues	Lip competence
	Upper lip length: 20 mm
	Naso-labial angle: Obtuse
Upper incisor show	At rest: 1 mm
	Smiling: 5 mm
Temporo-mandibular joint	Healthy with good range and co-ordination of movement

Intra-oral

Teeth present	7654321/1234567
	7654321/1234567
Dental health	Good
(restorations, caries)	No restorations or active caries
Oral hygiene	Good
Occlusion	Incisor relationship: Class III
	Overjet: Edge to edge
	Overbite: Reduced and incomplete
	Molar relationship: Class I bilaterally
	Canine relationship: ½ unit class II bilaterally
	Centre lines: Upper to right by 1 mm
	Functional occlusion: Group function
	Bilateral crossbite tendency with no displacement
Lower arch	Mild crowding
	Incisor inclination: Retroclined
	Curve of Spee: Flat
Upper arch	Severe crowding
	Incisor inclination: Average

Summary

A 13-year-old female presented with a class III malocclusion on a mild skeletal class III pattern with increased vertical dimensions complicated by an edge-to-edge incisor relationship, reduced incomplete overbite and severe crowding in the maxillary arch (Figures 6.12 and 6.13).

What factors influence the decision to treat a class III malocclusion with orthodontics alone?

Key factors are the existing skeletal relationship and degree of dento-alveolar compensation. The more severe the skeletal class III relationship, the less likely it is that camouflage treatment will be successful.

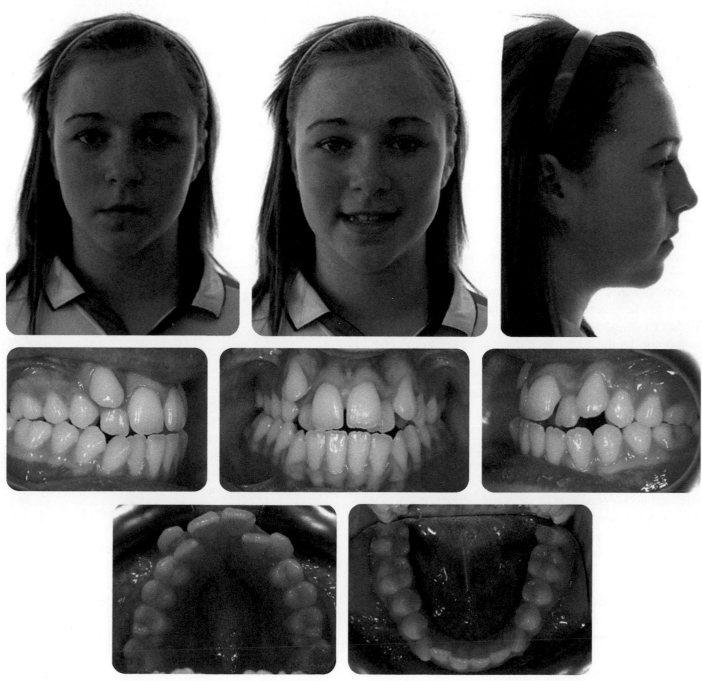

Figure 6.12

Similarly, the more retroclined the mandibular incisors and proclined the maxillary incisors, the less likely it is that camouflage will be possible.

Potential future growth is a key factor. In individuals with a class III malocclusion there is a tendency for mandibular growth to persist well beyond adolescent growth (Baccetti *et al.*, 2007; Battagel, 1993). Unlike class II malocclusions, where residual antero-posterior mandibular growth is beneficial and makes orthodontic treatment to camouflage the skeletal discrepancy more likely to be successful, in class III malocclusions supplemental mandibular growth is detrimental and may result in re-establishment of a reverse overjet either during or following treatment. Therefore, it is often better to delay orthodontic treatment (particularly when it involves extractions in the lower arch and retroclination of the lower labial segment) until late adolescence or early adulthood.

What are the potential risks of orthodontic camouflage?

The main risks are not being able to achieve a class I incisor relationship in more severe cases, or achieving correction of the incisor relationship only for post-orthodontic change to occur due to continued unfavourable growth. In these cases, if orthognathic surgery becomes necessary, the pre-surgical orthodontics will necessitate decompensation of incisor position, which in the mandibular arch can be difficult to do, particularly if extractions have been carried out, as there is a tendency for space to re-open as the incisors are advanced.

How is camouflage treatment achieved for a class III malocclusion?

Class III camouflage may be achieved with proclination of the maxillary incisors, retroclination of the mandibular incisors or a combination of these movements. Typically, maxillary incisors are already proclined and mandibular incisors are upright, in an attempt to compensate for the skeletal imbalance. The magnitude of movements permissible is governed by aesthetics, function, periodontal health and bone volume.

Which tooth movements are most favourable?

Retroclination of the mandibular incisors is usually preferable to excessive maxillary incisor advancement, as significant maxillary incisor proclination may be unaesthetic and may induce non-axial loading, resulting in abnormal mobility (fremitus). However, the amount of lower incisor retroclination may be limited by insufficient alveolar bone labial to the lower incisors and a thin gingival biotype. Excessive retroclination may, therefore, risk dehiscence, root resorption and gingival recession.

What are the limits for orthodontic treatment of a class III malocclusion?

The limits of camouflage treatment are determined by how far the dentition can be moved physically to produce an acceptable result both aesthetically and occlusally. In a class III malocclusion, this involves proclination of the maxillary incisors and retroclination of the mandibular incisors. Retrospective studies have attempted to identify cephalometric indicators of when camouflage treatment is possible, although these are of limited value (Burns *et al.*, 2010; Kerr *et al.*, 1992; Stellzig-Eisenhauer *et al.*, 2002). The limits of tooth movement are defined by the alveolar bone and gingival health. As a general rule, it is unwise to procline the upper incisors beyond 120 degrees to the maxillary plane or retrocline the lower incisors beyond 80 degrees to the mandibular plane.

The criteria for class III cases that can be successfully camouflaged are similar to those for successful interceptive treatment:
- Skeletal class I or mild class III
- Average to low maxilla to mandibular planes angle (MMPA)
- No or minimal existing dento-alveolar compensation
- Edge-to-edge incisor relationship in RCP
- Class I or up to ½ unit class III molar relationship in RCP.

In general, camouflage of a class III malocclusion is less successful than camouflage of a class II malocclusion, because even if an acceptable occlusal result can be achieved, retroclination of the lower incisors may increase the relative prominence of the chin and compromise the soft tissue profile further.

Summarize the principles of treatment when camouflaging a class III malocclusion

- Avoid extracting in the upper arch or extract as far back as possible in order to support the upper labial segment and allow for advancement of the maxillary incisors.
- Extract further forward in the lower arch to create space for retroclination of the lower incisors and relief of any (usually mild) crowding.

- Mechanics may be facilitated by the extraction of upper second premolars and lower first premolars.
- An alternative in a non-growing patient is extraction of a lower incisor, facilitating retroclination of the remaining incisors.
- Use of class III elastics during treatment will help correct the incisor relationship.
- Placing contra-lateral brackets on the lower canines when using a pre-adjusted edgewise appliance will reverse the angulation in the bracket and encourage retroclination of the mandibular incisors.
- Retroclination of the lower incisors is also promoted by avoiding using a full dimension wire in the lower arch, particularly during space closure.

Summarize the main cephalometric features of the malocclusion in Figure 6.13

There is maxillary and mandibular retrognathia, a mild skeletal class III pattern and increased vertical proportions. The maxillary incisors are slightly proclined and the mandibular incisors are slightly retroclined.

What features of this malocclusion suggest that camouflage treatment can be carried out?

The antero-posterior skeletal pattern is only mild class III, the existing incisor compensation is not excessive and there is no significant reverse overjet. In addition, the molar relationship is essentially class I bilaterally. One area of concern is the presence of increased vertical proportions and an openbite tendency, which might be difficult to address and correct with stability, particularly as there is a crossbite tendency requiring expansion to correct.

Why have all the first premolar teeth been extracted (Figure 6.14)?

First premolars were extracted in the maxillary arch to provide space for the severely crowded upper labial segment. In the mandibular arch, by extracting first premolars in a mildly crowded arch, maximal space is available to retract the lower incisors to correct the incisor relationship and attempt some increase in the overbite.

What tooth movements are being achieved in Figure 6.14? What is the purpose of the light elastic attached to the UR3?

Incisor alignment is being achieved with light round nickel–titanium archwires and the crossbite is being corrected with a fixed quadhelix appliance. This light elastic is retracting the UR3 into the extraction space, which will provide space to align the palatally crowded UR2.

What is happening in Figure 6.15?

The UR3 has been retracted and the UR2 attached to the archwire, and alignment is continuing in the maxillary arch. In the mandibular arch, alignment is at a more advanced stage and there has been some

SNA	72
SNB	71
ANB	1
SN Mx	12
Wits Appraisal	-3
FMA	36
MMPA	36
UI Mx	112
LI Md	88
Interincisor Angle	123
LI to APo	6
Upper lip E-plane	-3
Lower Lip E-Plane	-1
Nasolabial Angle	138
TAFH	120
UAFH	51
LAFH	69
% LAFH	57

Figure 6.13

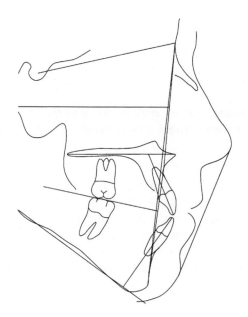

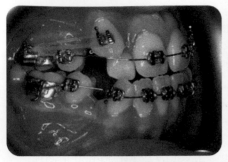
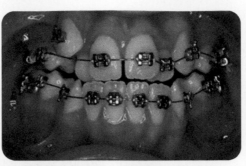
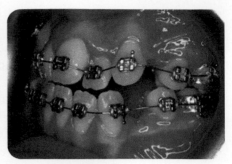

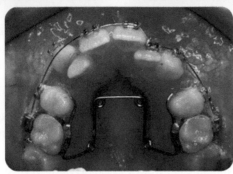
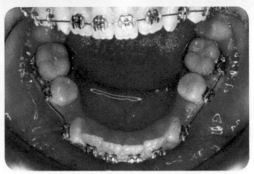

Figure 6.14

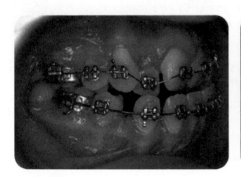
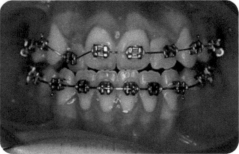
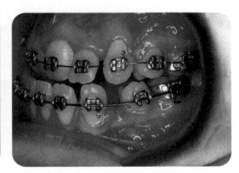

Figure 6.15

proclination of the lower incisors, which has resulted in a worsening of the reverse overjet.

How could the presence of a reverse overjet during alignment have been prevented?

The mandibular canine brackets could have been swapped, eliminating the mesial tip but maintaining the torque. Laceback stainless steel ligatures could have been applied from the first molars to canines, which will also reduce the mesial tip of the canines during alignment. In addition, the lower archwire could have been cinched back behind the first molars to prevent forward movement of the labial segment. However, these latter two interventions are anchorage demanding – encouraging forward movement of the first molars. In this case, as the lower arch is only

mildly crowded and most of the space will be used to retract the incisors, these interventions could have been used.

What mechanics are being used in Figure 6.16?

In both arches alignment is complete. In the maxillary arch, the quadhelix has been removed and all the extraction space has been used during alignment, because of the severe crowding that was present. Both upper lateral incisors are under-torqued at this stage, during alignment from their initial positions on the palatal side, and the crowns are now relatively more labial than the roots because the coronal portion of these teeth moves more effectively than the root. In the mandibular arch, some extraction space is left

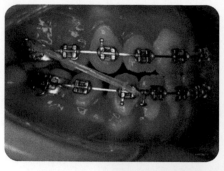
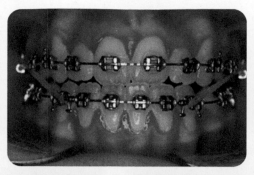
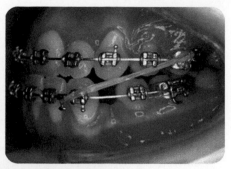
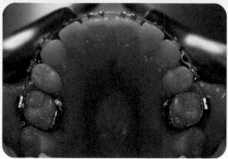
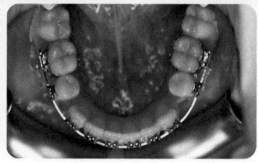

Figure 6.16

following alignment, which is essential as this is required to retract the lower labial segment and correct the incisor relationship.

Rigid rectangular stainless steel archwires are present and class III mechanics are being utilized to retract the lower labial segment, close the extraction spaces and procline the upper labial segment.

What are the disadvantages of using class III traction in this case?

The main disadvantage is the associated extrusive force, which will tend to worsen an already reduced overbite.

Figure 6.17 shows the final occlusion following removal of the fixed appliances. Describe the finish

The overbite is a little tenuous. Any late facial growth with a vertical element might result in further

reduction of the overbite, which in this case might lead to development of an open bite. The UL2 crown is slightly distally angulated and both upper lateral incisors could have their incisal edges a little higher in relation to the central incisors.

What additional torque was required for the maxillary lateral incisors and how can this be achieved?

These teeth required labial root torque. The maxillary incisor brackets can be inverted, which changes the torque prescription from negative to positive. Alternatively, individual torque can be placed on these teeth via third-order bends in the archwire. This can be done on a 19 × 25″ stainless steel or titanium–molybdenum alloy archwire (Thickett et al., 2007).

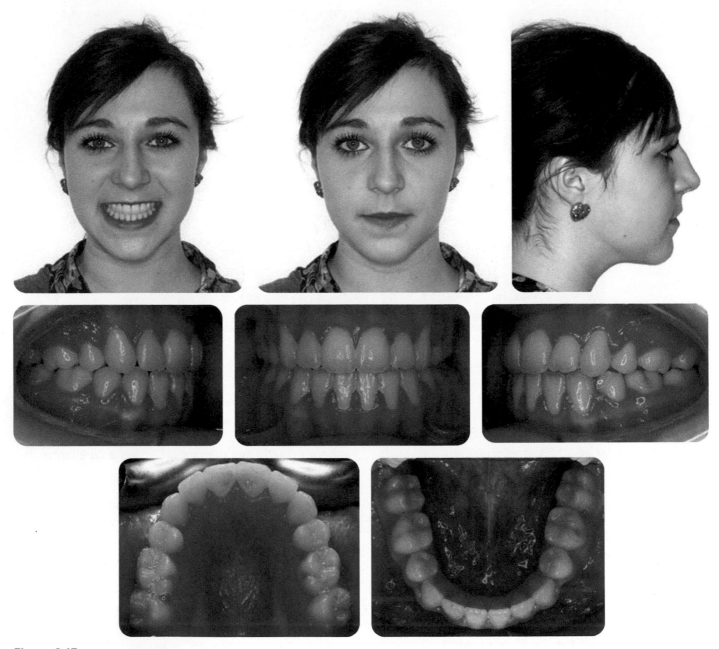

Figure 6.17

Case 6.5

This 15-year-old female was referred by her general dentist in relation to a class III malocclusion and concern about her incorrect bite. There was no relevant medical history.

Extra-oral

Skeletal relationship

Antero-posterior	Mild skeletal class III
Vertical	FMPA: Average
	Lower face height: Average
Transverse	Facial asymmetry: None
Soft tissues	Lip competence: Competent
	Naso-labial angle: Average Tranverse Chin point to the right
Upper incisor show	At rest: 2 mm
	Smiling: 6 mm
Temporo-mandibular joint	Healthy with good range and co-ordination of movement

Intra-oral

Teeth present	7654321/1234567
	7654321/1234567
Dental health (restorations, caries)	Good
Oral hygiene – periodontal	Good
Lower arch	Crowding: Mild
	Incisor inclination: Retroclined
	Curve of Spee: Increased
Upper arch	Crowding: Moderate
	Incisor inclination: Average
	Canine position: Buccal
Occlusion	Incisor relationship: Class III
	Overjet: –3 mm
	Overbite: Increased and complete
	Molar relationship: Class III bilaterally
	Canine relationship: Class III bilaterally
	Centre lines: Coincident with each other and the mid-facial axis
	Functional occlusion: Group function
	Other feature: An occlusal displacement from centric relation to centric occlusion

Summary

A 15-year old female presented with a class III malocclusion on a mild skeletal class III base with average vertical dimensions complicated by a reverse overjet, maxillary arch crowding and an increased overbite (Figure 6.18).

Treatment Plan

- Non-extraction treatment
- Upper and lower pre-adjusted edgewise appliances (Figure 6.19)
- Long-term retention

The final treatment result is shown in Figure 6.20.

Is the presence of a displacement a positive or negative prognostic indicator in class III cases?

It is a positive indicator. It suggests that the malocclusion may be less severe in RCP. Hence, less lower incisor retraction is required to correct the incisor relationship.

What other factors suggest the prognosis for orthodontic camouflage is favourable in this case?

- Mild skeletal discrepancy
- Favourable soft tissue profile
- Increased overbite
- Maxillary arch crowding
- Minimal mandibular crowding
- Upright maxillary incisors

Can you envisage any impediment to correction of the incisor relationship in this case? How might this be overcome?

The presence of the increased overbite could impede correction. The occlusion can be disengaged with bite blocks (using glass ionomer or composite) or with

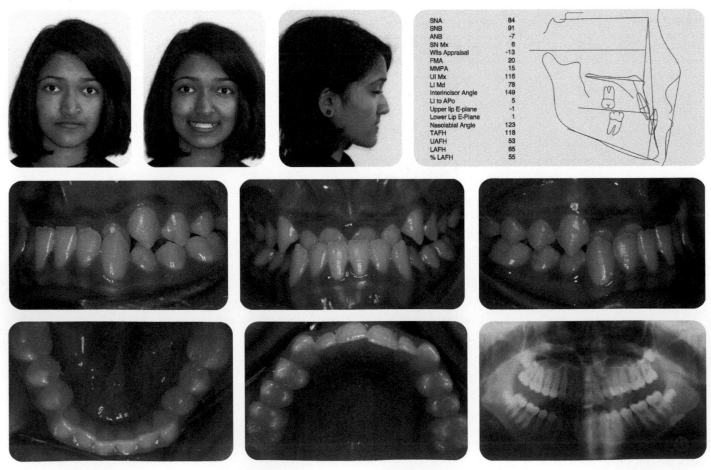

SNA	84
SNB	91
ANB	-7
SN Mx	6
Wits Appraisal	-13
FMA	20
MMPA	15
UI Mx	116
LI Md	78
Interincisor Angle	149
LI to APo	5
Upper lip E-plane	-1
Lower Lip E-Plane	1
Nasolabial Angle	123
TAFH	118
UAFH	53
LAFH	65
% LAFH	55

Figure 6.18

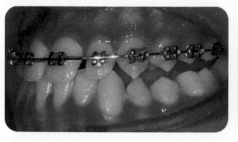 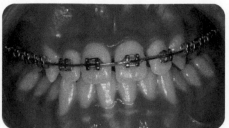 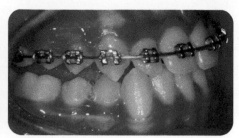

Figure 6.19

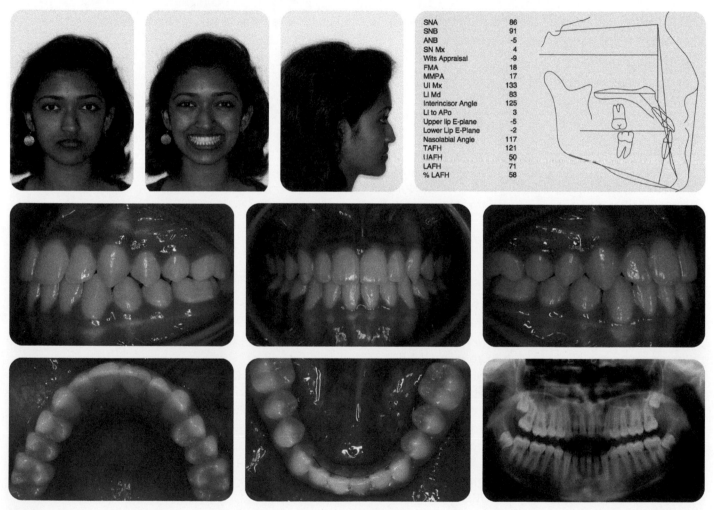

SNA	86
SNB	91
ANB	-5
SN Mx	4
Wits Appraisal	-9
FMA	18
MMPA	17
UI Mx	133
LI Md	83
Interincisor Angle	125
LI to APo	3
Upper lip E-plane	-5
Lower Lip E-Plane	-2
Nasolabial Angle	117
TAFH	121
UAFH	50
LAFH	71
% LAFH	58

Figure 6.20

removable appliances to facilitate unimpeded tooth movement.

Why was a lower fixed appliance placed in this case?

Following correction of the anterior crossbite, the increased curve of Spee in the lower arch resulted in lateral open bites. Therefore, a lower appliance was placed to allow proper seating of the buccal occlusion and enhance occlusal interdigitation. The lower appliance also permitted use of class III inter-arch traction.

Case 6.6

This 13-year-old female was referred by her general dental practitioner regarding unerupted second premolars. There was no relevant medical history.

Extra-oral

Skeletal relationship	
Antero-posterior	Mild skeletal class III
Vertical	FMPA average
	Lower anterior face height: Average
Tranverse	Chin point to the right
Soft tissues	Lip competence: Competent
	Naso-labial angle: Obtuse
Upper incisor show	At rest: 3 mm
	Smiling: 7 mm
Temporo-mandibular joint	Healthy with good range and co-ordination of movement

Intra-oral

Teeth present	6E4321/1234E6
	76 4321/1234E67
Dental health (restorations, caries)	Generalized enamel hypoplasia
Lower arch	Crowding: Mild
	Incisor inclination: Retroclined with the LR3 mesio-angular and the LL3 disto-angular
	Loss of the LRE (in the clinical photographs) with little space available for the LR5
Upper arch	Crowding: Mild
	Incisor inclination: Proclined with the upper lateral incisors mesio-palatally rotated and the upper canines mesially-angulated
	UR2 is in crossbite
	Both maxillary second primary molars are still present
Occlusion	Incisor relationship: Class III (edge to edge)
	Overbite: Decreased and complete
	Molar relationship: Class III on the right and class I on the left
	Centre lines: Lower centre line is displaced to the right by 3 mm
	Crossbites: Crossbite tendency on the right side.

Comment on the transverse relationship (Figure 6.21)

There is mild facial asymmetry, with the chin point and lower dental centre line to the right of the facial midline.

What are the main problems associated with this case (Figure 6.21)?

- Mild skeletal class III pattern and incisor relationship
- Mild facial asymmetry

- Congenitally absent: UR5, UL5 and LL5.
- Impacted LR5
- UR2 in crossbite
- Lower centre line discrepancy

What are the possible causes of the centre line discrepancy in this case?

- Mild facial asymmetry
- Occlusal displacement (although there was no displacement on closure in this case)
- Space loss in the lower right quadrant

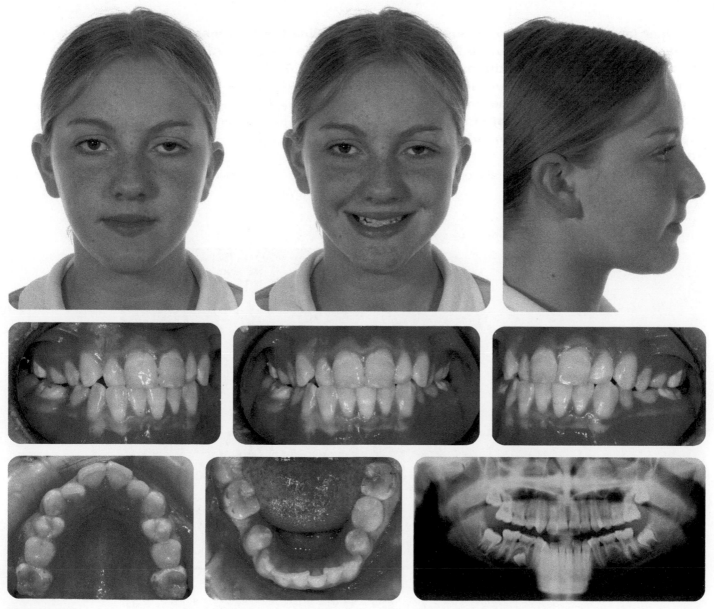

Figure 6.21

At presentation this patient was 13 years old. At this time a decision to monitor facial growth and request removal of the retained upper and lower left second primary molars was made. Discuss the rationale behind these decisions.

Removal of the remaining primary molars was performed at this stage to permit some spontaneous space closure in the quadrants with hypodontia.

In view of the mild facial asymmetry, it was felt appropriate to monitor growth, as future growth may result in the asymmetry becoming more marked, possibly requiring an orthognathic approach to address it.

One year later there was no obvious change in the facial asymmetry (Figure 6.22) and a decision was made to treat the patient orthodontically. Therefore, arrangements were made for removal of the impacted LR5 and treatment with pre-adjusted edgewise fixed appliances. List the aims of this treatment

- Expansion to correct the unilateral crossbite
- Levelling and alignment
- Space closure
- Correction of the lower centre line
- Correction of the anterior crossbite
- Obtain a class I incisor relationship

At the start of treatment, a quadhelix was fitted in the upper arch and a lingual arch in the lower arch. Discuss the rationale behind this

A quadhelix was fitted to address the transverse inter-arch discrepancy with a view to eliminating the unilateral crossbite.

The lingual arch was placed to reinforce anchorage in the lower arch whilst lower centre line correction was carried out.

Outline the treatment mechanics that would enable the centre line correction seen in Figure 6.23

- In the lower arch, reverse the lower canine brackets to prevent expression of mesial tip and resultant proclination of the lower labial segment
- Place a laceback in the lower left quadrant to aid centre line correction
- Proceed to 0.018-inch stainless steel archwires in the lower arch

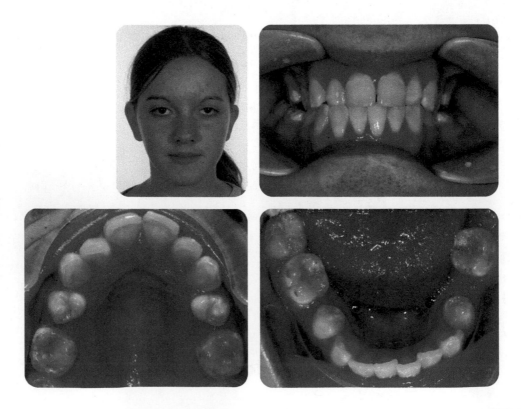

Figure 6.22

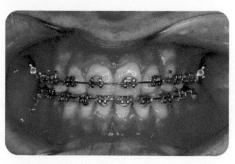

Figure 6.23

- Continue lower centre line correction with intra-arch mechanics in the left buccal segment, with elastomeric chain from a circle hook on the 0.018-inch stainless steel archwire to the hook on the lower first molar band.

The final occlusion is shown in Figure 6.24.

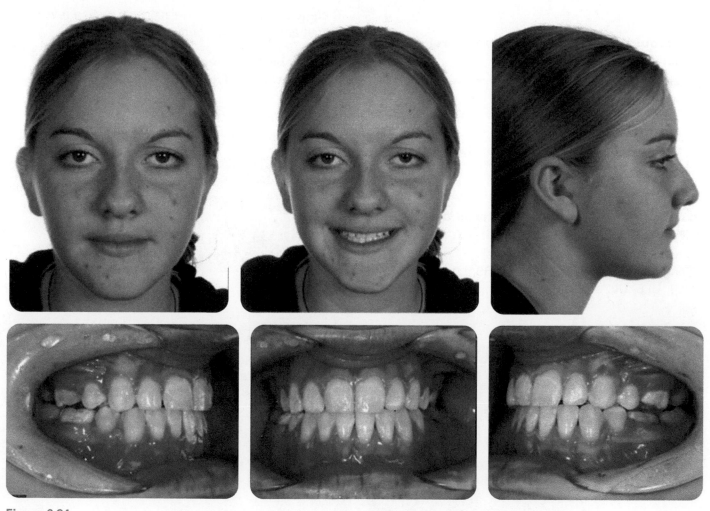

Figure 6.24

Case 6.7

This 15-year-old male presented complaining of the appearance of his teeth. He was medically fit and well.

How would you describe his extra-oral appearance (Figure 6.25)?

- Skeletal class II profile with increased vertical proportions
- Appears to be an increased FMPA and increased lower anterior face height
- Profile is retrusive, with an obtuse nasio-labial angle
- No evidence of facial asymmetry
- Lips appear competent at rest

Describe the radiographic features associated with the dentition (Figure 6.26)

- Severe tooth agenesis (oligodontia)
- Congenitally absent teeth: LR8, LR5, LR4; LL5, LL8; UL8, UL5, UL2; UR2, UR5

Retained teeth: LRE, LRD; LLD, LLE

- Lower Ds are soon to be exfoliated but the lower Es have reasonable root form

Describe the incisor relationship (Figure 6.27)

There is a class III incisor relationship, with a reverse overjet and increased overbite.

What does the lower right photograph demonstrate in Figure 6.27. Why is this helpful?

It demonstrates that the patient is able to achieve an edge-to-edge incisor relationship in RCP, and that the

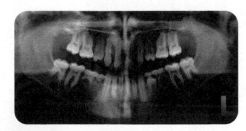

Figure 6.26

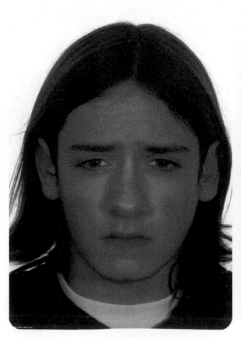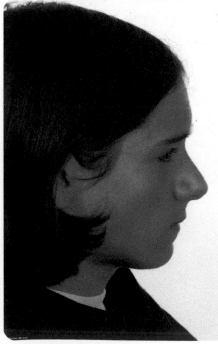

Figure 6.25

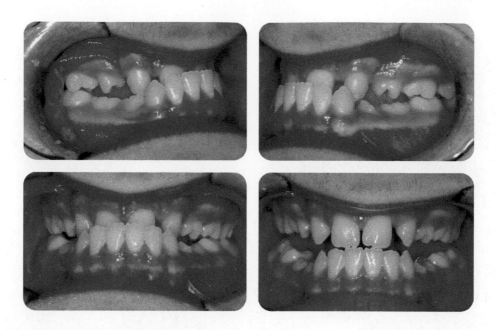

Figure 6.27

reverse overjet is the result of a mandibular anterior displacement. This is favourable, indicating that it may be possible to correct the incisor relationship by orthodontic camouflage.

How can you account for the differences between the patient's soft tissue profile clinically and the radiographic appearance (Figure 6.28)? The radiograph has been taken in RCP.

It is likely that the patient is not in occlusion in the profile photograph. The cephalogram taken in the undisplaced position confirms that he has a skeletal class I pattern.

Discuss the aetiology of this patient's malocclusion

The extra-oral examination and radiographic examination confirm that a sagittal skeletal discrepancy is not contributing to the class III malocclusion.

There has been some evidence of compensation in the lower arch with the lower incisors retroclined. In the maxillary arch the incisors are of average inclination, indicating there is some scope for further compensation.

The aetiology of this malocclusion is related to the oligodontia, resulting in a significant tooth size-to-arch length discrepancy, which contributes to the inability to achieve a positive overjet and overbite.

What has been undertaken in Figure 6.29?

A diagnostic wax-up or Kesling set-up has been undertaken. In cases with tooth agenesis, treatment planning can be aided by carrying out the proposed tooth movements on study models and evaluating the spatial relationships.

In the maxillary arch a decision was made to open space for replacement of the absent lateral incisors and to close the remaining space in the buccal segments. What factors will have been taken into account when reaching this decision?

A significant component of the class III incisor relationship is the tooth size-to-arch length discrepancy created by the tooth agenesis in this arch. In view of this, space opening for the congenitally absent upper lateral incisors will help to produce a class I incisor relationship. Closing space in the buccal segments reduces the restorative commitment required in the maxillary arch.

What are the differences between the two options presented with regard to the lower arch? What factors will be taken into account when choosing between these options?

Option 1 involves removal of the LLE and closing the remaining space in the lower left quadrant. In the

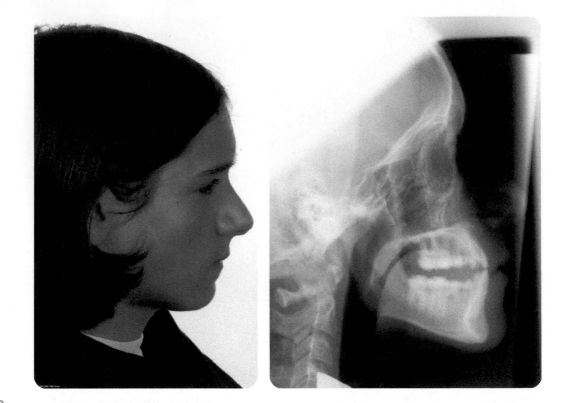

Figure 6.28

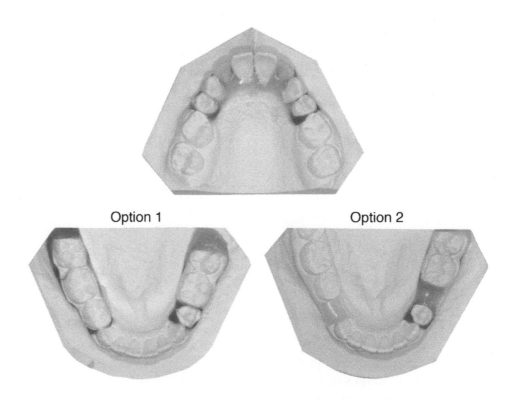

Option 1   Option 2

Figure 6.29

lower right quadrant, the LRE has been retained and the LR4 space has been closed.

In option 2 the LRE has also been retained but the LR4 space has been maintained for restorative replacement. In the lower left quadrant the LLE space has been reduced to 1 unit with a view to being restored.

Option 1 minimizes the long-term restorative commitment; however, the ability to achieve this will depend on the ease of space closure. Both options rely on retaining the LRE, which has an average long-term prognosis. However, whilst *in situ* this tooth will help to maintain bone levels. A major limitation of option 1 is the amount of space closure required in the lower right quadrant, which, while achievable, may have a detrimental effect on the long-term prognosis for the LRE.

Describe the mechanics illustrated in the mid-treatment photographs (Figure 6.30)

Space has been created for replacement of the upper lateral incisors and is being maintained with closed coil. Class II elastics are being used on 19 × 25-inch stainless steel archwires to reduce the overjet and overbite. On the right, the class II elastic is aiding mesial movement of the LRE.

How has the space for replacement of the maxillary lateral incisors been calculated?

The ideal dimension for the replacement lateral incisors has been based on the width of the central incisors. The aim was to create space for the lateral incisor such that this was in 'golden proportion' to the central incisor.

The occlusion on removal of the fixed appliances is shown in Figure 6.31. Upper and lower Hawley retainers were provided. How would these be designed and how should they be worn?

The upper Hawley retainer should have pontics to maintain the upper lateral incisor spaces and metal

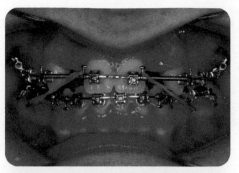

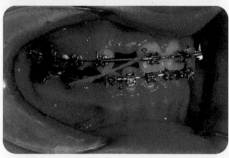

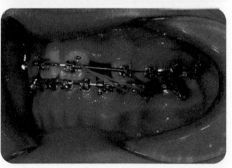

Figure 6.30

stops mesial and distal to these pontics to ensure that space is maintained should the prosthetic tooth fracture. A conventional design would be appropriate for the lower retainer. These retainers should be worn on a full-time basis until definitive replacement of the missing teeth following periodontal reorganization (usually 6 months). New retainers should then be constructed and worn part-time.

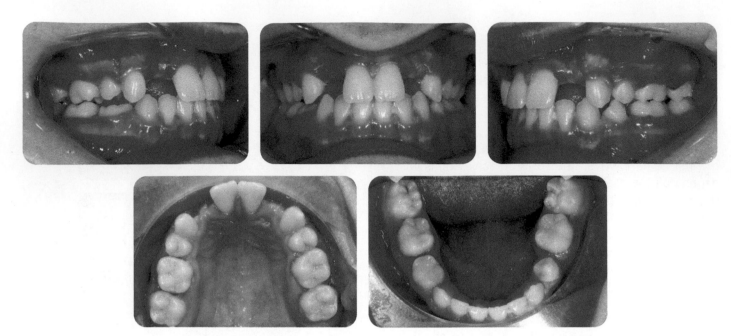

Figure 6.31

Case 6.8

This 15-year-old female was referred by her general dental practitioner complaining about the appearance of her teeth.

Summarize this malocclusion (Figure 6.32 and Figure 6.33)

A class III incisor relationship on a mild skeletal class III pattern with increased vertical dimensions complicated by:

- Crowding of both arches
- Buccally-displaced UL3
- Bilateral buccal crossbites
- Reduced overbite
- Centre line discrepancy.

How could the transverse issue be addressed?

The posterior crossbites could be corrected by maxillary arch expansion and limited constriction of the mandibular arch. As the degree of transverse discrepancy is greater than 8 mm, skeletal expansion is indicated to correct the crossbites. As this patient was 14 years old, rapid maxillary expansion to achieve sutural expansion was undertaken (Figure 6.34). Constriction of the mandibular arch could be promoted with removal of second premolars.

What overall treatment plan could be considered?

- Rapid maxillary expansion
- Upper and lower pre-adjusted edgewise appliances with removal of four second premolars

Extractions were justified in this case in view of the severe crowding, reduced overbite, class III tendency and posterior crossbites. In particular, space was required in the maxillary arch for relief of crowding. In the mandibular arch, space was required to relieve crowding, to constrict the arch and to aid retraction of the lower labial segment to achieving a positive overjet and overbite.

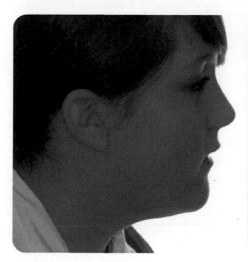
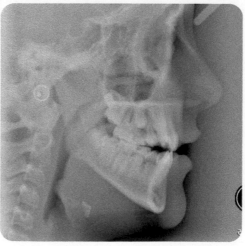

Figure 6.32

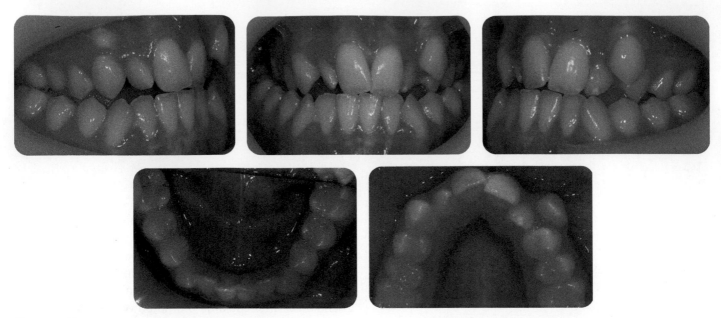

Figure 6.33

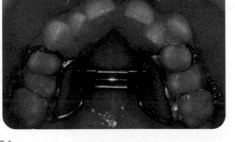

Figure 6.34

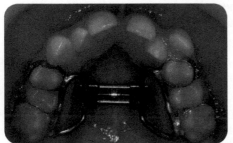

Figure 6.35

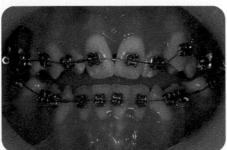

Figure 6.36

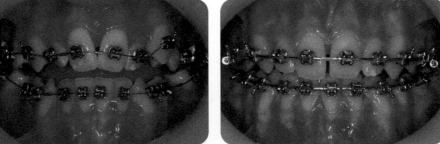

During the expansion phase the overbite reduced with an anterior open bite developing (Figure 6.35). Why has this occurred?

This is likely to be related to buccal flaring of the maxillary first molars following expansion. Some degree of tipping is inevitable irrespective of the modality of expansion, although the degree of tipping is thought to be less with RME than with gradual forms of expansion.

During the fixed phase of treatment the anterior open bite was corrected. How has this been brought about (Figure 6.36)?

Orthodontic space closure has resulted in protraction of the buccal segments; the 'counter-wedge' effect with protraction of these teeth leads to an increase in overbite. Furthermore, extrusion of the anterior teeth is likely with orthodontic space closure.

Case 6.9

This 15-year-old female was referred by her general dental practitioner complaining about her crowded upper front teeth.

Summarise this malocclusion (Figure 6.37)

A class III incisor relationship on a mild skeletal class III pattern with increased vertical dimensions complicated by:

- Crowding of both arches
- Palatally-excluded UR2
- Bilateral buccal crossbites
- Reduced overbite.

What treatment options would you consider in this case?

The initial treatment decision revolves around whether the malocclusion can be camouflaged orthodontically. If a surgical solution were deemed necessary, this would likely have involved maxillary advancement with removal of two maxillary premolars to relieve the maxillary arch crowding and facilitate decompensation to permit antero-posterior skeletal change.

However, the skeletal discrepancy was mild and the patient was happy with her facial profile; therefore, orthodontic camouflage was attempted with upper and lower fixed appliances. Camouflage may have been undertaken with removal of both maxillary second premolars and both mandibular first premolars, creating sufficient space to relieve the crowding and retract the lower labial segment. In this case, the maxillary arch was treated on a non-extraction basis, aligning UR2 and allowing the upper labial segment to advance slightly. A mandibular incisor was then removed and the space generated utilized to retract the mandibular incisors to produce a positive overjet and overbite (Figure 6.38).

What bracket variations may have been considered in this case?

The UR2 bracket could have been inverted. This would have reversed the torque imparted on the tooth, promoting labial movement of the root as the tooth was palatally-displaced at the outset.

The mandibular canine brackets could have been reversed, changing the inherent mesial crown tip to a distal crown tip to facilitate retraction of the mandibular incisors. This, however, was not considered necessary following space analysis.

Are centre lines likely to be coincident following treatment?

The maxillary centre line should be coincident with the mid-facial plane. However, the middle of the remaining (right) mandibular central incisor will become the new lower dental centre line. Consequently, there will be an apparent centre line discrepancy of 2.5–3 mm.

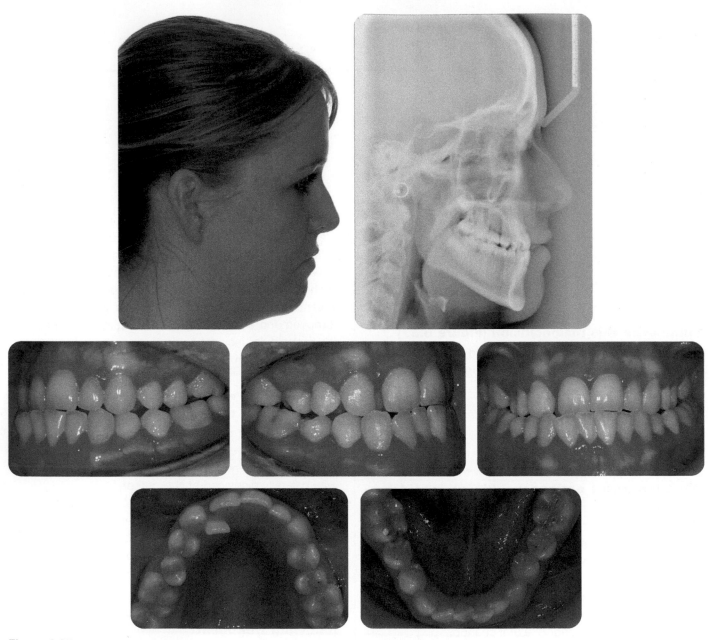

Figure 6.37

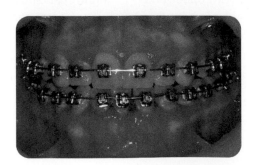

Figure 6.38

Case 6.10

This 22-year-old female presented complaining about the appearance of her front teeth. There was no relevant medical history.

Summarize the clinical findings associated with this malocclusion (Figure 6.39)

A 22-year-old female presents with a class III incisor relationship on a skeletal class I base with increased lower anterior face height. The lips appear to be competent and the soft tissue profile is good. All permanent teeth are present intra-orally, with the exception of the UR3 and the third molars. There is a retained URC. The dentition is heavily restored, with the LR6 and UL6 restored with large cast gold restorations.

There is mild crowding in the mandibular arch, with the LL3 crowded and distally angulated. In the maxillary arch there is severe crowding, with the UR3 unerupted and impacted.

In occlusion, there is a class III incisor relationship associated with an anterior open bite of 1 mm. The molar relationship is ¼ unit class III bilaterally and the lower centre line is displaced 1 mm to the left.

Comment on the radiographic findings (Figure 6.40)

The cephalometric radiograph confirms a skeletal class I pattern with increased MMPA. The incisor relationship is class III, with both upper and lower incisors at a normal inclination to the maxillary and mandibular planes.

The UL6 and LR6 are root canal treated, whilst the UL4, UR6, LL7 and LR7 have amalgam restorations.

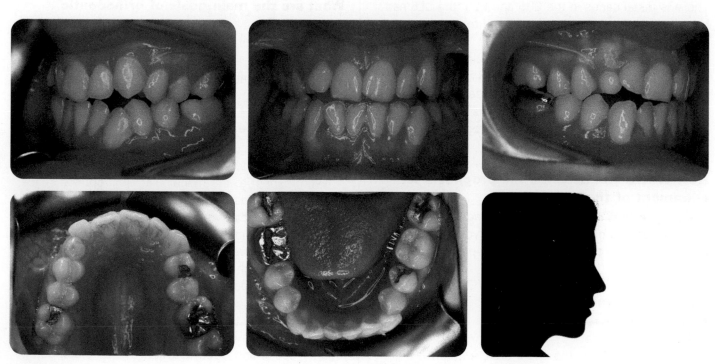

Figure 6.39

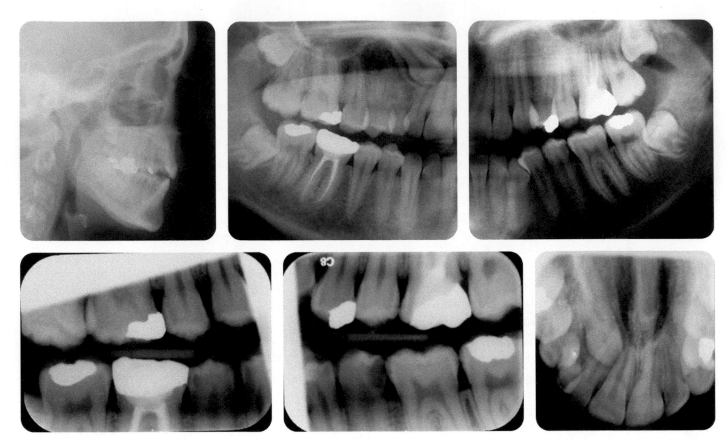

Figure 6.40

There is distal caries in the LR5 and LL5 (the LL5 had been restored by the time the clinical records were taken).

The UR3 is impacted, mesially angulated and displaced medially (adjacent to the UR1 root) and high. Parallax suggests that this tooth is essentially in the line of the arch. The root of the URC is long and this tooth appears to have a reasonable prognosis, certainly in the short-term.

How would you describe the prognosis for alignment of the UR3?

The prognosis is not good. This is an adult patient and the position of this tooth is not favourable, particularly given that it is high and displaced towards the midline.

What is the main problem list?

- Class III incisor relationship
- Anterior open bite
- Severe crowding in the upper arch, with an impacted UR3

What are the main goals of orthodontic treatment?

- Obtain a class I incisor relationship with a positive overbite
- Align the dental arches

How can these objectives be achieved?

Fixed orthodontic appliances will be required and space will need to be generated.

With respect to the mandibular arch, optimal space would be provided by extraction of the lower first premolars, providing space to align the lower labial segment, retrocline it and help obtain a class I incisor relationship. However, the LL5 has a large amalgam restoration, which encroaches on the pulp and therefore has a poor long-term prognosis. In addition, the LR6 is root canal treated and has a full gold crown. Therefore, the extraction of these teeth is justified in the lower arch, even though they will not provide optimal space and treatment time will be prolonged by the requirement for closure of space in the lower right quadrant. The distal caries in the LR4 was restored with composite.

In the maxillary arch, to align the UR3 would require extraction of the URC, surgical exposure of the UR3 and orthodontic traction. In addition, space would be required to achieve this as the URC crown is smaller than the UR3, there is already crowding amongst the erupted teeth in the upper arch and applying traction to the UR3 will be anchorage demanding. Several factors make orthodontic alignment of the UR3 unfavourable, namely the poor position of this tooth (high and displaced toward the midline) and the patient's age. Moreover, the extraction of a healthy UR4 to provide enough space for this tooth to be aligned is a potentially risky strategy if the UR3 does not move under traction. Attempting to erupt the canine will also significantly increase treatment time. In this case, it was therefore decided to extract the UR3 and URC. With the loss of two permanent tooth units in the lower arch and one unit in the upper right quadrant, it will be necessary to extract in the upper left quadrant. In this case there are really two candidates; either the restored UL4 or the UL6. Given the large restoration of the UL6, it was decided to extract this tooth. Following these extractions, fixed appliances were placed.

The final occlusion is shown in Figure 6.41.

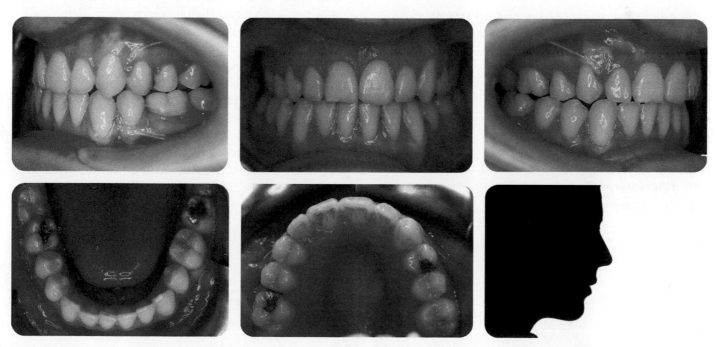

Figure 6.41

Case 6.11

This 16-year-old girl was referred by her general dental practitioner and was unhappy with the appearance of her teeth.

Summarize this malocclusion (Figure 6.42)

A class III incisor relationship on a mild skeletal class III pattern with increased vertical dimensions complicated by:

- Upper and lower arch crowding
- Bilateral buccal crossbites
- Reduced overbite
- Previous loss of UL4
- Centre line discrepancy.

Is there anything unusual about the centre line discrepancy?

Yes. The unilateral loss of the UL4 would increase the chances of the upper centre line being displaced to the left; however, in this girl the lower centre line is actually to the left of the upper by 2 mm. There are several things to consider during the clinical examination.

If the upper dental centre line is displaced to the left relative to the facial midline because of the absent UL4 (and indeed, the crowded UL2) this means that the lower dental centre line is quite markedly displaced, either due to a left-sided mandibular displacement on closing or a left-sided mandibular asymmetry. The LL3 is more crowded than the LR3, which might result in the lower dental centre line moving to the left a little, but this is unlikely to be by enough to explain a lower centre line that is more displaced to the left than the upper. If the upper dental centre line is coincident with the face, then the left-sided displacement of the lower is less severe and could be explained by the crowded LL3.

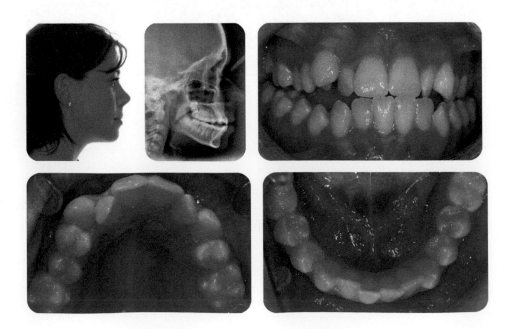

Figure 6.42

In reality, the upper dental centre line was essentially coincident with the face; space for the absent UL4 had been lost from behind.

What treatment options would you consider in this case?

The initial decision is to assess whether the malocclusion may be camouflaged. The patient was anxious to avoid a surgical solution and had no concerns in relation to her facial aesthetics. Consequently, a decision was made to treat the malocclusion orthodontically. Several clinical features of this malocclusion suggest that it can be treated orthodontically: an edge-to-edge incisor relationship can be achieved, there is no obvious pre-existing dento-alveolar compensation for the skeletal pattern and the skeletal class III pattern is mild.

The bilateral posterior crossbites were initially addressed with a quadhelix appliance to expand the buccal segments over a period of 4 months. This was followed by upper and lower fixed appliances in combination with extraction of the UR5 and both lower first premolars.

Comment on the extraction pattern

Lower first premolars provide maximum space to retract the lower incisors, correct the centre line and achieve a positive overbite. Extraction of the UR5 provides some space to align the upper arch, but allows the upper incisors to be kept in a forward position, which helps to achieve a class I incisor relationship.

What do you notice about the bracket on the LR3 in the left-hand panel of Figure 6.43?

A LL3 bracket has been used on the LR3 tooth. Consequently, the LR3 has assumed a distal crown angulation. This approach favours retraction of the mandibular incisors to correct the incisor relationship. In the right-hand panel of Figure 6.43, the bracket has been re-orientated; the tooth is now upright as the crown has moved mesially. The decision to change the bracket back was made as the incisor relationship had been fully corrected and some advancement of the lower anteriors was permissible to reduce the overjet and improve the canine intercuspation.

Is this result likely to be stable (Figure 6.44)?

Correction of the anterior crossbite should be stable as there is a positive overjet and overbite; little unfavourable growth arose during treatment and further unfavourable growth is unlikely. Maxillary arch expansion will require retention to limit constriction following active treatment. Alignment of the teeth will be maintained with upper and lower bonded retainers. These will be supplemented with an upper Hawley retainer to preserve the transverse increase, and a lower Essix-type retainer.

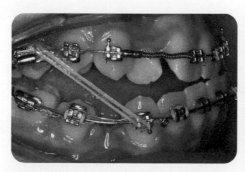 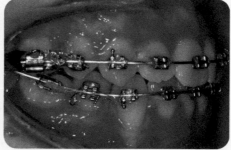

Figure 6.43

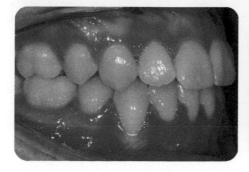 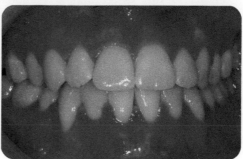

Figure 6.44

Case 6.12

This 16-year-old female was referred by her dentist as she was concerned about her crooked teeth that "stuck out". There was no relevant medical history.

Extra-oral

Skeletal relationship	
Antero-posterior	Mild skeletal class II
Vertical	Increased
Transverse	No asymmetry
Soft tissues	Lip competence: Incompetent but habitually held together
	Naso-labial angle: Average
Upper incisor show	Rest: 6 mm
	Smiling: 12 mm
Temporo-mandibular joints	No signs/symptoms. Good range of movements

Intra-oral

Teeth present

$$\frac{7654321/1234567}{7654321/1234567}$$

Dental health (restorations/caries)	Good
Lower arch	Crowding: Mild
	Incisor inclination: Proclined
	Curve of Spee: Flat
	Canines: Upright
Upper arch	Crowding: Mild
	Incisor inclination: Proclined
	Canines: Upright
Occlusion	Incisor relationship: Class III
	Overjet: 1 mm
	Overbite: Reduced and incomplete
	Molar relationship: Class 1 bilaterally
	Canine relationship: ¼ unit class II on the left; class I on the right
	Centre lines: Mandibular to left due to asymmetry of crowding
	Functional occlusion: Group function left and right

Summary

A 16-year-old female presented with a class III malocclusion on a mild skeletal class II base with increased vertical dimensions complicated by mild crowding and bi-maxillary protrusion (Figures 6.45 and 6.46).

Treatment Plan

The aims of treatment were to relieve crowding and reduce the bi-maxillary protrusion.

All four first bicuspids were extracted to create space and a pre-adjusted edgewise appliance was placed. After initial alignment with round nickel–titanium wires, rectangular stainless steel wires were placed and the labial segments were retracted using intra-arch elastics supported using short class II elastics (Figures 6.47, 6.48 and 6.49).

What is bi-maxillary protrusion?

Bi-maxillary dento-alveolar protrusion or proclination refers to anterior positioning and proclination of the upper and lower incisors in relationship to the underlying dental bases and soft tissues, often resulting in procumbency of the lips. It is more prevalent in patients of Afro-Caribbean and Asian descent. It is usually associated with a flat curve of Spee and reduced overbite or even frank anterior open bite resulting from the proclination of the incisors.

The dentition erupts and establishes itself in a zone of balance between the lips and cheeks on one side

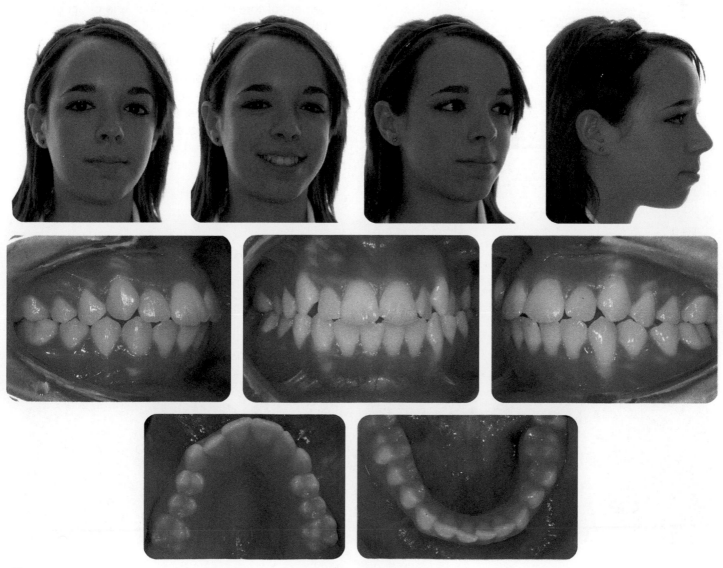

Figure 6.45

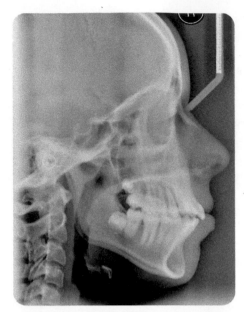

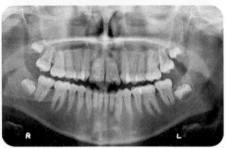

Figure 6.46

and the tongue on the other (Proffit, 1978); bi-maxillary protrusion is therefore often regarded to be in harmony with normal physiognomy and ethnicity. However, treatment is often sought due to concerns about perceived protrusion of the dentition and everted incompetent lip morphology.

How is it treated?

The aim of treatment is to retract the incisors and lips. Lip form is partly defined by the position of the underlying dentition and therefore, by moving the teeth, the soft tissue lip profile can be altered. However, this is not a simple, proportionate relationship with soft tissue responses notoriously difficult to predict and subject to large individual and ethnic variability (Talass et al., 1987). Indeed, in the presence of lip competence at the start of treatment, movement of the incisors will have little effect on the soft tissues. However, in cases of bi-maxillary protrusion, a predictable improvement in the profile can be achieved following extraction of premolars and fixed appliances (Leonardi et al., 2010).

To retract the incisors, space needs to be created. The decision as to whether extractions and anchorage are required depends on the extent to which the labial segments are to be moved. Generally, if the dental health is good, either the first or second bicuspids are

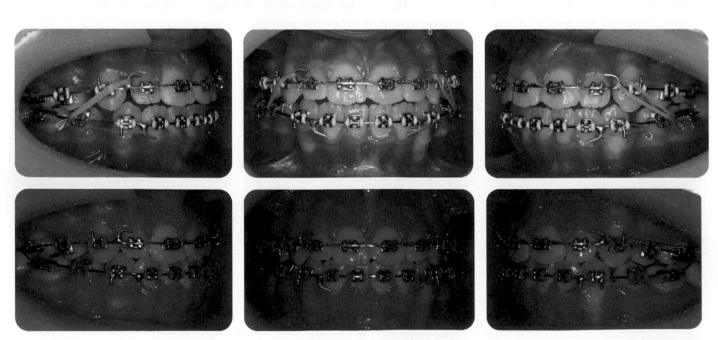

Figure 6.47

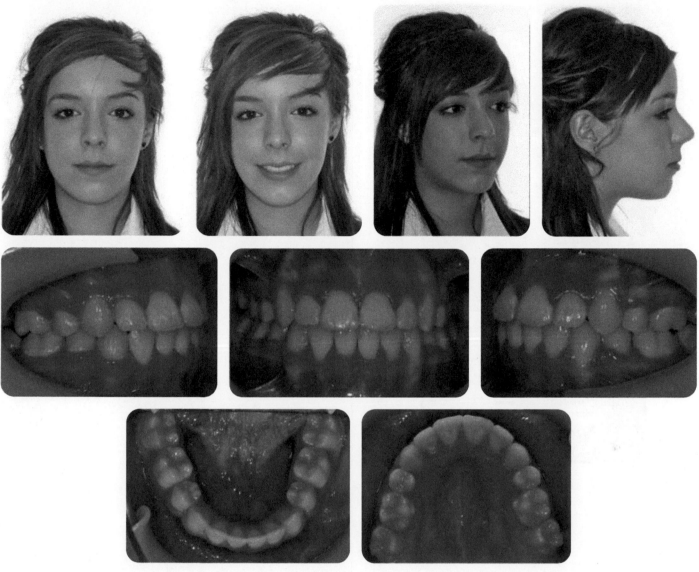

Figure 6.48

extracted and fixed appliances are used to retract the incisors. If maximum anchorage is required, headgear can be used, although skeletal anchorage, including temporary anchorage devices or mini-plates, now offers an attractive alternative. Inter-maxillary traction can also be used in the form of class II or III elastics.

How stable is the treatment?

Teeth erupt into a zone of balance between the soft tissues; disruption can result in an imbalance of forces, culminating in tooth movement. This is classically seen in adult patients with periodontal disease and drifting of the maxillary incisors labially. This is due to a

reduction of periodontal support of teeth, making them more susceptible to movement with lighter forces, and a change in the lip morphology with age as the lower lip moves inferiorly and no longer controls the upper incisors. The soft tissues, therefore, partly define the limits of tooth movement and in cases of bi-maxillary protrusion, by retracting the incisors out of this zone of balance, they will encroach on the space occupied by the tongue (Ackerman and Proffit, 1997). Retraction may therefore be unstable, necessitating permanent retention to prevent relapse in most cases.

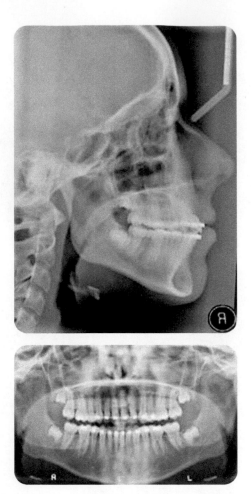

Figure 6.49

Case 6.13

This adult patient presented with a class III malocclusion.

What features of this malocclusion suggest that an orthognathic approach (orthodontics and jaw surgery) may be indicated (Figure 6.50)?

Extra-oral examination reveals a skeletal class III pattern, with a hypoplastic maxilla and prognathic mandible. There is a facial asymmetry with the chin point to the left of the facial midline.

If the patient is concerned about her facial features, in particular her mandibular asymmetry, this can only be addressed with a joint orthodontic–surgical approach.

Intra-orally, there is evidence of dento-aveolar compensation, with significant retroclination of the lower incisors and proclination of the upper incisors. There is a reduced overbite, with the upper and lower incisors almost edge to edge.

It would be difficult to achieve an ideal occlusion, with a positive overjet and overbite, with orthodontic camouflage alone.

There is a centre line discrepancy in this case, with the lower dental centre line to the left of the facial midline. What is the likely aetiology of this centre line discrepancy?

The lower dental centre line is coincident with the midline of the chin, which has deviated to the left as a result of the mandibular asymmetry. Therefore, the centre line discrepancy is skeletal in origin.

At what stage in treatment will centre line correction be achieved?

If this case is to be treated in conjunction with orthognathic surgery, with correction of the skeletal asymmetry, the lower dental centre line needs to be maintained in the middle of the chin during the pre-surgical orthodontics. Correction of the centre line will be achieved by surgery as a result of the correction of the mandibular asymmetry.

What factors need to be taken into account when planning the pre-surgical orthodontics in this case?

The pre-surgical orthodontics is planned around the surgery required to achieve optimal aesthetics and occlusion.

What factors need to be taken into account when planning the surgery?

The required surgery is planned around the aetiology of the skeletal discrepancy. In this case, the maxilla is hypoplastic and the mandible is prognathic. An assessment of the relative discrepancy in both jaws, taking into account facial aesthetics, allows the decision to made regarding whether the maxilla is to be advanced or the mandible set back, or a combination of these.

In this case, in order to address the mandibular asymmetry, a mandibular procedure is required. The surgical plan was made to advance the maxilla and set the mandible back, with rotation of the mandible to correct the mandibular asymmetry.

The upper incisor show at rest is minimal. It is recognized that advancing the maxilla will improve the incisor show.

The pre-treatment overbite is tenuous. In order to address this, the maxilla can be posteriorly impacted in addition to advancement, improving the overbite post surgically.

What occlusal factors need to be taken into account at pre-surgical planning?

- **Expansion:** Assessment of arch co-ordination using the pre-treatment models in a class I position will identify the extent of any required expansion of the maxillary arch.

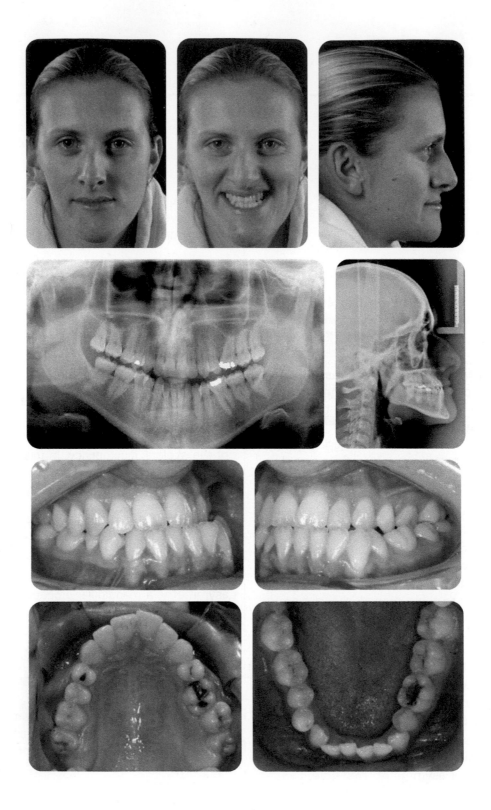

Figure 6.50

If minimal expansion is required, as in this case, this can be achieved using the orthodontic archwires during pre-surgical orthodontics. In this case, there is mild crowding in the upper arch and space will be created by the expansion required for arch co-ordination to alleviate the crowding. The expansion in the upper arch will help decompensate the upper arch, with some uprighting of the upper labial segment.

- **Reverse overjet:** The planned surgical moves for optimal aesthetics dictate the reverse overjet required pre-surgically. In this case, the patient has a minimal reverse overjet pre-treatment. In order to achieve the reverse overjet required to optimize the surgical moves, the crowding in the lower arch is addressed by proclination (decompensation) of the lower incisors.

Case 6.14

This malocclusion is to be treated with a combination of orthodontics and orthognathic surgery. The surgical plan in this case is maxillary advancement with anterior and posterior impaction; and mandibular set-back, with rotation to the right.

What features of the extra-oral appearance lead to this treatment plan (Figure 6.51)?

The patient has a skeletal class III pattern with a hypoplastic maxilla and a prognathic mandible, which is slightly to the left. She has increased vertical proportions, with minimal incisor show at rest and complete incisor crown show on smiling. Advancement of the maxilla will address the para-nasal hollowing, and result in further increase in incisor show, indicating the possible need for anterior impaction of the maxilla. Posterior impaction of the maxilla (greater than the anterior impaction, i.e. differential impaction) is required to address the reduced overbite and anterior open bite tendency. Mandibular set back with rotation to the right will address the prognathic mandible and mandibular asymmetry.

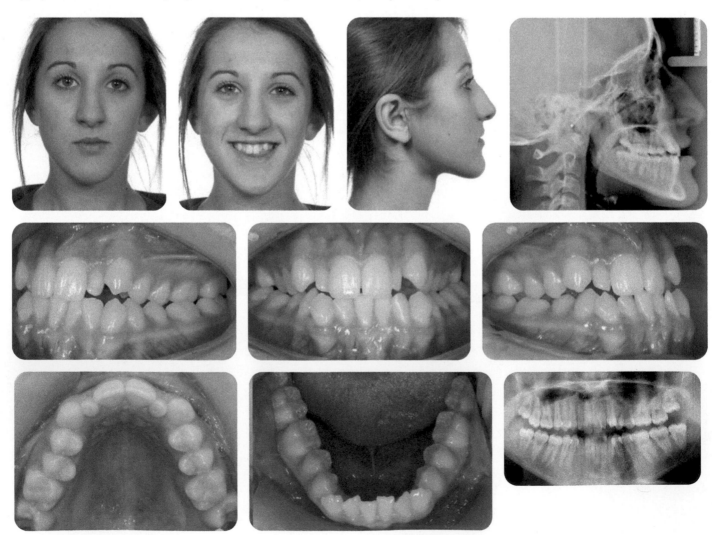

Figure 6.51

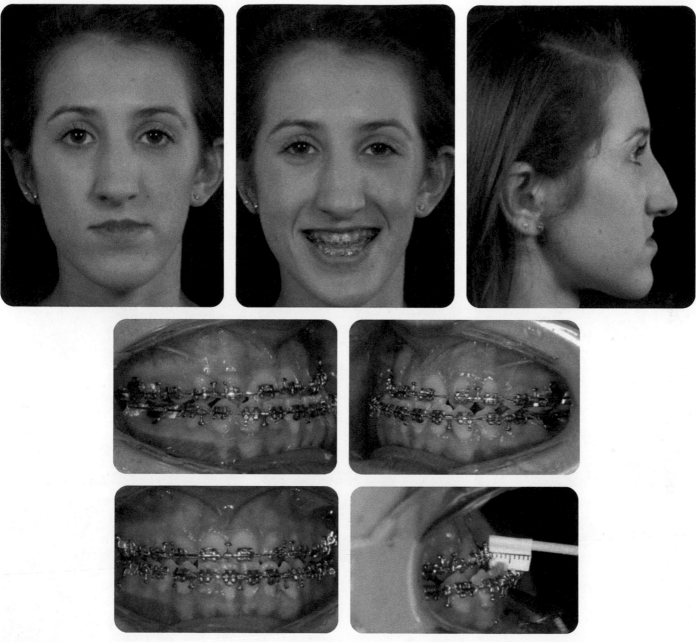

Figure 6.52

What are the aims of the pre-surgical orthodontics? How have these been achieved in this case (Figure 6.52)?

- **Levelling and alignment of the arches:** Alignment of the aches has occurred using flexible archwires at the start of pre-surgical orthodontics. Levelling occurs mainly in stainless steel archwires.
- **Arch co-ordination:** Assessment of future arch co-ordination is made from the pre-treatment study models. In this case, the required expansion of the upper arch could be achieved in a rectangular stainless steel archwire.
- **Decompensation:** In this case, decompensation of the upper and lower arches was required to produce an appropriate reverse overjet pre-surgically and allow the desired surgical movements to be carried out to promote the desired facial change. Decompensation of the upper arch requires

uprighting of the upper labial segment. This was carried out by extraction of the diminutive upper lateral incisors to create the appropriate space. In the lower arch, decompensation was carried out by proclination of the lower incisors.

- **Maintenance of the lower centre line with the mid-point of the chin:** In this case, the lower arch was treated on a non-extraction basis. As the lower centre line was coincident with the chin at the start of the pre-surgical orthodontics, this was maintained during levelling and aligning of the lower arch.

The final result is shown in Figure 6.53.

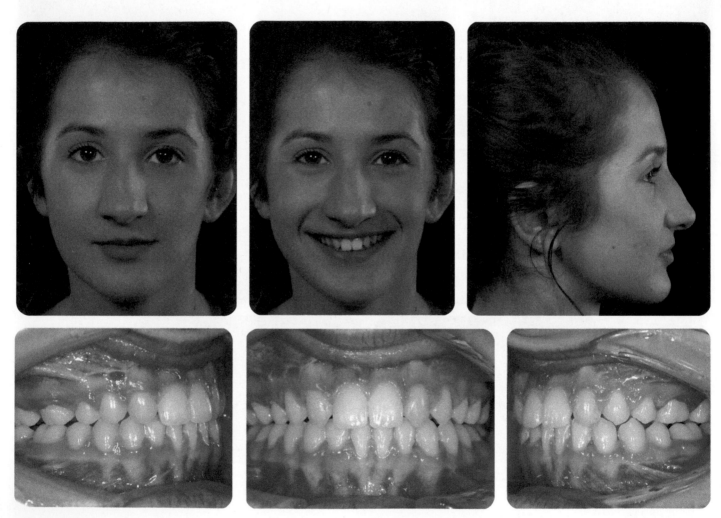

Figure 6.53

Case 6.15

This 9-year-old female presented with concerns in relation to her reversed bite and spacing between her upper front teeth. Cephalometric analysis confirmed the presence of a mild-to-moderate skeletal class III deformity (with some maxillary retrusion and mandibular protrusion) with average vertical skeletal proportions. The maxillary incisors were of average inclination (108 degrees). The panoramic view confirmed that dental development was in keeping with her chronological age. The maxillary second premolars were developing. There was no mandibular displacement.

Summarize the malocclusion (Figure 6.54)

A 9-year-old female presented with a class III malocclusion on a mild-to-moderate skeletal class III pattern in the mixed dentition complicated by:
- Reverse overjet (−3 mm)
- Crowding of both arches (but severe in the maxillary arch due to early loss of the Es)
- Palatally-displaced and crowded maxillary lateral incisors
- Space loss in the maxillary second premolar region.

What is the aetiology of the malocclusion?

- **Skeletal:** There is a skeletal class III deformity with both maxillary retrusion and mandibular prognathism. This has contributed to the class III incisor relationship and negative overjet.
- **Dento-alveolar:** There is a tooth size-to-arch length mismatch in both arches, resulting in crowding and palatal displacement of the maxillary lateral incisors. Dento-alveolar compensation has contributed to uprighting of the mandibular incisors, limiting the extent of the reversed overjet, but increasing the space deficiency in the mandibular arch.

- **Local factors:** Premature loss of the maxillary second primary molars has exacerbated the underlying dento-alveolar disproportion with severe crowding in the maxillary second premolar region. This will lead to their eventual impaction or palatal displacement.

Is treatment necessary in this case?

Treatment is not essential as there is no displacement associated with the anterior crossbite. Consequently, there is no likelihood of pathological tooth wear, gingival recession or temporo-mandibular joint symptoms. Nevertheless, treatment would be beneficial to facilitate eruption of the maxillary second premolars and for cosmetic reasons to address the class III incisor relationship.

In the short-term, eruption of the UL2 needs to be monitored. In this case, this tooth was close to eruption, erupting in a similar palatal position to the UR2 within 2 months.

What treatment could be considered in this case?

Treatment should be geared towards addressing the two most salient problems: reverse overjet and space loss in the maxillary second premolar region. Consequently, an upper sectional pre-adjusted edgewise appliance could be used to redistribute space in the upper arch, permit eruption of the second premolars and achieve upper anterior alignment. In addition, protraction headgear could be added to the fixed appliance to facilitate correction of the incisor relationship. The protraction headgear will need to be worn for a minimum of 14 hours per day to produce significant change.

Is there a disadvantage to using protraction headgear in this case?

Other than the generic disadvantages of using headgear, protraction headgear will tend to worsen the buccal segment crowding.

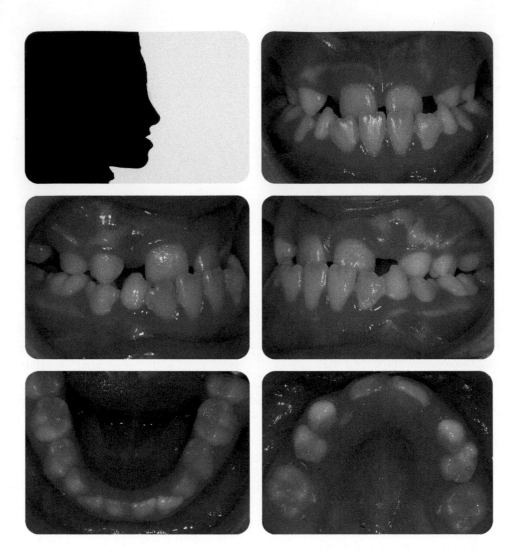

Figure 6.54

Are there any other treatment options?

A treatment alternative would include the use of a reverse functional appliance to correct the malocclusion. However, effects of this type of appliance are likely to be predominantly dento-alveolar in nature. Consequently, this approach is unlikely to be successful given the magnitude of the skeletal discrepancy, the large reverse overjet and absence of a displacement.

Similarly, while an upper fixed appliance in isolation would be capable of upper arch alignment and space redistribution to permit eruption of the second premolars, correction of the incisor relationship would not be possible with this approach. Addition, of reverse headgear, however, would allow all treatment objectives to be achieved, with 60% of the overjet increase attributable to skeletal changes (Gu *et al.*, 2000).

Alternatively, following eruption of the UL2, a simple removable appliance could be used to procline the upper incisors and correct the incisor relationship. This should be achievable within a few months and the presence of an overbite should prevent relapse. Further growth and development of the jaws and dentition could then be monitored. If this is favourable, fixed appliances could be used in the early permanent dentition to align the teeth and co-ordinate the dental arches, almost certainly in conjunction with premolar extractions. If the skeletal class III relationship worsens, then a combined orthodontic–surgical option should be considered. In this case, this would probably involve maxillary advancement and mandibular set-back with the loss of two premolars in the maxillary arch.

What are the likely effects of protraction facemask therapy?

A recent multi-centre randomized controlled trial in the UK has reported interim results on the effectiveness of early protraction facemask treatment for class III malocclusion in children under the age of 10 years. After 15 months of treatment, children undergoing early facemask therapy had 1.3 degrees more forward movement of SNA, almost 2 degrees less forward movement of SNB and an overall ANB improvement of around 2.6 degrees when compared to the control group. In addition, the overjet improved by more than 4 mm and the relative PAR score by more than 40% in the facemask compared to the control group. Thus, early class III protraction facemask treatment in patients under 10 years of age would seem to be skeletally and dentally effective in the short-term (Mandall et al., 2010).

Would you expect any difference in treatment outcome in an older patient?

There is believed to be a difference in outcome between subjects treated before the age of 10 years compared to more mature subjects. In particular, modification of maxillary position appears to be less easily carried out in older subjects. This advantage is counter-balanced by the likelihood of longer treatment and a greater premium on compliance and co-operation with early treatment (Franchi et al., 2004). Consequently, although correction of the incisor relationship may be attempted in older subjects, it is very important that the severity of the underlying skeletal pattern is taken into account when trying to achieve this.

What measure could have been performed to improve the alignment of the upper arch without recourse to active orthodontics?

Interceptive removal of the primary canines could have been undertaken. This would likely have improved the alignment of the incisors. This improvement is likely to be temporary, however, with crowding likely to appear as the canines erupt. In addition, there is evidence from prospective research that interceptive removal of primary canines actually exacerbates space conditions in the permanent dentition (Kau et al., 2004).

Treatment was carried out with a simple upper sectional fixed appliance and reverse headgear. The maxillary second premolars erupted into a good position (Figure 6.55). What definitive treatment is now likely to be required?

The residual occlusion has some mild crowding. In particular, there is underlying crowding in the maxillary canine region. Therefore, while it may be possible to complete treatment with upper and lower pre-adjusted edgewise appliances, given that the maxillary incisors have proclined quite significantly during the initial treatment phase, consideration should be given to premolar extractions to achieve alignment, a class I incisor relationship and normal axial inclination of these teeth. Final decisions will be made as the permanent dentition is established.

What other information is required at this stage?

The position of the maxillary canine teeth needs to be known and also of the mandibular second premolars.

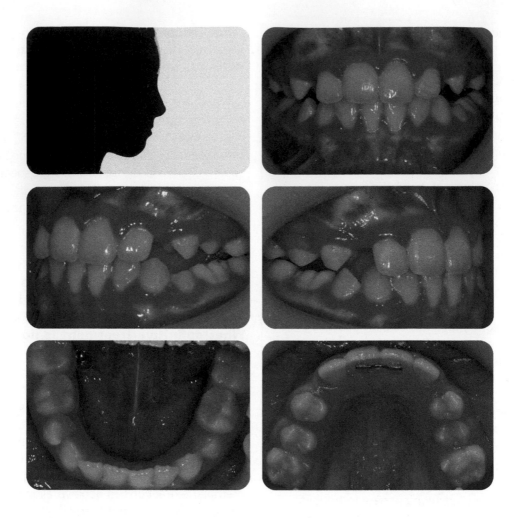

Figure 6.55

Case 6.16

This 12-year-old female was referred by her dentist due to crowding; however, she did not like the space between her front teeth.

Extra-oral

Skeletal relationship

  Antero-posterior   Mild skeletal class III

  Vertical   Average FMPA and lower face height

  Transverse   No asymmetry

Soft tissues   Lip competence: Competent

                              Naso-labial angle: Average

Upper incisor show   Rest: 6 mm

                              Smiling: 10 mm

Temporo-mandibular joints   No signs/symptoms

                              Good range of movements

Intra-oral

Teeth present

$$\frac{654\ \ 21/12\ \ 4E6}{6E\ \ 321/1234E6}$$

Dental health   Good

(restorations/caries)   Generalized mottling, probably due to fluorosis

Lower arch   Crowding: Mild

                              Incisor inclination: Average

                              Curve of Spee: Normal

                              Canines: Distally angulated

Upper arch   Crowding: Severe

                              Incisor inclination: Average

                              Canines: Palpable buccally but short of space.

Occlusion   Incisor relationship: Class III

                              Overjet: 2 mm

                              Overbite: Reduced and complete to upper central incisors

                              Molar relationship: Angle class I left; ½ unit class II right

                              Centre lines: Central and coincident

                              Functional occlusion: Group function left and right

Radiographic examination   All teeth except third molars were present with maxillary canines in the line of the arch

                              Cephalometric assessment confirmed a mild skeletal class III relationship with average maxillary–mandibular planes angle and incisor inclination

Summary

This 12-year-old female presented with a class III malocclusion on a mild skeletal class III base with average vertical dimensions complicated by severe crowding (Figures 6.56 and 6.57).

Treatment Plan

The aims of treatment were to relieve the crowding and create space for the maxillary canines, align the arches and achieve a class I incisor and buccal segment relationship.

Space was created in the maxillary arch using a Hilger's pendulum appliance (Figure 6.58). Once the maxillary first molars had been moved distally, a palatal arch with a Nance button was fitted and self-ligating pre-adjusted edgewise appliances (Innovation R) were placed. Open coil spring was used to re-allocate space in the maxillary arch, allowing the maxillary canines to erupt, at which point brackets were bonded to align them (Figure 6.59). Finally, a posterior cross-elastic was used to correct a crossbite on the right first molars and brackets were placed on the second molars to align them. Following removal of the fixed appliances, a lower bonded retainer was placed, and upper and lower vacuum-formed r etainers were provided for night-only wear (Figure 6.60). Active treatment time was 28 months.

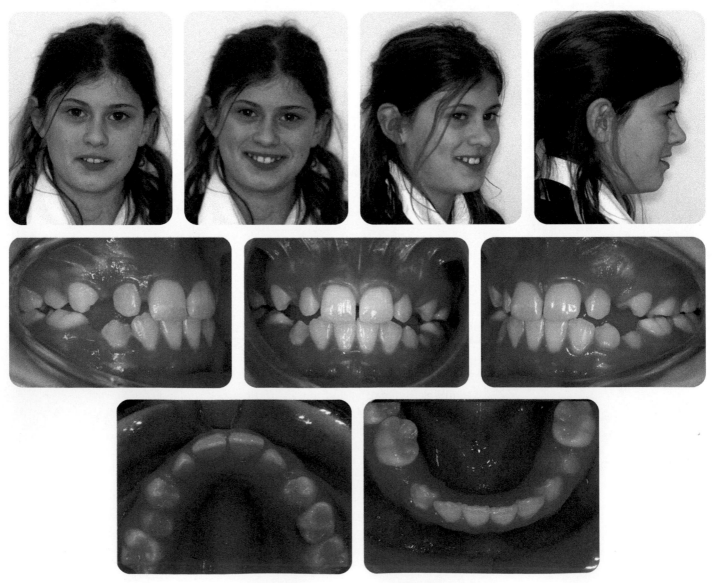

Figure 6.56

How does the pendulum appliance work?

The pendulum appliance is designed to move maxillary first molars distally (Hilgers, 1992). It uses the palate for anchorage through a large Nance palatal arch. Force is applied directly to the maxillary first molars using 'pendulum' helical TMA springs extending from the distal of the Nance button engaged into sleeves on the lingual aspect of bands on the first molars. The tendency for the molars to move palatally is countered by opening the U loop in the spring. If expansion is required, the Nance button can have an in-built screw which the patient activates.

It is one of a number of non-compliance appliances designed to create space without the need for extra-oral traction or headgear, thus reducing the reliance on compliance. Other appliances described have used compressed nickel–titanium springs or repelling magnets, again utilizing the palate for anchorage (Gianelly *et al.*, 1991; Bondemark and Kurol, 1992). The main problem is that, despite the incorporation of a palatal button, some anchorage loss is inevitable and the upper incisors will tend to advance; however, in the case presented this was desirable as there was a reduced overjet. Also, as force is applied to the molars, they will tip distally, risking anchorage loss as they are uprighted later in treatment (Bylott and Daendeliler, 1997). To address this, a passive Nance palatal arch was placed following distal molar movement (Figure 6.58, right panel). More recently, mini-implants and mini-plates have been used to provide skeletal anchorage against which teeth can be distalized (Kinzinger *et al.*, 2006).

Why was a lingual arch used (Figure 6.61)?

The combined mesio-distal width of the primary canine and molars is greater than that of the permanent canine and premolars. This excess is known as the leeway space. In the maxilla it amounts to approximately 1.5 mm per side, while in the mandible it is closer to 2.5 mm due to the greater size of the mandibular second primary molar. Usually this space allows mesial migration of the mandibular first permanent molar, establishing a class I relationship as

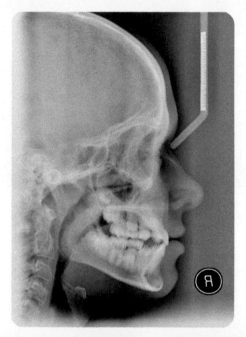

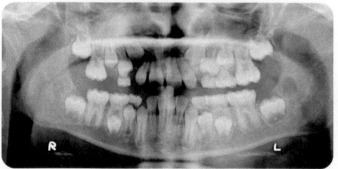

Figure 6.57

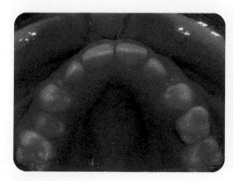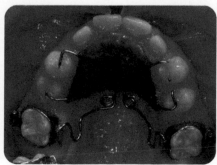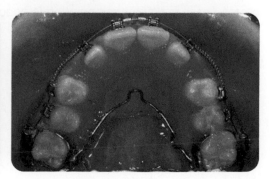

Figure 6.58

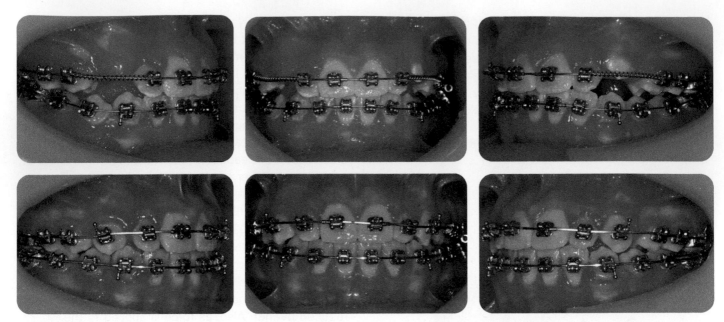

Figure 6.59

the primary molars are exfoliated and the permanent dentition becomes established. However, if the position of the permanent molar is maintained using a lingual arch, this space is available for the relief of labial crowding (Brennan and Gianelly, 2000). In this case, the lower first primary molars had been lost prematurely. The lingual arch was placed prior to loss of the second primary molars to maintain the arch length. Problems can arise from this as placement of a lingual arch can prevent the establishment of a class I molar relationship: the mandibular first molar does not migrate mesially and may necessitate subsequent distal movement of the maxillary molars, as in this case.

What alternative mechanics can be used to create space in the lower arch?

In the maxilla, headgear can be a very effective way to create space if patient co-operation is good. In the mandible, while headgear can be used, this is more problematic without restricting the mandibular movement and function.

An alternative technique is the use of a lip bumper. This utilizes the soft tissue pressure of the lower lip lying anterior to the lower incisors. This force is transferred to the lower molars via a rigid wire, uprighting them and promoting distal movement, particularly if the second molars are unerupted. As the lip bumper displaces the lips and cheeks away from the lower teeth, it will also result in passive expansion of the lower arch and proclination of the lower incisors under the unopposed influence of the tongue, which like all expansion of the lower labial segment tends to be unstable (O'Donnell et al., 1998). Despite this, the lip bumper is a popular adjunct in non–extraction-based orthodontic treatment (Cetlin and Ten Hoeve, 1983).

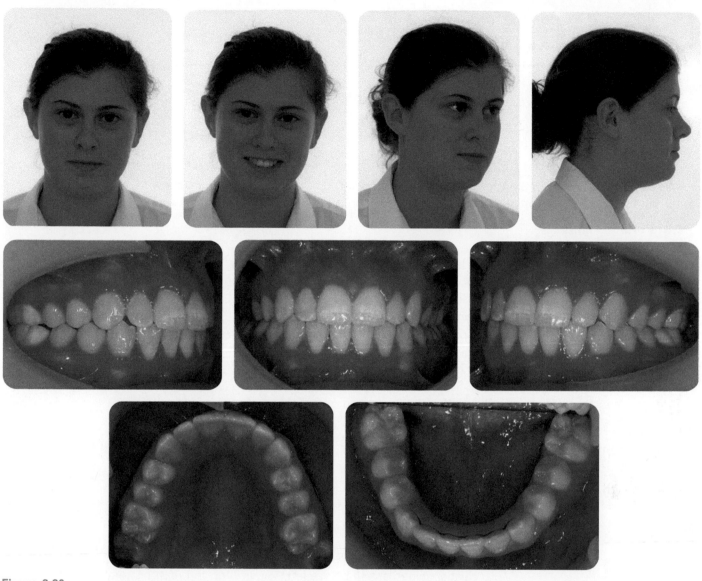

Figure 6.60

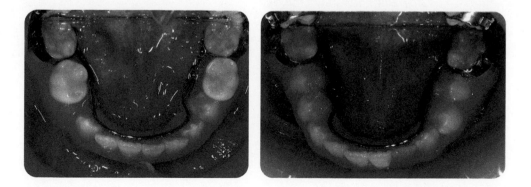

Figure 6.61

Case 6.17

This 10-year-old female was referred by her orthodontic specialist as she was unhappy with the appearance of her dentition and had masticatory difficulty.

Extra-oral

Skeletal relationship

Antero-posterior	Mild skeletal class III
Vertical	FMPA: Average
	Lower face height: Average
Transverse	Facial symmetry: None
Soft tissues	Lip competence: Competent with protrusive lower lip
	Naso-labial angle: Normal
Upper incisor show	At rest: 2 mm
	Smiling: 5 mm
Temporo-mandibular joint	Healthy with good range and co-ordination of movement

Intra-oral

Teeth present

6 4 21/12 456
654321/123456

Dental health (restorations, caries)	Good
	No active caries and excellent oral hygiene
Occlusion	Incisor relationship: Class III
	Overjet: −3 mm
	Overbite: Average and complete
	Molar relationship: Class III on the left; ½ unit II on the right bilaterally
	Anterior displacement on closing from RCP to ICP
Lower arch	Crowding: Spaced
	Incisor inclination: Retroclined
Upper arch	Crowding: Severely crowded
	Incisor inclination: Upright
	Canine position: Palpable buccally

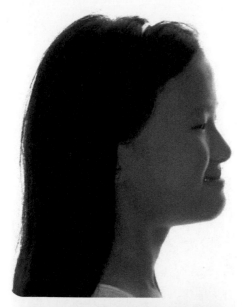

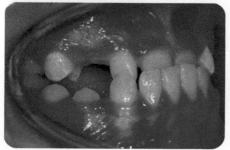

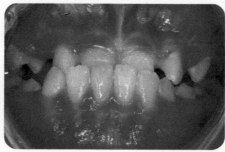

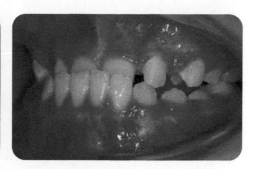

Figure 6.62

Summary

A 10-year-old female presented with a class III malocclusion on a mild skeletal class III base with average lower face height, well-aligned arches and an anterior crossbite with displacement, in the early permanent dentition (Figure 6.62). The malocclusion was complicated by an impacted UR5 and unerupted maxillary canines (with the UL3 crowded).

Treatment Plan

The primary aim was to correct the anterior crossbite and eliminate the occlusal displacement. Thereafter, comprehensive treatment would be directed at managing the impacted UR5, facilitating eruption of UL3 by consolidating space in the upper anterior region, aligning the arches and detailing the occlusion.

A reverse Twin Block was used to address the incisor relationship over a period of 7 months (Figure 6.63). Thereafter, a modified Nance palatal arch was fitted in conjunction with a sectional upper fixed appliance to initiate distal movement of the UR6. Subsequent, complete upper and lower fixed appliances were placed to complete space recreation for the impacted teeth and to complete arch alignment.

Comment on the active and retentive components of the reverse Twin Block

- **Active components:** Advancement of the maxillary incisors was promoted by cantilever springs palatal to the upper incisors. The acrylated lower labial bow could also be activated to retrocline the mandibular incisors. A midline screw was also included in the upper component to facilitate expansion.
- **Retentive components:** These keep the appliance securely in place during function, while resisting forces delivered by the active components. Adams cribs were placed on all first molars and maxillary first premolars as the lower first premolars had not erupted sufficiently to provide useful retention. An acrylated lower labial bow provided further retention

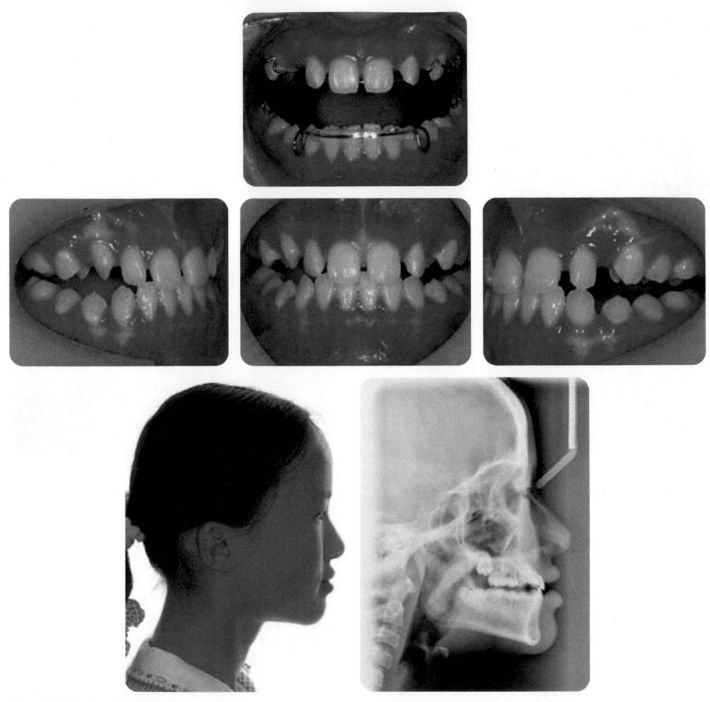

Figure 6.63

for the lower block. The intersecting blocks also enhance retention, making the appliances self-seating.

What alternatives may have been considered during the first phase of treatment?

- **Protraction headgear:** This approach would have facilitated a greater degree of skeletal change; however, the patient was reluctant to wear this appliance.

- **Removable appliance:** The effects of this appliance would be purely dento-alveolar in nature. This may well have been sufficient to address the malocclusion; however, retention of the appliance would have been problematic due to the number of teeth in crossbite.

- **Upper sectional fixed appliance (2 × 4 appliance):** This option would have permitted simultaneous correction of the crossbite and relocation of space for eruption of the impacted teeth. However, retraction of the lower incisors would not have been possible without recourse to a lower appliance, and elimination of the displacement may therefore have been impossible early in treatment.

What alternative plan may have been considered in the second treatment phase?

Consideration may have been given to removal of the impacted UR5. Consequently, the final molar relationship would have been class II on the right and class I on the left side. The premolar could have been removed prior to commencing treatment, which would have necessitated a surgical extraction. Alternatively, the procedure could be simplified by postponing removal until the premolar erupted in a palatal position.

What is the rationale for avoiding maxillary arch extractions in class III cases?

Upper arch extractions are limited in class III subjects to maintain a 'large' maxillary arch. This increases the likelihood of correcting the incisor relationship without recourse to either lower arch extractions or even a combined orthodontic–surgical approach. In essence, orthodontic camouflage may be promoted by both lower incisor retraction and maxillary incisor advancement.

In this case, the UR7 had yet to erupt, facilitating distal movement of the UR6 to permit space recreation for the impacted UR5 (Figure 6.64). There was also ample space between the upper incisors to allow relocation and encourage eruption of the UL3. The final occlusion is shown in Figure 6.65.

What alternatives could have been considered to effect distal movement of UR6?

- **Removable appliance:** A removable appliance with a palatal finger spring or split-plate and screw may have been used to distalize UR6. This feature could have been included in the design of the reverse Twin Block. A possible disadvantage of this approach is the potential for anchorage loss resulting in excessive advancement of the maxillary incisors. In addition, movement of the molar would have occurred by tipping; consequently, significant distal root movement would have been needed during the subsequent fixed phase.
- **Headgear:** Headgear may have been useful to reopen space for the premolar, particularly in view of the unerupted first molar. However, the use of headgear is contra-indicated in class III due to the potential of exacerbating the malocclusion.
- **Temporary anchorage devices:** The use of a mini-implant in the maxillary canine–premolar region could have been considered. The implant would then be used for indirect anchorage while applying a force to the first molar using open coil spring. This approach would best be deferred until the maxillary canine had erupted completely.
- **Other fixed distalizers:** A variety of other fixed distalizers could have been used as alternatives to the modified Nance palatal arch. In particular, a pendulum-type appliance may have been useful as a unilateral distalizer. A Jones' jig could also have been used in conjunction with a Nance palatal arch. Reciprocal advancement of the maxillary incisors is likely with any of these appliances unless they are implant-supported (Bolla *et al.*, 2002; Patel *et al.*, 2009). However, in this class III case some advancement of the incisors was desirable.

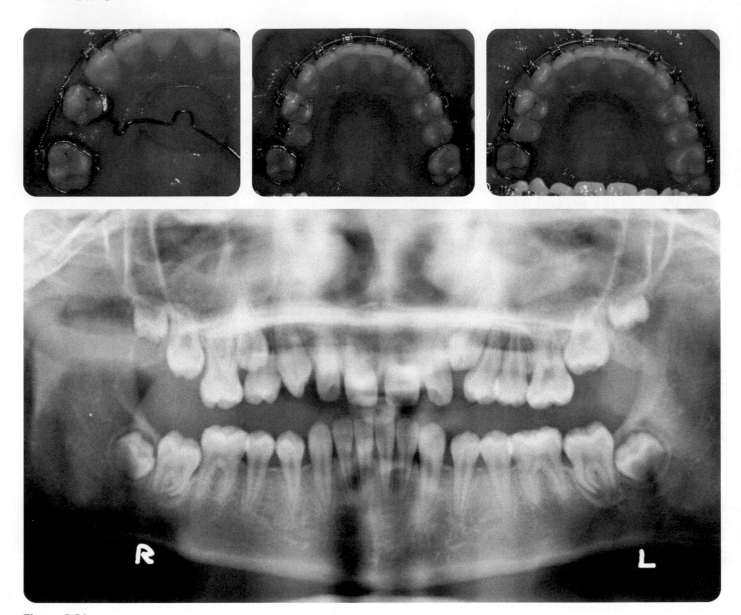

Figure 6.64

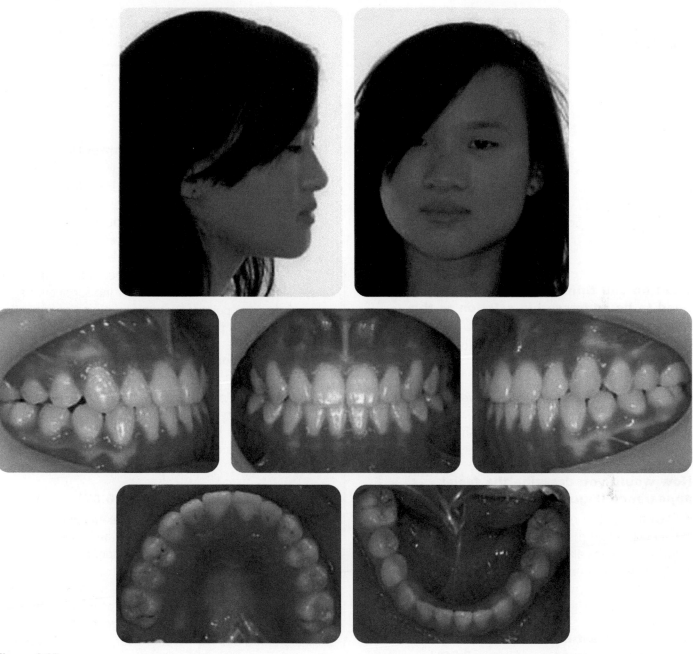

Figure 6.65

Case 6.18

This 18-year-old student was unhappy with her bite and the appearance of her teeth. She was medically fit and well and happy to undertake fixed appliance orthodontic treatment.

What do you think are the major issues that need to be addressed in relation to this malocclusion (Figure 6.66)?

- Class III incisor relationship (edge to edge)
- Anterior open bite (around 1 mm)
- Bilateral posterior crossbite
- Lower centre line discrepancy (lower off to the right by ½ incisor tooth unit)
- Class III molar and canine relationship
- Severe crowding in the upper arch

How would you describe the facial appearance (Figure 6.66)?

- Skeletal class III relationship with maxillary hypoplasia and mandibular hyperplasia
- Increased vertical proportions
- Mandibular asymmetry with the chin point over to the right
- Maxillary incisor tooth show a little reduced

Do the pre-treatment radiographs provide any additional information (Figure 6.66)?

- All four third molars are present and unerupted
- UR7 is unerupted in the panoramic radiograph but has erupted clinically
- Antero-posterior skeletal pattern is not severe
- Vertical proportions are increased
- Minimal incisor compensation for the skeletal pattern

How would you treat this case?

There are two options:
- Orthodontic camouflage
- Orthodontics and orthognathic surgery.

What are the limitations of camouflage?

It would probably be possible to align the teeth and obtain a class I incisor relationship using fixed appliances in conjunction with the extraction of four first premolar teeth. However, correcting the bilateral crossbite would require some arch expansion and this would make achieving a positive overbite difficult.

Camouflage would not correct the underlying skeletal pattern, increase the upper incisor show or correct the chin point, although dental centre line correction would probably be achievable.

What would combined treatment achieve?

Combined orthodontics and surgery would allow definitive correction of the occlusion and skeletal pattern, aiming to increase the upper incisor show, reduce the lower face height, bring the maxilla forward, take the mandible back and correct the chin point.

What has happened in Figure 6.67?

Orthodontic decompensation with fixed appliances has occurred. In particular, the maxillary arch has been aligned following extraction of the upper first premolars. It has been expanded to eliminate the crossbites, whilst the upper incisors have been maintained in their antero-posterior position. In the lower arch, the teeth have been aligned and the lower incisors proclined. The reverse overjet has increased and the centre line discrepancy maintained. The open bite has also been maintained.

The post-surgical occlusion is shown in Figure 6.68 and the radiographic changes in Figure 6.69. What surgical movements do you think have taken place and what have they achieved?

The maxilla has been moved forwards and impacted posteriorly. The mandible has been moved backwards and to the left. This has allowed dental centre line correction, and generation of a positive overbite and a class I incisor relationship. It has also improved the

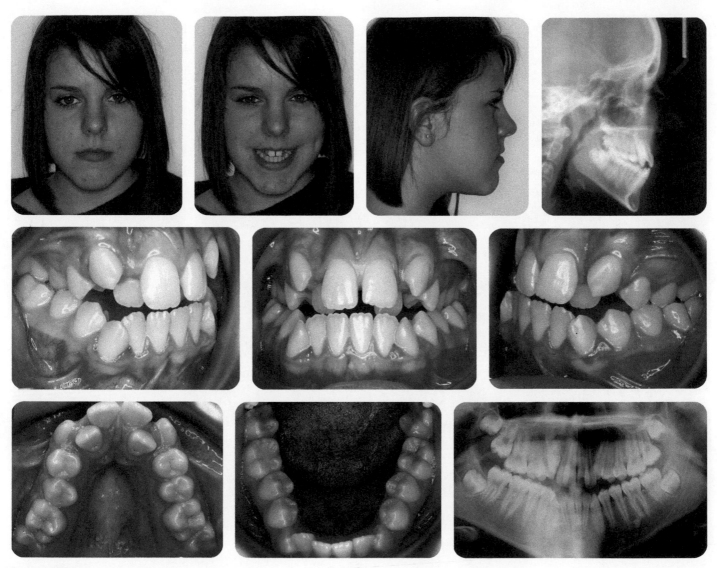

Figure 6.66

upper incisor show, and achieved a class I profile and facial asymmetry.

The occlusion 1 year post-treatment is shown in Figure 6.70. The patient is still wearing her Hawley retainers a few nights per week. What do you notice about the occlusion?

Dental alignment has been maintained but there has been some change in the occlusal position. In particular, the incisor and buccal segment relationship is a little more class III. The centre lines remain coincident.

What do you think has happened?

There has probably been some surgical relapse and the mandible has moved forward by about 1 mm bilaterally.

What would you advise?

Reassurance and continued part-time retainer wear. Mandibular set-back can be associated with some relapse and another 1 mm (in 50% of patients) or 2 mm (in 20%) of movement might occur.

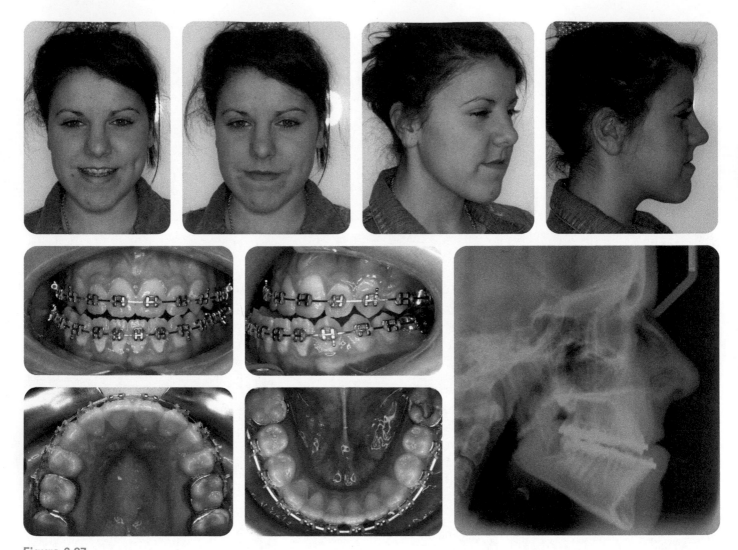

Figure 6.67

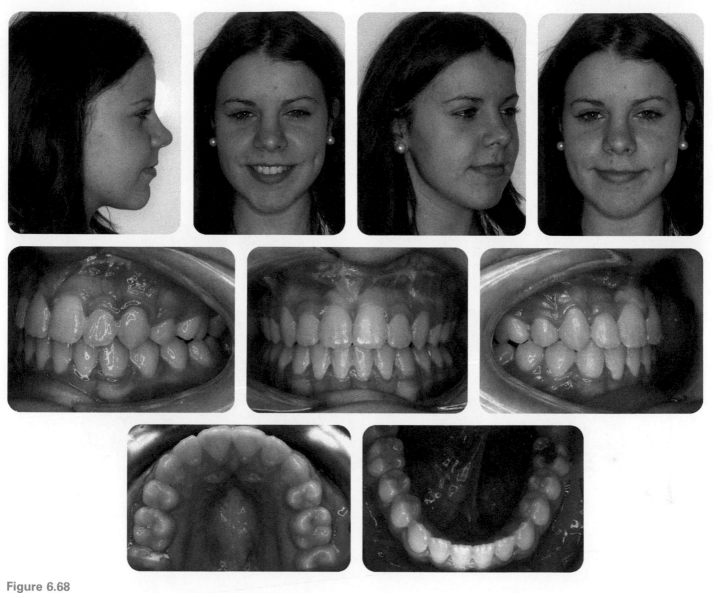

Figure 6.68

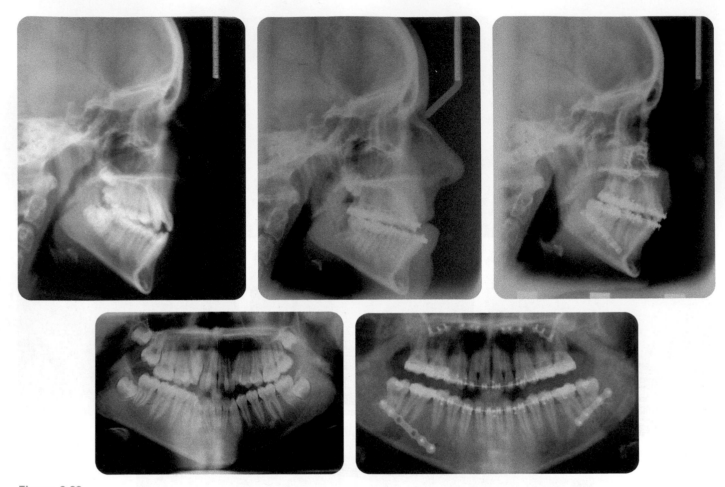

Figure 6.69

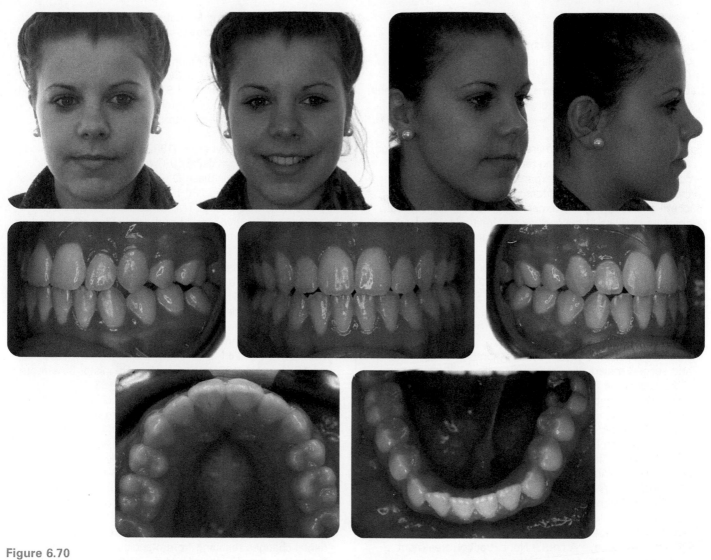

Figure 6.70

References

Ackerman JL, Proffit WR (1997) Soft tissue limitations in orthodontics: Treatment planning guidelines. *Angle Orthodontist* 67:327–336.

Baccetti T, Franchi, L, McNamara JA Jr (2000) Treatment and posttreatment craniofacial changes after rapid maxillary expansion and facemask therapy. *Am J Orthod Dentofacial Orthop* 118:404–413.

Baccetti T, Franchi L, McNamara JA Jr (2004) Cephalometric variables predicting the long-term success or failure of combined rapid maxillary expansion and facial mask therapy. *Am J Orthod Dentofacial Orthop* 126:16–22.

Baccetti T, Reyes BC, McNamara JA Jr (2007) Craniofacial changes in Class III malocclusion as related to skeletal and dental maturation. *Am J Orthod Dentofacial Orthop* 132171:e1–171 e12.

Battagel JM (1993) The aetiological factors in Class III malocclusion. *Eur J Orthod* 15:347–370.

Bolla E, Muratore F, Carano A, Bowman SJ (2002) Evaluation of maxillary molar distalization with the distal jet: a comparison with other contemporary methods. *Angle Orthod* 72:481–494.

Bondemark L, Kurol J (1992) Distalisation of maxillary first and second molars simultaneously with repelling magnets. *Eur J Orthod* 14:264–272.

Brennan MM, Gianelly AA (2000) The use of the lingual arch in the mixed dentition to resolve incisor crowding. *Am J Orthod Dentofac Orthop* 117:81–85.

Burns NR, Musich DR, Martin C, Razmus T, Gunel E, Ngan P (2010) Class III camouflage treatment: what are the limits? *Am J Orthod Dentofacial Orthop* 137:9 e1–9 e13; discussion 9–11.

Byloff FK, Ali Darendeliler M (1997) Distal molar movement using the pendulum appliance. Part 1: Clinical and radiological evaluation. *Angle Orthod* 67:249–260.

Cetlin NM, Ten Hoeve A (1983) Nonextraction treatment. *J Clin Orthod* 17:396–413.

Franchi L, Baccetti T, McNamara JA (2004) Postpubertal assessment of treatment timing for maxillary expansion and protraction therapy followed by fixed appliances. *Am J Orthod Dentofacial Orthop* 126:555–568.

Fudalej P, Kokich VG, Leroux B (2007) Determining the cessation of vertical growth of the craniofacial structures to facilitate placement of single-tooth implants. *Am J Orthod Dentofacial Orthop* 131(4 Suppl):S59–67.

Gu Y, Rabie AB, Hägg U (2000) Treatment effects of simple fixed appliance and reverse headgear in correction of anterior crossbites. *Am J Orthod Dentofacial Orthop* 117:691–699.

Gianelly AA, Bednar J, Dietz VS (1991) Japanese NiTi coils used to move molars distally. *Am J Orthod Dentofac Orthop* 99:564–566.

Guyer EC, Ellis EE 3rd, McNamara JA Jr, Behrents RG (1986) Components of class III malocclusion in juveniles and adolescents. *Angle Orthod* 56:7–30.

Haas AJ (1973) Rapid palatal expansion: A recommmended prerequisite to Class III treatment. *Trans Eur Orthod Soc* 311–318.

Hagg U, Tse A, Bendeus M, Rabie AB (2003) Long-term follow-up of early treatment with reverse headgear. *Eur J Orthod* 25:95–102.

Hilgers JJ (1992) The Pendulum appliance for class II non-compliance therapy. *J Clin Orthod* 16:706–714.

Kau CH, Durning P, Richmond S, Miotti FA, Harzer W (2004) Extractions as a form of interception in the developing dentition: a randomized controlled trial. *J Orthod* 31:107–114.

Kerr WJ, Miller S, Dawber JE (1992) Class III malocclusion: surgery or orthodontics? *Br J Orthod* 19:21–24.

Kidner G, DiBiase A, DiBiase D (2003) Class III Twin Blocks: a case series. *J Orthod* 30:197–201.

Kim JH, Viana MA, Graber TM, Omerza FF, BeGole EA (1999) The effectiveness of protraction face mask therapy: a meta-analysis. *Am J Orthod Dentofacial Orthop* 115:675–685.

Kinzinger GS, Diedrich PR, Bowman SJ (2006) Upper molar distalization with a miniscrew-supported Distal Jet. *J Clin Orthod* 40:672–678.

Leonardi R, Annunziata A, Licciardello V, Barbato E (2010) Soft tissue change following the extraction of premolars in non-growing patients with bimaxillary protrusion. *Angle Orthodontist* 80:211–216.

Loh MK, Kerr WJ (1985) The Function Regulator III: effects and indications for use. *Br J Orthod* 12:153–157.

Mandall N, DiBiase A, Littlewood S, et al. (2010) Is early Class III protraction facemask treatment effective? A multicentre, randomized, controlled trial: 15-month follow-up. *J Orthod* 37:149–161.

McKeown HF, Sandler J (2001) The two by four appliance: a versatile appliance. *Dent Update* 28:496–500.

Ngan P, Yiu C, Hu A, Hagg U, Wei SH, Gunel E (1998) Cephalometric and occlusal changes following maxillary expansion and protraction. *Eur J Orthod* 20:237–254.

O'Donnell S, Nanda RS, Ghosh J (1998) Perioral forces and dental changes resulting from mandibular lip bumper treatment. *Am J Orthod Dentofac Orthop* 113:247–255.

Patel MP, Janson G, Henriques JF, et al. (2009)_Comparative distalization effects of Jones jig and pendulum appliances. *Am J Orthod Dentofacial Orthop* 135:336–342.

Proffit WR (1978) Equilibrium theory revisited. *Angle Orthod* 48:175–186.

Schuster G, Lux CJ, Stellzig-Eisenhauer A (2003) Children with class III malocclusion: development of multivariate statistical models to predict future need for orthognathic surgery. *Angle Orthod* 73136–145.

Severt TR, Proffit WR (1997) The prevalence of facial asymmetry in the dentofacial deformities population at the University of North Carolina. *Int J Adult Orthod Orthognath Surg* 12:171–176.

Skeggs RM, Sandler PJ (2002) Rapid correction of anterior crossbite using a fixed appliance: a case report. *Dent Update* 29:299–302.

Stellzig-Eisenhauer A, Lux CJ, Schuster G (2002) Treatment decision in adult patients with Class III malocclusion: orthodontic therapy or orthognathic surgery? *Am J Orthod Dentofacial Orthop* 122:27–37; discussion 37–38.

Suda N, Ishii-Suzuki M, Hirose K, Hiyama S, Suzuki S, Kuroda T (2000) Effective treatment plan for maxillary protraction:

is the bone age useful to determine the treatment plan? *Am J Orthod Dentofacial Orthop* 118:55–62.

Sugawara J, Asano T, Endo N, Mitani H (1990) Long-term effects of chincap therapy on skeletal profile in mandibular prognathism. *Am J Orthod Dentofacial Orthop* 98:127–133.

Talass MF, Talass L, Baker RC (1987) Soft-tissue profile changes resulting from retraction of maxillary incisors. *Am J Orthod Dentofacial Orthop* 91:385–394.

Thickett E, Taylor NG, Hodge T (2007) Choosing a pre-adjusted orthodontic appliance prescription for anterior teeth. *J Orthod* 34:95–100.

Ulgen M, Firatli S (1994) The effects of the Frankel's function regulator on the Class III malocclusion. *Am J Orthod Dentofacial Orthop* 105:561–567.

Vaughn GA, Mason B, Moon HB, Turley PK (2005) The effects of maxillary protraction therapy with or without rapid palatal expansion: a prospective, randomized clinical trial. *Am J Orthod Dentofacial Orthop* 128:299–309.

Wells AP, Sarver DM, Proffit WR (2006) Long-term efficacy of reverse pull headgear therapy. *Angle Orthod* 76:915–922.

Xue F, Wong RW, Rabie AB (2010) Genes, genetics, and Class III malocclusion. *Orthod Craniofac Res* 13:69–74.

7

Tooth Impaction

Introduction

Failure of eruption or impaction of a tooth is a commonly encountered problem in orthodontics and affects almost 20% of the general population. With the exception of third molars, the most commonly impacted permanent teeth occur in the maxilla and include canines, second molars, central incisors and first molars (Kurol and Bjerklin, 1982; Bishara, 1992; Bondemark and Tsiopa, 2007). General causes of failed eruption include mechanical obstruction, ectopic dental development with the tooth assuming an abnormal position, or a failure of the eruption process itself.

Causes of mechanical obstruction include crowding, resulting in insufficient space to accommodate the tooth in the dental arch, and the presence of supernumerary teeth physically blocking the tooth from erupting; the latter being the main cause of the failure of eruption of maxillary central incisors. Manifestations of ectopic dental development include palatally displaced maxillary canines, maxillary first molars impacted against the second primary molar and, less commonly, dental transpositions.

The reasons for tooth ectopia remain poorly understood. While there is a definite genetic component to true transpositions (Ely *et al.*, 2006), the aetiology of ectopic eruption of palatally impacted maxillary canines is less clear. Epidemiologically, there are racial and gender differences, implying a degree of familial inheritance (Peck *et al.*, 1994). There is also an association with aberrant or missing lateral incisors, implying that eruption of the canine is guided by the root of the lateral incisor and indicating a mechanical cause for the ectopia (Brin *et al.*, 1986). However,

given that tooth size and form is also under genetic control, ectopic maxillary canines in conjunction with absent or diminutive lateral incisors also implicates an inherited pattern in ectopia. Failure of the eruptive process is also seen in teeth that have become ankylosed following trauma and in cleidocranial dysplasia.

Occasionally, teeth can fail to erupt or to erupt fully, with no obvious cause for the defective eruption. This rare condition may affect a group of teeth (primary failure of eruption) or may be confined to one tooth (mechanical failure of eruption) with teeth posterior to the affected tooth erupting normally (Proffit and Vig, 1981; Frazier-Bowers *et al.*, 2007). Specific mutations leading to primary failure of eruption have been identified (Frazier-Bowers *et al.*, 2010).

Correct diagnosis of unerupted teeth requires comprehensive records, often involving radiographs to locate the tooth and identify any associated pathology. Location usually involves two radiographs taken at different angles to the impacted tooth using the principle of parallax, whereby apparent movement of an impacted tooth will occur due to movement of the X-ray tube. The advent of cone beam computed tomography (CT) scanning has helped in accurately locating impacted teeth, highlighting higher levels of root resorption of adjacent teeth than are apparent on normal films (Walker *et al.*, 2005). Three-dimensional imaging is also becoming increasingly useful in planning treatment and mechanics, permitting visualization of the potential path of eruption, particularly for palatally ectopic canines (Ericson and Kurol, 1987, 2000a).

Clinical Cases in Orthodontics, First Edition. Martyn T. Cobourne, Padhraig S. Fleming, Andrew T. DiBiase, and Sofia Ahmad.
© 2012 Martyn T. Cobourne, Padhraig S. Fleming, Andrew T. DiBiase, and Sofia Ahmad. Published 2012 by Blackwell Publishing Ltd.

Whilst asymptomatic impacted third molars may be routinely left untreated, problems may arise with unerupted teeth, including dentigerous cyst formation and pathological resorption of adjacent teeth. Active management varies depending upon the presentation, particularly the position of the impacted tooth and the underlying malocclusion. Treatment may range in complexity from simple interceptive removal of the overlying primary tooth to mechanical eruption, surgical removal or even auto-transplantation of the impacted tooth (Ericson and Kurol, 1988a). With profound failure of the eruptive process, the options are more limited, as these teeth are invariably not amenable to orthodontic tooth movement. In general, however, optimal treatment usually involves space redistribution to accommodate the impacted tooth in the dental arch, followed by surgical exposure if the tooth fails to erupt with mechanical traction via an orthodontic fixed appliance. Thus, the management of impacted teeth routinely necessitates a multidisciplinary approach involving both orthodontist and oral and maxillofacial surgeon.

Case 7.1

This 13-year-old female was referred by her orthodontic specialist in relation to an ectopic lower premolar. There was no relevant medical history.

Extra-oral

Skeletal relationship

    Antero-posterior   Skeletal class II

    Vertical   FMPA: Average

                                 Lower face height: Average

    Transverse   Facial asymmetry: None

Soft tissues   Normal protrusion

                                 Lip competence: Competent

                                 Naso-labial angle: Obtuse

Upper incisor show   At rest: 3 mm

                                 Smiling: 7 mm

Temporo-mandibular joint   Healthy with good range and co-ordination of movement

Intra-oral

Teeth present

654321/123456
7654321/1234E67

Dental health   Good
(restorations, caries)

Oral hygiene   Good

Lower arch   Crowding: Moderate

                                 Incisor inclination: Average

                                 Curve of Spee: Average

Upper arch   Crowding: Moderate

                                 Incisor inclination: Average

                                 Canine position: Buccal

Summarize the occlusal features (Figure 7.1)

- Incisor relationship: Class I
- Overjet: 2 mm
- Overbite: Reduced and complete
- Canine relationship: Class I on left; ½ unit class II on right
- Molar relationship: Class I on right; ½ unit class II on left
- Centre lines: Co-incident with each other and facial midline

What additional information does the panoramic radiograph provide (Figure 7.2)?

The LL5 is ectopic, being horizontally orientated. The follicle surrounding this tooth is slightly enlarged. Some minor root resorption of the LLE has occurred; however, the form and length of the roots are good, and there is no caries or coronal restoration.

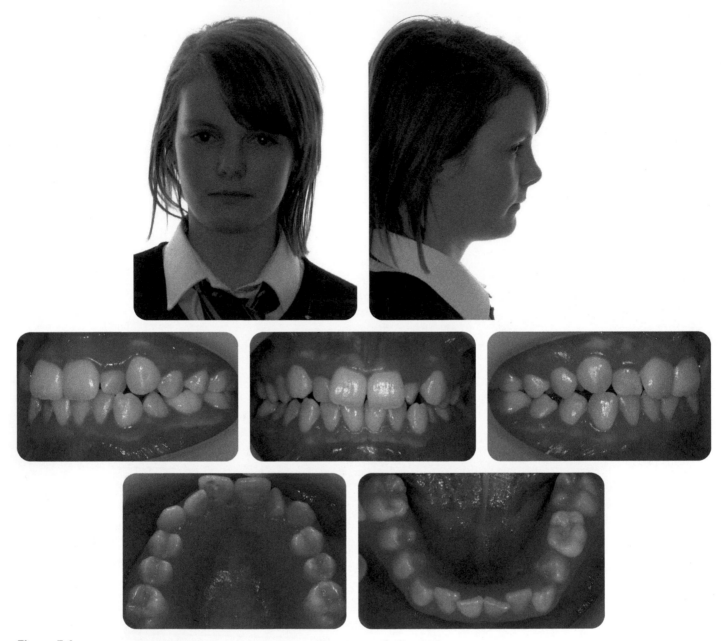

Figure 7.1

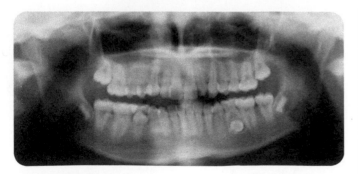

Figure 7.2

Summary

A 13-year-old female presented with a class I incisor relationship on a mild skeletal class II base complicated by the presence of an impacted LL5 in a poor developmental position and a retained LLE (Figure 7.1).

Treatment Plan

- Surgical removal of the LL5 and extraction of the UR4, UL4, LR5 and LLE
- Upper and lower pre-adjusted edgewise appliances
- Long-term retention
  The final occlusal result is shown in Figure 7.3.

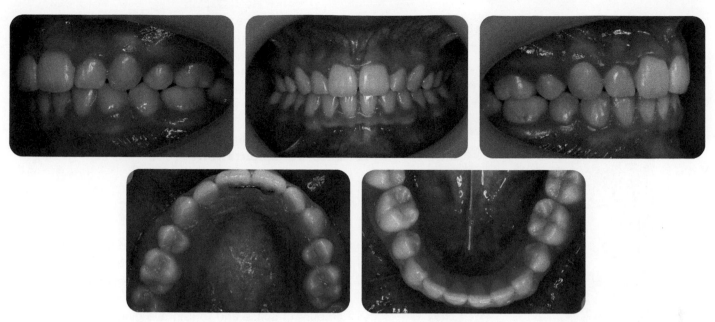

Figure 7.3

Why are the LL5, UR4, UL4, LR5 and LLE being extracted?

The ectopic position of the LL5 tooth is not favourable for surgical exposure and accommodation in the lower arch. The presence of moderate crowding in both arches means that space is required for alignment and this is provided by loss of the LLE, LL5 and three further premolar units.

Could this patient have been treated without extractions? If so, comment on the relative merits of such an approach in this case

Yes. This approach would have allowed advancement of the labial segments to provide additional soft tissue support and improve the facial profile. This would have placed a premium on permanent fixed retention in the lower labial segment to limit relapse potential. Furthermore, mechanical eruption and alignment of the LL5 would have been complex and prolonged, extending treatment time significantly. If mechanical eruption of the LL5 were unsuccessful, prosthetic replacement of the LL5 would have been necessary. Therefore, an alternative plan may have involved removal of the LL5 only, with indefinite preservation of the LLE. However, surgical removal of the LL5 without causing any damage to the LLE might be difficult to achieve.

Is there any association between an enlarged dental follicle and dentigerous cyst formation?

The follicular sizes of unerupted canines developing ectopically and those developing normally have been compared (Ericson and Bjerklin, 2001). Little difference in follicle size was noted between the groups. Follicles developing into cysts were also indistinguishable on CT scans from those that had been enlarged physiologically.

Could auto-transplantation of the LL5 have been considered?

Yes. If this approach were undertaken, the malocclusion would have been treated on a non-extraction basis. However, this approach was not considered viable, as auto-transplantation requires successful atraumatic removal. As the LL5 was severely displaced, this would not have been possible. Furthermore, the ideal time had passed, as in excess of two-thirds of the root of the LL5 had formed.

How successful is auto-transplantation of teeth?

Success rates of up to 98% have been reported in Scandinavia (Andreasen *et al.*, 1990; Czochrowska *et al.*, 2002). However, success is related to careful

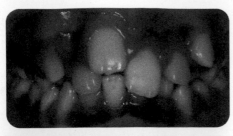

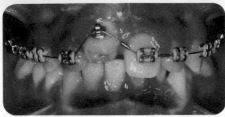

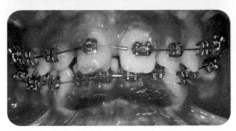

Figure 7.4

surgical technique and experience. Transplants are performed less frequently in the UK and North America. However, a recent retrospective analysis of maxillary canine transplantation carried out in a UK hospital setting has suggested a mean survival period for transplants of over 14 years (Patel *et al.*, 2011).

What factors influence the success rate of auto-transplantation?

- Surgical technique
- Degree of root maturity
- Donor tooth and site
- Size of the apical foramen

Transplantation of mandibular second premolars to the maxillary central incisor region is particularly successful (Kvint *et al.*, 2010). The second premolar is rotated 90 degrees to occupy the correct amount of space and to improve gingival aesthetics. In Figure 7.4 a mandibular second premolar has been autotransplanted to replace a UR1.

Case 7.2

This 26-year-old female was referred by her orthodontic specialist due to concerns in relation to her mobile primary canine teeth.

Extra-oral

Skeletal relationship

Antero-posterior	Skeletal class I
Vertical	FMPA: Average
	Lower face height: Average
Transverse	Facial asymmetry: None
Soft tissues	Lip competence: Competent
	Naso-labial angle: Average
Upper incisor show	At rest: 3 mm
	Smiling: 8 mm
Temporo-mandibular joint	Healthy with good range and co-ordination of movement

Intra-oral

Teeth present

7654C21/12C4567
7654321/1234567

Dental health (restorations, caries)	Good
	Restorations in first permanent molars
Oral hygiene – periodontal	Good
Lower arch	Crowding: Mild
	Incisor inclination: Average
	Curve of Spee: Average
Upper arch	Crowding: Mild
	Incisor inclination: Average
	Canines unerupted

Summarize the occlusal features in Figure 7.5

- Incisor relationship: Class I
- Overjet: 3 mm
- Overbite: Average and complete
- Canine relationship: Both primary maxillary canines retained
- Molar relationship: Class I on left; ¼ unit class II on right
- Centre lines: Upper 2 mm to left and lower 1 mm to right of facial midline
- Functional occlusion: Group function

Describe the position of the maxillary canines (Figure 7.6)

Both maxillary canines are ectopic. The UR3 is vertically-orientated, with the tip overlying the lateral incisor. The UL3 is severely displaced. On the panoramic view, the canine tip has crossed the midline of the central incisor, has a mesial angulation and is also vertically displaced. There is no evidence of associated pathology.

The position of the UL3 can also be assessed using vertical parallax. The tooth appears to move upwards

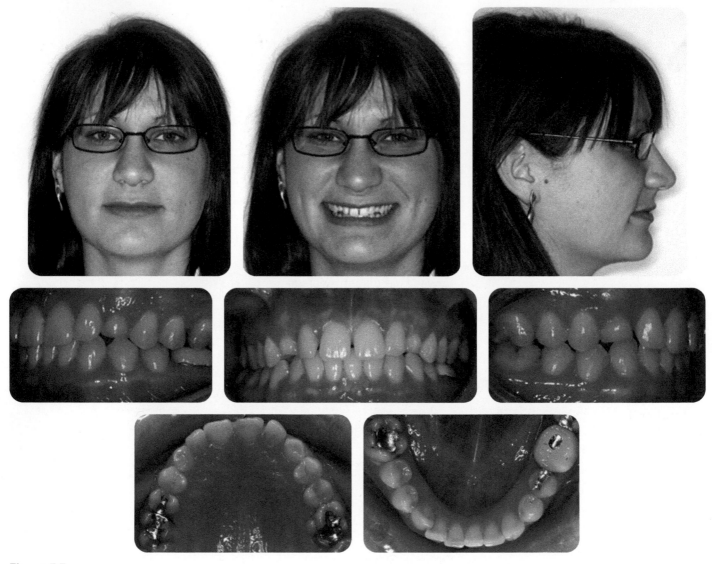

Figure 7.5

on the anterior occlusal view relative to the adjacent central incisor when compared to its relationship to this tooth on the panoramic view. As the tooth has appeared to move in the direction of the tube-shift, it is palatally placed.

Summary

A 26-year-old female presented with a class I malocclusion on a skeletal class I pattern with average vertical dimensions complicated by ectopic palatal maxillary canines (Figures 7.5 and 7.6).

Treatment Plan

- Extraction of the primary canines and surgical open exposure of the maxillary permanent canines
- Upper and lower pre-adjusted edgewise appliances to align the teeth and accommodate the canines
- Long-term retention

List the reasons for the high prevalence of impacted maxillary canines

- Long, tortuous eruption path
- Displacement of developing tooth germ
- Congenital absence of maxillary lateral incisors
- Diminutive maxillary lateral incisors
- Commonly erupts after the maxillary first premolar, making it susceptible to crowding
- Retention of primary canines
- Ankylosis
- Trauma
- Pathology

What appliances may be used to mechanically erupt maxillary canines?

Although upper or lower removable appliances may be used as adjuncts to permit eruption of canines, the mainstay of treatment involves fixed appliances.

What auxiliaries may be used in conjunction with fixed appliances to permit mechanical eruption?

- Elastomeric traction
- Piggy-back archwires
- Customized auxiliaries

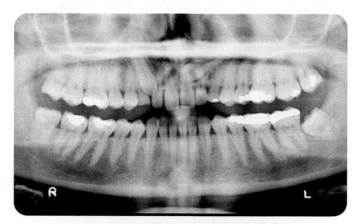

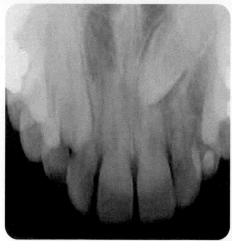

Figure 7.6

What was used in this case (Figure 7.7)?

A trans-palatal arch with two auxiliary springs was fitted. This has the advantage of re-enforcing anchorage and providing a means of applying a distally-orientated extrusive force on the canines.

What reactionary forces may arise during treatment?

A reactionary intrusive force on the adjacent teeth may arise. Mesial tipping of the maxillary buccal segments and narrowing of the maxillary arch may also occur.

How are unfavourable reactionary forces minimized during eruption of the canine?

Mesial tipping of the buccal segments and constriction of the maxillary arch may be limited by the use of a trans-palatal arch. Vertical anchorage may be augmented using rigid stainless steel base archwires (0.018 or 0.019 × 0.025 inch) while applying vertical traction to the displaced tooth. Temporary anchorage devices may also be used to facilitate distal and vertical canine movement while resisting reactionary forces.

What type of surgical exposure of impacted canines may be undertaken?

- Open exposure
- Apically-repositioned flap
- Closed exposure and bonding

What factors govern the choice of exposure type?

Exposure type is governed primarily by the position of the tooth and individual preferences of the treating clinicians. Superficial palatally-displaced canines lend themselves to open surgical exposure; deeper impactions and those in the line of the arch are more

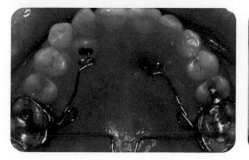

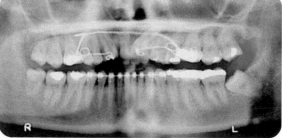

Figure 7.7

suited to closed exposure and bonding to avoid excessive bone removal and damage to adjacent teeth, respectively. Apically-repositioned flaps may be considered with teeth lying labially or in the line of the dental arch where the crown is covered by a band of attached gingiva.

What is the expected duration of treatment to align an ectopic canine?

Treatment duration varies considerably for canine ectopia, with more severe impactions likely to require an extended period of treatment. An average treatment duration of almost 29 months has been reported to align an impacted canine prior to commencing finishing procedures (Iramaneerat et al., 1998).

Is there a difference in overall treatment duration with different exposure types?

Research in this area would suggest little difference in treatment time, although these studies have all been retrospective in design. One study reported a time saving of 4 months with open exposure (Wisth, 1976), whilst another described open exposure taking 4 months longer (Pearson et al., 1997). A further study has reported no difference in treatment duration (Iramaneerat et al., 1998).

Outline the risks of treatment involving mechanical eruption of impacted canines

Most canines are treated successfully without deleterious consequences. However, specific risks include:
- Root resorption of neighbouring teeth
- General root resorption
- Pulpal obliteration with discolouration of the crown
- Crestal bone loss
- Decalcification
- Poor compliance
- Treatment failure.

Are the positions of these canines likely to be stable following their mechanical eruption (Figure 7.8)?

Post-treatment changes are likely following any orthodontic intervention with inadequate retention. Following alignment, maxillary canines can be more prone to changes, including mesial rotation, lingual displacement and intrusion (Woloshyn et al., 1994).

What other options exist in this case if the patient is not prepared to wear fixed appliances?

- No treatment. However, the impacted canines should be periodically reviewed for any signs of pathology; the long-term prognosis for the ULC and URC is poor.
- Extraction of the impacted canines and primary canines followed by restorative replacement.
- Extraction of the primary canines and auto-transplantation of the impacted canines. This strategy is complicated by the fact that the coronal width of the primary canines is less than that of the permanent canines, which in the absence of any orthodontic treatment means that transplantation can be difficult, although the transplanted canines can be rotated slightly to take up less space. In addition, the position of the UL3 is not conducive to atraumatic removal.

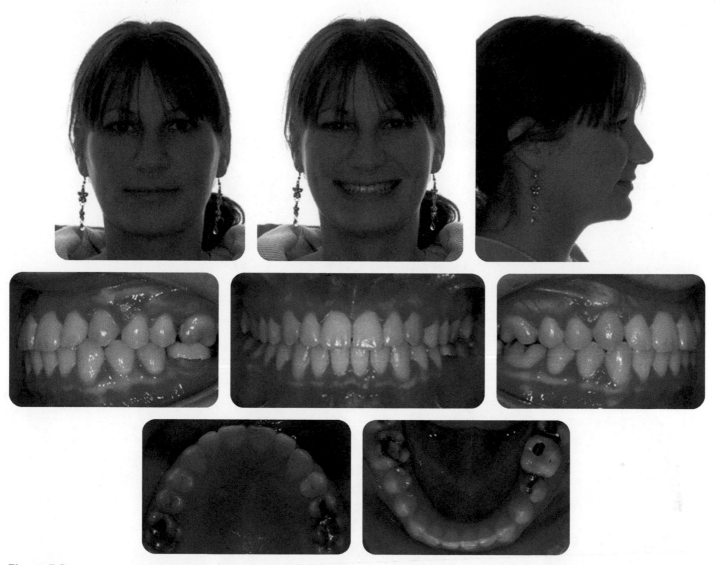

Figure 7.8

Case 7.3

This 15-year-old male was referred by his orthodontic specialist in relation to an unerupted incisor. He was concerned about the spacing between his front teeth. There was no relevant medical history.

His clinical and radiographic records are shown in Figure 7.9.

Extra-oral

Skeletal relationship	
Antero-posterior	Skeletal class II
Vertical	FMPA: Average
	Lower face height: Average
Transverse	Facial asymmetry: None
Soft tissues	Lip competence: Competent
	Naso-labial angle: Average
Upper incisor show	At rest: 2 mm
	Smiling: 6 mm
Temporo-mandibular joint	Healthy with good range and co-ordination of movement

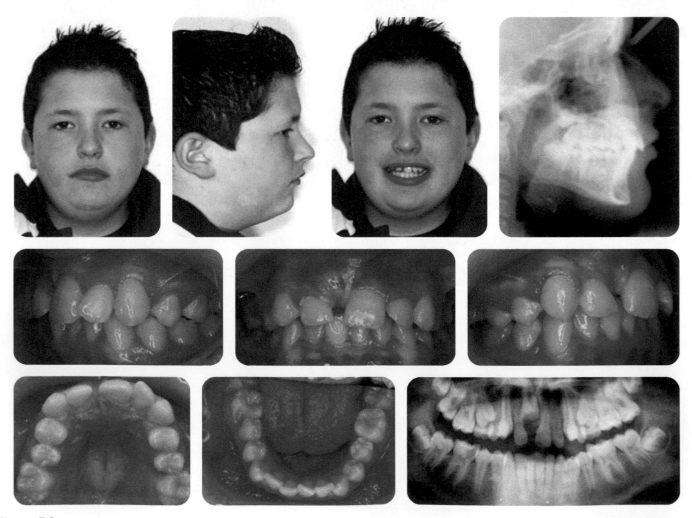

Figure 7.9

Describe the intra-oral findings

- Teeth present $\dfrac{765432 \,/\, 1234567}{7654321 \,/\, 1234567}$

  UR1 is unerupted
- Dental health (restorations, caries): Active caries in LR6
- Oral hygiene: Reasonable, some gingival inflammation associated with the UR3
- Lower arch:
  - Crowding: Moderate
  - Incisor inclination: Average
  - Curve of Spee: Average
- Upper arch:
  - Crowding: Potentially moderately crowded
  - Incisor inclination: Average

Summarize the occlusal features

- Incisor relationship: Class II division 1 (the UR1 is unerupted)
- Overjet: increased (to 5 mm)
- Overbite: Increased and complete
- Molar relationship:
  - Class II on right side
  - Class I on left side
- Centre lines:
  - Upper 2 mm to right side
  - Lower correct to facial midline

Are there any other features of note from the clinical examination?

The maxillary incisors and mandibular second premolars are significantly enlarged, introducing a Bolton tooth-size discrepancy.

What are the radiographic findings (Figure 7.9)?

- All teeth are present, including the UR1 and third molars
- UR1 is vertically-orientated, crowded, with complete root development and no evidence of dilaceration or associated pathology
- UL1 had a short root form
- LR6 is grossly carious
- An unerupted conical supernumerary is present in the lower right premolar region, with no associated pathology

Summary

A 15-year-old male presented with a class II division 1 incisor relationship on a mild skeletal class II base, complicated by the presence of:

- Impacted UR1
- LR6 of poor long-term prognosis
- Potentially moderate crowding in both dental arches
- An unerupted supernumerary tooth in the lower right quadrant.

Treatment Plan

- Oral hygiene instruction
- Exposure and bonding of UR1. Removal of the unerupted supernumerary in the lower right quadrant was suggested; however, the patient decided against this due to the risk of surgical morbidity. Therefore upper and lower pre-adjusted edgewise appliances were used in conjunction with the extraction of upper first premolars and lower first permanent molars. The unerupted supernumerary was left in situ
- Long-term retention

  The final treatment result is shown in Figure 7.10.

What are the possible causes of impacted central incisors?

- Supernumerary teeth
- Dilaceration
- Trauma
- Retained primary tooth
- Ankylosed primary tooth
- Systemic causes

Comment on the anchorage demands in this case

The anchorage demand was high in the upper right quadrant, necessitating inter-maxillary class II traction and individual retraction of the UR1 into a class I relationship prior to consolidation of space in the maxillary arch. Vertical anchorage was also necessary to allow mechanical eruption of the UR1; this was provided by a rigid 0.018-inch steel-base archwire in conjunction with a nickel–titanium piggy-back archwire.

Are there any problems associated with the use of fixed appliances in this case?

The UL1 has a short root form. Short, tapered, thin and pipette-shaped roots are predisposed to further root resorption during appliance therapy. The risk of resorption during treatment is related to longer treatment times and greater apical movement. In

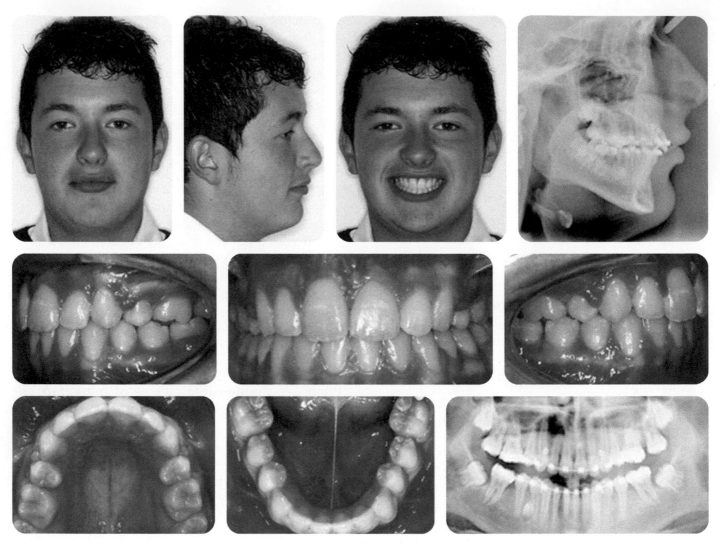

Figure 7.10

particular, the following should be undertaken with caution:

- Inter-arch elastics
- Torque application
- Intrusion.

What factors govern the likelihood of spontaneous eruption of a central incisor following removal of the supernumerary?

- Adequate space
- Position of the incisor and displacement of the apex
- Morphological type of supernumerary (Ashkenazi et al., 2007)
- Chronological age (Leyland et al., 2006)

How likely is spontaneous eruption following the removal of a supernumerary alone, without resort to orthodontic treatment?

Retrospective studies have suggested spontaneous eruption occurs in up to 92% of cases, although other studies have demonstrated lower success rates (DiBiase, 1969; Mitchell and Bennett, 1992; Leyland et al., 2006). In many of these, orthodontic alignment is required to improve the final position of the impacted tooth. As a general anaesthetic is often required to remove the supernumerary, concurrent exposure of the unerupted incisor is usually performed to avoid the risk of a further anaesthetic.

Does spacing in the anterior region have an impact on oral health-related quality of life (OHrQoL)?

A significant association has been demonstrated between impaired OHrQoL and both visible spacing and increased overjet. In one study, the OHrQoL of parents of affected children was also impaired (Johal et al., 2007). Consequently, successful management of impacted incisors is of benefit to dental, social and psychosocial health.

What measures may be taken to identify and manage progressive resorption of the central incisor?

A mid-treatment radiograph is advocated to assess root resorption during treatment, as a significant correlation between resorption arising during the first 6 months of treatment and overall root resorption has been demonstrated (Smale et al., 2005). If significant progressive resorption is noted, consideration may be given to pacifying the appliance for 2–3 months (Levander et al., 1994).

Case 7.4

This 14-year-old female was referred by her orthodontic specialist in relation to multiple unerupted teeth. There was no relevant medical history.

Extra-oral

Skeletal relationship

  Antero-posterior   Mild skeletal class III

  Vertical   FMPA: Average

                             Lower face height: Average

  Transverse   Facial asymmetry: None

Soft tissues   Retrusive

                             Lip competence: Competent

                             Naso-labial angle: Average

Upper incisor show   At rest: 2 mm

                             Smiling: 6 mm

Temporo-mandibular joint   Healthy with good range and co-ordination of movement

Intra-oral

Teeth present

76	321 / 1234	67
76	321 / 123	67

Dental health   Good

(restorations, caries)

Oral hygiene   Poor with plaque deposits and marginal gingivitis

Lower arch   Crowding: Severe

                             Incisor inclination: Retroclined

                             Curve of Spee: Average

Upper arch   Crowding: Severe

                             Incisor inclination: Retroclined

                             Canine position: In line of the arch

Occlusion   Incisor relationship: Class III

                             Overjet: 0 mm

                             Overbite: Reduced and complete

                             Molar relationship: ½ unit class II on right; class I on left

                             Centre lines: Mandibular centre line has deviated 2 mm to the right

                             Functional occlusion: Group function

Summarize the radiographic findings (Figure 7.11)

The panoramic view confirms the developmental absence of UL5 and UR5. The mandibular premolars are developing but impacted, with no evidence of associated pathology.

Summary (Figure 7.11)

A 14-year-old female presented with a class III incisor relationship on a mild skeletal class III pattern complicated by:

- Multiple unerupted premolar teeth
- Hypodontia of maxillary second premolars
- Severe crowding of both arches.

Treatment Plan

- Surgical removal of the LR4 and LL4
- Exposure and bonding of the LR5 and LL5
- Upper and lower pre-adjusted edgewise appliances (Figure 7.12)
- Long-term retention

What is the most common cause of second premolar impaction?

Premature loss of second primary molars is the most likely cause of second premolar impaction. This typically results in mesial migration and mesial tipping of the first permanent molars. However, the severity of the problem in this case suggests that there is also underlying dento-alveolar disproportion in the mandibular arch. This has culminated in the impaction of all four mandibular premolars.

How common is agenesis of maxillary second premolars?

Maxillary second premolars are the third most frequently absent tooth (Polder et al., 2004) with a prevalence of around 1.5%.

What do you notice about the lower second premolars (Figure 7.12)?

There is a mismatch in tooth size between these teeth. The LR5 is diminutive and hypoplastic. The consequences of a significant tooth-size discrepancy include a non-ideal occlusion and the potential for residual spacing following orthodontic treatment. This tooth would, therefore, benefit from restorative build-up to achieve an ideal occlusal result.

How common is a tooth-size discrepancy?

A discrepancy of 2mm or more in tooth size is considered significant. The prevalence of tooth-size disproportion of this order in an orthodontic population is around 24% in the mandibular arch and 28% in the maxillary arch (Othman and Harradine, 2007).

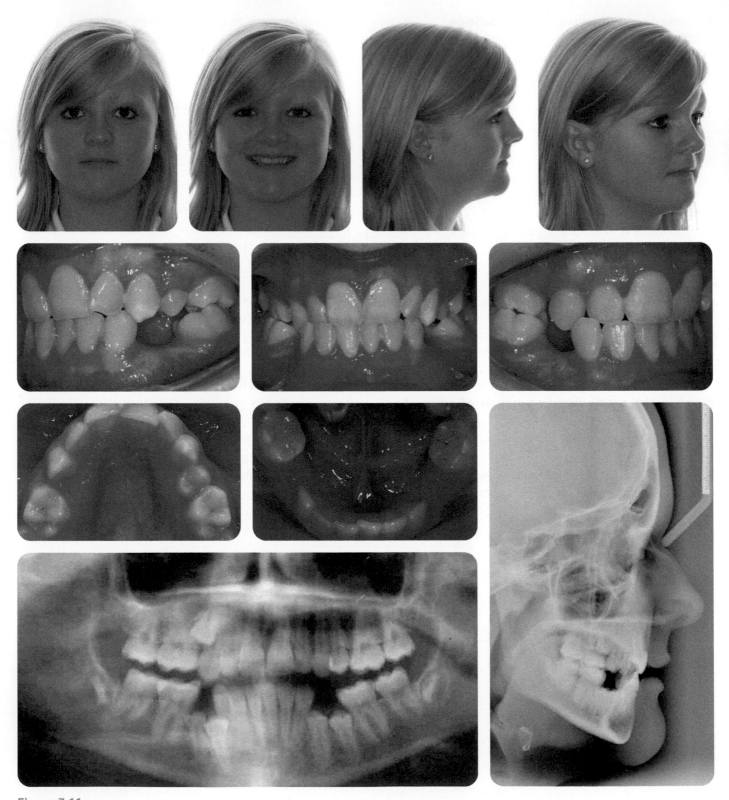

Figure 7.11

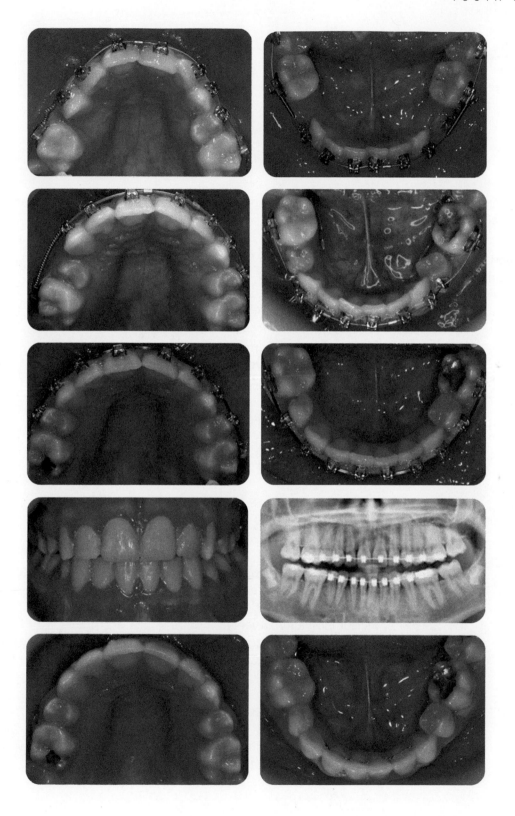

Figure 7.12

Case 7.5

This 12-year-old female was referred by her orthodontic specialist in relation to misplaced teeth. There was no relevant medical history.

Extra-oral

Skeletal relationship
  Antero-posterior   Mild skeletal class II
  Vertical   FMPA: Average
                          Lower face height: Average
  Transverse   Facial asymmetry: None
Soft tissues   Lip competence: Competent
                          Naso-labial angle: Average
Upper incisor show   At rest: 3mm
                          Smiling: 7mm
Temporo-mandibular joint   Healthy with good range and co-ordination of movement

Intra-oral

Teeth present

76 4C21/1234E67
76E4321/123 67

Dental health   Good
(restorations, caries)
Oral hygiene   Good
Lower arch   Crowding: Moderate
                          Incisor inclination: Retroclined
                          Curve of Spee: Average
Upper arch   Crowding: Mild
                          Incisor inclination: Average
                          Canine position: Buccal on right side and erupted on left side
Occlusion   Incisor relationship: Class II division 1
                          Overjet: 5mm
                          Overbite: Average and complete
                          Molar relationship: Class II on right; class I on left
                          Centre lines:
                              Upper 2mm to right
                              Lower 1mm to left of facial midline
                          Functional occlusion: Group function

Summarize the clinical and radiographic features of this case (Figure 7.13)

A 12-year-old female presented with a class II division 1 incisor relationship on a mild skeletal class II pattern complicated by:

- Impacted UR3 (which is palpable buccally) and UR5
- Crowding of the lower arch and a retrusive soft tissue profile.

The UR3 has a reasonable prognosis for orthodontic alignment; however, there is some evidence of external root resorption affecting the UR2. The UR5 is

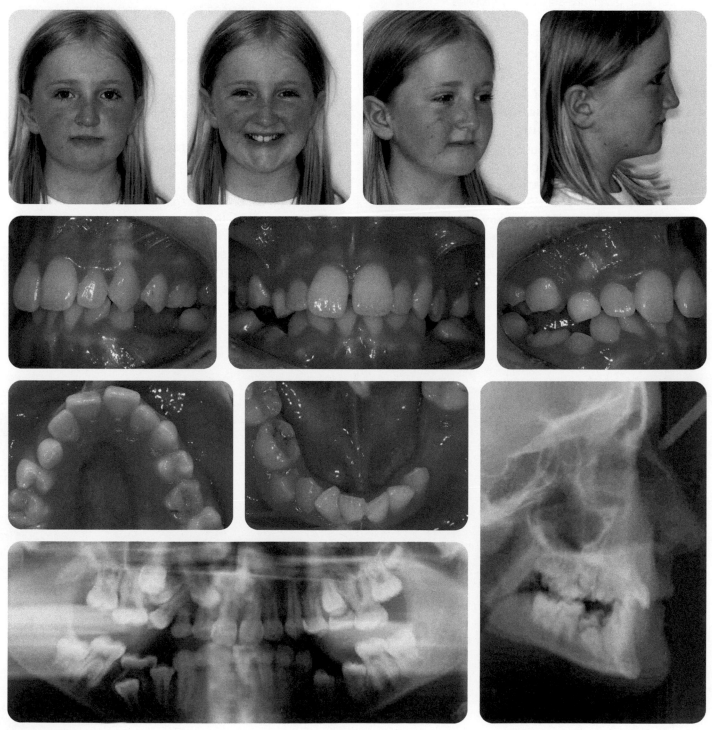

Figure 7.13

markedly ectopic, with a poor prognosis for orthodontic alignment, with an infra-occluded URE in close proximity.

Treatment Plan

- Surgical exposure and bonding of the UR3, extraction of the UR5, URE and LLE
- Upper and lower pre-adjusted edgewise appliances
- Long-term retention
  The final result is shown in Figure 7.14.

What is the aetiology of buccal canine ectopia and why can the management of these teeth be challenging?

The majority of unerupted buccal maxillary canines are displaced due to dental crowding. However, buccal ectopia may also develop. This is less frequent than palatal displacement (1:5). Management of buccally ectopic canines may be very complex. Difficulty may be encountered in moving the canine past the root of the adjacent lateral incisor to align the canine, particularly if the canine is high. In addition, unlike palatally displaced canines, those impacted on the buccal side often lie under non-keratinized mucosa and require an apically repositioned flap.

What problems may be encountered during mechanical eruption of an ectopic buccal canine?

Controlling the vector of tooth movement may be difficult. Movement may be impeded by the adjacent lateral incisor, delaying treatment and risking resorption of either tooth.

What is the aetiology of buccal ectopia?

- Poorly understood
- Often but not exclusively associated with crowding
- Lateral incisor anomalies (Chaushu *et al.*, 2009)

How common is root resorption affecting maxillary lateral incisors adjacent to ectopic canines?

- This depends on the imaging modality.
- Early research with intra-oral radiographs indicated a prevalence of 12.5% (Ericson and Kurol, 1988b).
- Conventional CT scanning (Ericson and Kurol, 2000a, b) and cone beam CT scanning (Walker *et al.*, 2005) have demonstrated levels of 48% and 67%, respectively.

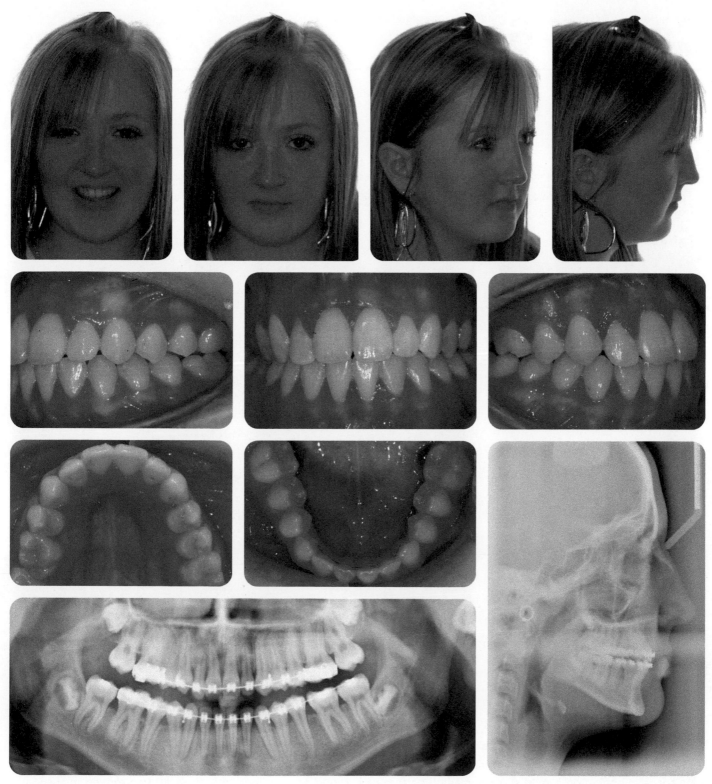

Figure 7.14

Case 7.6

This 12-year-old female was referred by her general dentist in relation to crowding. There was no relevant medical history.

Extra-oral

Skeletal relationship
 Antero-posterior — Mild skeletal class II
 Vertical — FMPA: Average
  Lower face height: Average
 Transverse — Facial asymmetry: None
Soft tissues — Lip competence: Competent
  Naso-labial angle: Average
Upper incisor show — At rest: 5 mm
  Smiling: 10 mm
Temporo-mandibular joint — Healthy with good range and co-ordination of movement

Intra-oral

Teeth present

7654321/12 4567
———————————
7654321/1234567

Dental health — Good
(restorations, caries) — Hypoplastic first permanent molars with right first molars most severely affected
Oral hygiene — Good
Lower arch — Crowding: Mild
  Incisor inclination: Average
  Curve of Spee: Increased
Upper arch — Crowding: Severe
  Incisor inclination: Average
  UL3 ectopic

Summarize the clinical findings (Figure 7.15)

A 12-year-old female presented with a class II division 1 incisor relationship on a mild skeletal class II pattern complicated by an ectopic UL3 and crowding of both arches. The overjet is increased to 5 mm, the overbite is increased and complete, and both dental centre lines are to the left of the facial midline (2 mm). The molar relationship is class I on the right side and a full-unit class II on the left side.

Localize the UL3

Using vertical parallax between the panoramic and peri-apical radiographs, the UL3 has moved in the same direction as the tube when viewed on the peri-apical radiograph, and is therefore palatal.

Treatment Plan

- Surgical removal of the UL3 and extraction of the UR4

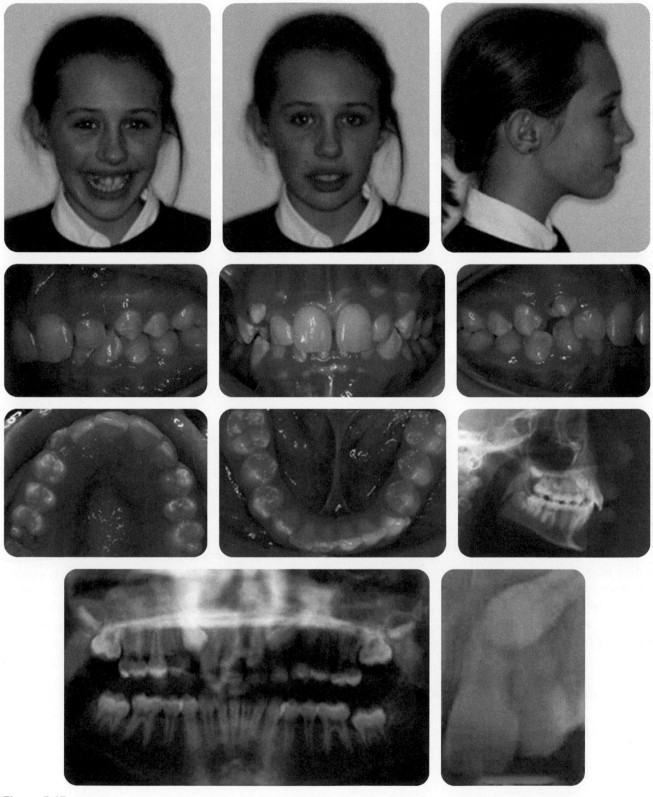

Figure 7.15

- Upper and lower pre-adjusted edgewise appliances with a trans-palatal arch
- Long-term retention
  The final result is shown in Figure 7.16.

What influences the decision to extract a maxillary canine?

The decision to remove an ectopic maxillary canine is influenced by local and general factors. Surgical removal is recommended in the following instances:

- Poor oral hygiene, poor co-operation
- Reluctance to wear orthodontic appliances
- Early resorption of adjacent teeth or dentigerous cystic change
- Patient too old for interception
- Good contact between adjacent lateral incisors and the first premolar or treatment to achieve this is predictable
- Degree of displacement is excessive.

What modifications may be necessary to the first premolar during treatment to substitute for a maxillary canine?

- Rotate the first premolar mesio-palatally to occupy more space and hide the palatal cusp. This may be achieved by intentional distal bracket placement and archwire bends.
- Palatal cusp reduction to improve aesthetics and eliminate occlusal interferences.
- Introduction of buccal root torque.
- Levelling of gingival margins. This may be required in the presence of a high smile line and may necessitate labial veneering to restore crown height if intrusion was required.
- Occasionally, mesio-distal build-up of the premolar or lateral incisor may be required. This should be assessed prior to treatment using a tooth-size analysis.

On what grounds can an ectopic canine be left *in situ*?

Generally, if orthodontics is planned and the impacted tooth is likely to interfere with treatment, the canine should be removed. When no orthodontics is planned the canine may be left *in situ* in the following circumstances:

- The patient does not want treatment
- There is no evidence of resorption of adjacent teeth or cystic degeneration
- There is either a good contact between the lateral incisor and first premolar or the primary canine has a good prognosis
- Regular radiographic review of the impacted tooth is possible.

What is the expected lifespan of a retained primary canine?

Research in this area is exclusively retrospective and usually focuses on persistence of primary molars associated with the developmental absence of premolars. In general, retained primary canines tend to persist until the fourth decade, although there is individual variation. There is some evidence that mandibular primary canines have an improved lifespan (Haselden *et al.*, 2001).

Why was the lower arch treated on a non-extraction basis?

- Space requirements were minimal
- Reduces antero-posterior anchorage demands
- Facilitates overbite reduction

Comment on the outcome of this case

Lower incisor proclination has contributed to overbite and overjet reduction, placing a premium on prolonged retention to maintain ideal alignment. Therefore, consideration may have been given to removal of two mandibular second premolars. Indeed, whilst there was minimal crowding in the lower arch prior to treatment, the curve of Spee was increased, both lower canines were distally angulated and the second permanent molars were unerupted; all of these factors have associated space and therefore anchorage requirements.

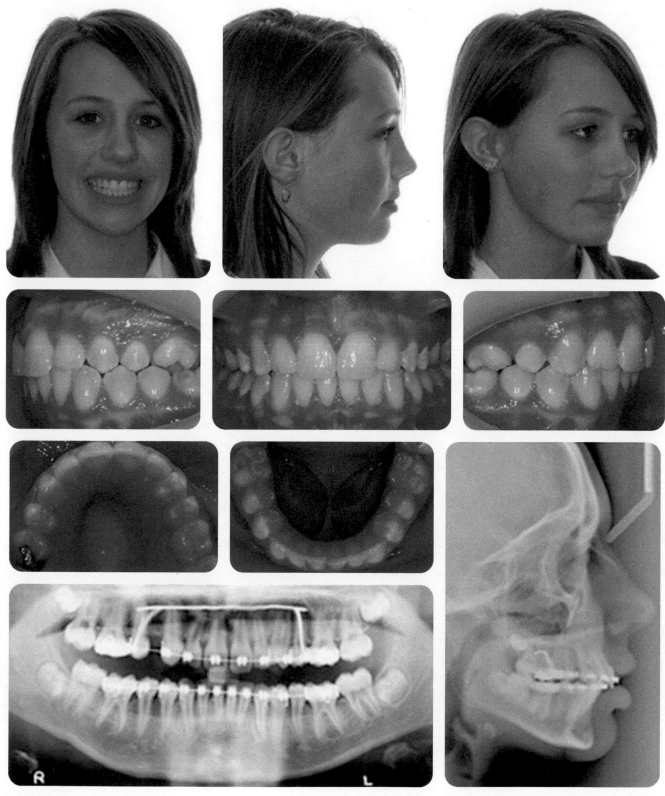

Figure 7.16

Case 7.7

This 14-year-old male was referred by his orthodontic specialist in relation to missing teeth. There was no relevant medical history.

Extra-oral

Skeletal relationship	
Antero-posterior	Mild skeletal class III
Vertical	FMPA: Average
	Lower face height: Average
Transverse	Facial asymmetry: None
Soft tissues	Lip competence: Competent
	Naso-labial angle: Average
Upper incisor show	At rest: 3 mm
	Smiling: 7 mm
Temporo-mandibular joint	Healthy with good range and co-ordination of movement

Intra-oral

Teeth present

76 4 21/123 67
76 4321/1234E67

Dental health (restorations, caries)	Good
Oral hygiene	Good
Lower arch	Crowding: Mild
	Incisor inclination: Average
	Curve of Spee: Average
Upper arch	Crowding: Mild
	Incisor inclination: Average
	UR3 ectopic
Occlusion	Incisor relationship: Class III
	Overjet: 0 mm
	Overbite: Average and complete
	Molar relationship: ½ unit class II on right; class I on left
	Centre lines:
	Upper 2 mm to right side
	Lower correct to facial midline
	Functional occlusion: Group function

Summary (Figure 7.17)

A 14-year-old male presented with a class III incisor relationship on a mild skeletal class III pattern complicated by:
- Unerupted UR3, UR5, UL5 and LL5
- Mild lower labial segment crowding
- Rotation of UR4.

Comment on the radiographic findings (Figure 7.18)

The UR3 is palatally impacted with a favourable prognosis for orthodontic alignment. There is some follicular enlargement of this tooth but no root resorption of the UR2. The UL5, UR5 and LL5 are congenitally absent. All third molars are developing.

Treatment Plan

- Surgical exposure and bonding of UR3
- Upper and lower pre-adjusted edgewise appliances with removal of the LR5 and LLE
- Long-term retention

The final result is shown in Figure 7.19.

What is the prognosis for successful orthodontic eruption of a palatally-displaced maxillary canine?

The prognosis for successful orthodontic eruption of palatally-displaced maxillary canines is influenced primarily by age and the position of the developing tooth. In adult patients, a significant risk of ankylosis of the displaced tooth exists with one study suggesting

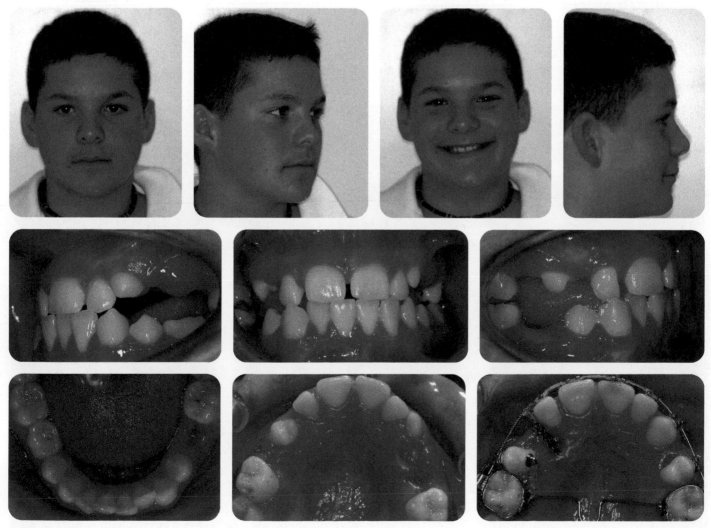

Figure 7.17

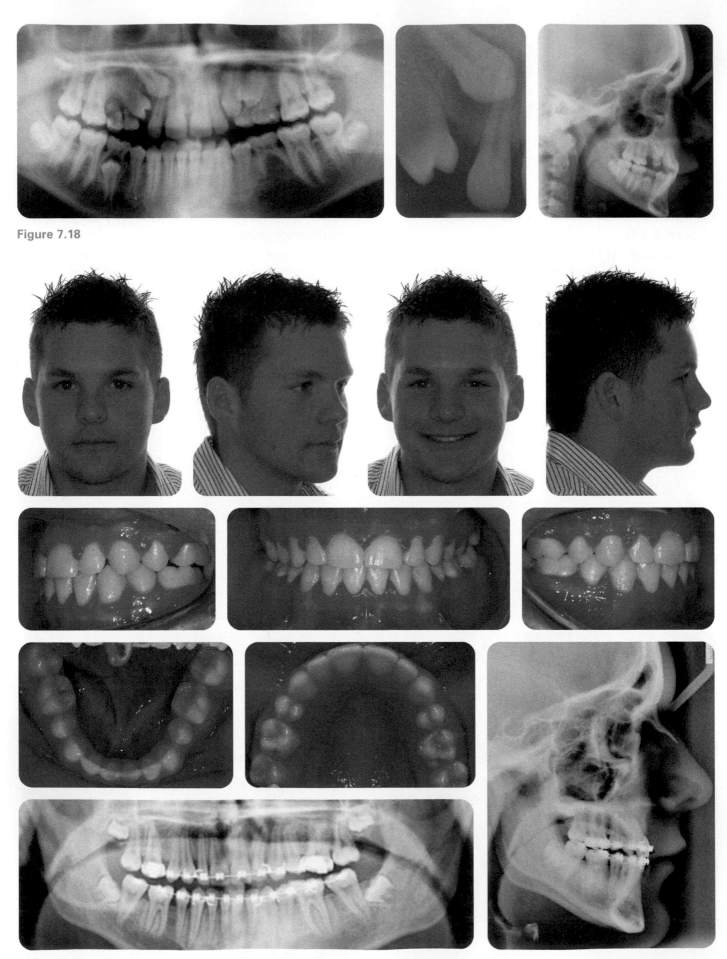

Figure 7.18

Figure 7.19

30% of impacted canines are not erupted successfully in subjects over 30 years of age (Becker and Chaushu, 2003).

The position of the canine is usually gauged on a panoramic radiograph. The average time taken to mechanically erupt the impacted tooth is governed by mesio-distal displacement, vertical displacement and angulation of the impacted tooth. In particular, increased treatment time has been attributed to greater mesial (Fleming *et al.*, 2009) and vertical (Stewart *et al.*, 2001) displacement of the canine.

How is the progress of canine eruption monitored?

With open surgical exposures, progress can be monitored clinically and using repeated photography. With closed exposures, the visible links on the gold chain can be counted as they are progressively removed to assess movement.

Where little discernible movement has occurred over a period of 6 months, a repeat radiograph is warranted.

Is there an association between tooth agenesis and canine ectopia?

Yes. In particular, developmental absence of maxillary lateral incisors often co-exists with ectopic development. The reason for this is unclear; absence of lateral incisors may interfere with normal guidance of the adjacent canine (Becker, 1995). However, others contend that the concurrence of these features is an expression of a genetic predisposition; the association between canine ectopia and remote hypodontia lends support to this theory (Peck *et al.*, 1994).

How is sufficient labial root torque applied to the ectopic canine?

Supplementary labial root torque is often necessary after alignment of the canine crown to optimize dental aesthetics and to facilitate stability. Torque is augmented by altering bracket prescription to deliver labial root torque (up to −7 degrees). The bracket prescription is expressed by using large dimension rectangular wires (0.019 × 0.025-inch or 0.021 × 0.025-inch stainless steel in a 0.028-inch slot) for prolonged periods. Localized torque may be added using artistic wire bends or using torqueing auxiliaries.

Case 7.8

This 10-year-old female was referred by her general dentist in relation to her asymmetric eruption pattern and concern for the spacing between her front teeth. There was no relevant medical history.

Extra-oral

Skeletal relationship
- Antero-posterior   Mild skeletal class II
- Vertical   FMPA: Average
        Lower face height: Average
- Transverse   Facial asymmetry: None

Soft tissues   Lip competence: Competent
      Naso-labial angle: Average

Upper incisor show   At rest: 2 mm
      Smiling: 6 mm

Temporo-mandibular joint   Healthy with good range and co-ordination of movement

The intra-oral appearance is shown in Figure 7.20.

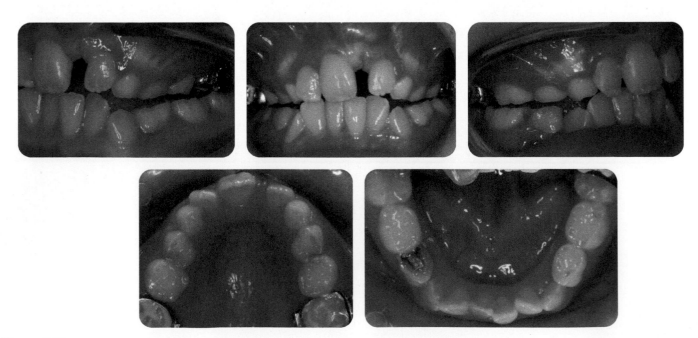

Figure 7.20

Which teeth are present?

6EDC21/ 2CDE6
6ED321/123DE6

Summary (Figure 7.20)

A class I incisor relationship (the mandible is postured anteriorly in the photographs) with a normal overjet and reduced but complete overbite. The UCL is displaced to the left by 2 mm and the molar relationship is ½ unit class II on the right side and a full unit class II on the left. There is a bilateral posterior crossbite.

Summarize the radiographic findings (Figure 7.21)

All teeth are present, including the UL1 and the third molars. The UL1 is horizontally orientated with complete root development. There is no evidence of pathology. A cone beam CT (CBCT) scan confirmed the UL1 to be dilacerated, but with a good prognosis for mechanical eruption.

Treatment Plan

Phase 1

- Maxillary arch expansion: Quadhelix appliance
- Surgical exposure and bonding of the UL1

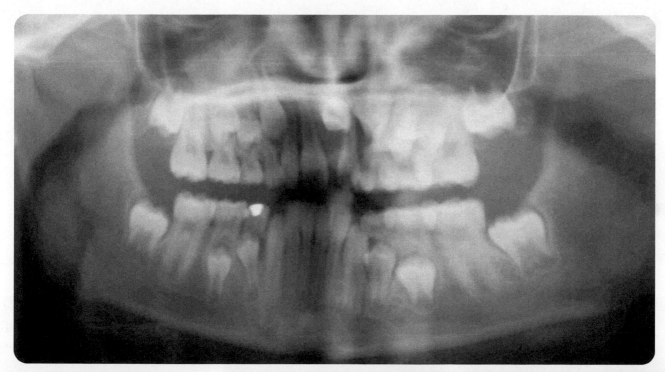

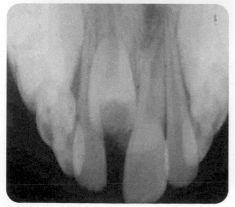 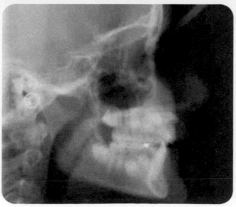 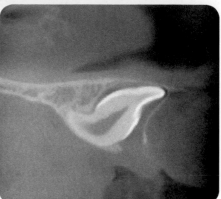

Figure 7.21

• Mechanical eruption of the UL1 with an upper pre-adjusted edgewise appliance (Figure 7.22)

Phase 2
• Review in relation to a lower pre-adjusted edgewise appliance
• Long-term retention (Figure 7.23)

Comment on the use of CBCT in the diagnosis of impacted teeth

CBCT is a useful three-dimensional imaging technique with particular application in the localization of unerupted teeth, permitting assessment of associated pathology and the prognosis for orthodontic alignment, and identifying resorption related to impacted teeth and bone dimensions for mini-implant placement. At present, routine use of CBCT in orthodontics is not recommended due to the risks of ionizing radiation (Isaacson *et al.*, 2008).

For the localized assessment of an impacted tooth, including consideration of resorption of an adjacent tooth where the current imaging method of choice is conventional dental radiography, CBCT may be used when the information cannot be obtained adequately

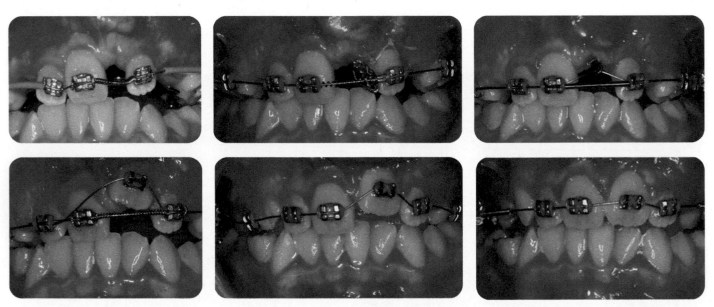

Figure 7.22

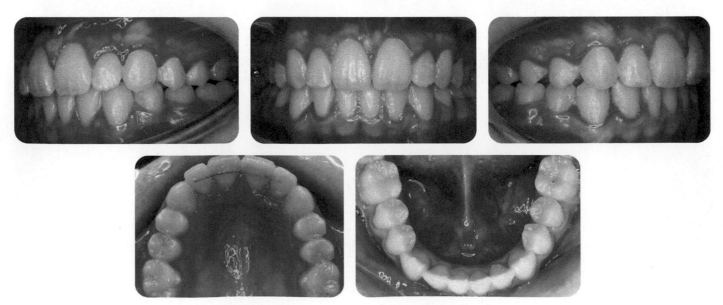

Figure 7.23

by lower dose conventional radiography. With further dose limitation, CBCT is likely to become the routine imaging technique of choice.

Outline the main differences between conventional CT and CBCT

Unlike the fan-shaped X-ray beam used in CT scans, CBCT uses a cone-shaped beam to record projection data via a flat detector, during a single 360-degree rotation. CBCT is capable of higher spatial resolution (with isotropic voxels as small as 0.125 mm^3) than conventional CT. Scanning time is comparable to that of state-of-the-art conventional CT (10–40 s). However, although the radiation dosage encountered in a typical CBCT scan is higher than in conventional radiographic imaging, it is significantly lower than dosages associated with a multi-slice CT. CBCT units are generally smaller and cheaper than conventional CT scanners.

How do CBCT images compare to conventional plain film lateral cephalograms for orthodontic diagnosis?

Thick multi-planar, perspective or orthogonal reconstructions of CBCT scans can be used to produce lateral and frontal cephalometric images without distortion or magnification for orthodontic assessment. Landmark identification is considered easier with synthetic cephalograms derived from CBCT due to greater contrast (Grauer et al., 2010). Consistency between measurements generated from a CBCT scan with actual measurements on a skull have been confirmed with the NewTom 3G™ (Lascala et al., 2004) with readings being smaller with CBCT images, but largely insignificant. In a further study, skulls were scanned with i-CAT™ and compared with the anatomic truth and with various plain-film radiographic images (Hilgers et al., 2005). With the exception of some outliers, the 3D radiographic reconstructions provided accurate and reliable linear measurements.

List the main potential applications of CBCT in orthodontics?

- Localization of impacted teeth
- Measurement of bone volume, root length and periodontal support
- CBCT cephalometry
- Digital model production, removing the need for impressions and plaster models

Comment on the final occlusal result in this case (Figure 7.23); How could this have been improved?

The final occlusion is imperfect, with the upper centre line remaining to the left. This could have been addressed with the extraction of a maxillary premolar unit in the upper right quadrant to allow distalization of the canine into a class I relationship and alignment of the centre lines. It was decided not to pursue this course of treatment as the centre line shift was not of concern to the patient and more incisor movement would have prolonged the treatment and risked further root resorption.

What are the causes of dilaceration?

Dilaceration is typically developmental in origin with a female predilection. Based on a study of 41 dilacerated unerupted maxillary central incisors, 71% were developmental in origin, 22% resulted from trauma to the deciduous predecessor and the remaining 7% were associated with cysts or supernumerary teeth (Stewart, 1978).

What are the options for treating a dilacerated tooth?

- Complete orthodontic alignment. Elective root filling and apicectomy may be necessary in the presence of severe labial root dilaceration.
- If the malformation is severe, extraction or acceptance of partial orthodontic alignment may be necessary.

If extraction of the incisor is required, should space be maintained for long-term replacement?

Space can be maintained initially with a fixed or removable prosthesis; implants will provide a definitive solution at cessation of vertical growth (Iseri and Solow, 1996). Prolonged space maintenance can lead to significant alveolar bone loss in the affected region, making implant placement reliant on bone grafting procedures. Therefore, spontaneous space closure can be facilitated in the labial segment. In the long-term, space can be re-created with fixed appliances prior to definitive restoration (Kokich and Crabill, 2006).

Case 7.9

How would you describe the incisor relationship?

The lower incisor edges are occluding on the cingulum plateau of the maxillary incisors, reflecting a class I incisor relationship. However, the overbite is increased and a rotation associated with the UR1 has produced an increased overjet in association with this tooth.

How would you describe the skeletal pattern?

The antero-posterior skeletal pattern appears class II when viewing the clinical profile. However, the cephalometric analysis suggests a skeletal class I

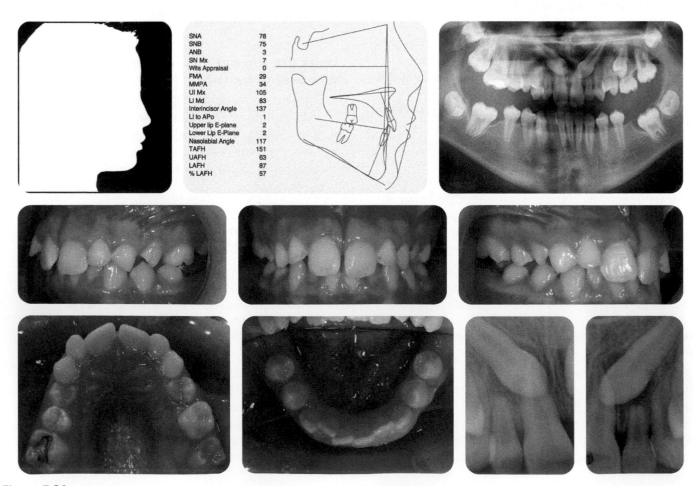

SNA	78
SNB	75
ANB	3
SN Mx	7
Wits Appraisal	0
FMA	29
MMPA	34
UI Mx	105
LI Md	83
Interincisor Angle	137
LI to APo	1
Upper lip E-plane	2
Lower Lip E-Plane	2
Nasolabial Angle	117
TAFH	151
UAFH	63
LAFH	87
% LAFH	57

Figure 7.24

pattern (ANB 3 degrees; Wits 0 mm). The vertical proportions are slightly increased (MMPA 34 degrees; % lower face height 57%).

Describe the intra-oral features

- Oral hygiene: Good
- Occlusal amalgam restoration in the UR6 and previous extraction of the UL6, LL6 and LR6
- Teeth present: $\dfrac{654C21 / 12C4E\ 7}{54321 / 12345}$

What further diagnostic information is required?

The position of the unerupted maxillary canines needs to be elucidated. Clinical palpation of the anterior buccal sulcus and anterior maxilla should be carried out. In addition, further radiographic analysis of the upper canines should be undertaken.

Describe the occlusion

- Mild crowding in the lower arch, with the mandibular second molars unerupted bilaterally
- Lower incisors are retroclined and both canines distally angulated
- Maxillary arch is reasonably well-aligned, with both maxillary primary canines retained and the permanent canines unerupted
- Incisor relationship is class I with an increased overjet on the UR1
- Molar relationship cannot be defined.
- Canine relationship is class I, although the upper canines are primary teeth
- Centre lines are coincident

What information does the panoramic radiograph provide?

The panoramic radiograph confirms the previous extraction of the UL6, LL6 and LR6. There is no caries and the occlusal restoration in the UR6 is sound. The mandibular second molars are erupting and all four third molars are developing. The UL5 is potentially crowded, although the ULE is undergoing normal physiological root resorption. The maxillary lateral incisors are microdont. Both maxillary permanent canines are impacted, mesially angulated and displaced toward the midline.

What additional information do the periapical radiographs provide?

The position of both upper permanent canines has changed little relative to adjacent structures on the panoramic view and they appear to be buccally displaced. There is some evidence of resorption affecting the apex of the UR2 and the follicles of both maxillary canines are enlarged.

Comment on the prognosis for successful eruption of the canines

These teeth are in a poor position, primarily because of the mesial displacement. The UR3 in particular is markedly displaced to the midline of the maxilla and is also displaced vertically.

Comment on the timing of first molar extraction in this case

It is likely that these teeth were extracted at a later stage than is desirable for optimal occlusal outcome. Whilst the UL7 is erupting into a good position, both lower second molars are mesially-angulated and there is spacing. It is likely that they will erupt with a mesial crown tip.

What is the main problem list for this patient?

- Ectopic maxillary canines
- Retained primary maxillary canines
- Unerupted UL5
- Resorption associated with the UL2
- Previous loss of three first permanent molars

What are the main treatment options?

Orthodontic treatment with fixed appliances could be carried out to align and co-ordinate the dental arches. If this is to be undertaken, the main decision would be whether to extract the maxillary canines or attempt to erupt them mechanically.

What are the difficulties of accommodating the permanent canines in the maxillary arch?

This option will require surgical exposure of the canines; the degree of displacement dictates that a general anaesthetic will probably be required. The retained maxillary primary canines and the ULE should also be extracted. The UL5 is likely to erupt unaided.

The main difficulty will be associated with bringing the canines into occlusion. A closed exposure and placement of gold chains is probably most appropriate because of the severity of the vertical displacement. In addition, space redistribution will be required in the maxillary arch because the permanent canines have larger crowns than their primary predecessors.

Anchorage will also be an important consideration; there is some available space in the upper left quadrant because of the presence of the ULE and small amount of space between the erupting UL7 and the ULE. However, there is a shortage of space in the upper right quadrant.

What extraction pattern may be considered in the maxillary arch?

Space could be created by extracting the UR6 as there is an occlusal restoration in this tooth and the other three first permanent molars have been extracted; however, the UR7 is currently unerupted. This would mean that placement of fixed appliances may need to be deferred as vertical anchorage is required to resist extrusive forces on the impacted canines. The loss of the UR6 would also provide more space than is required, necessitating a protracted period of space closure.

Alternatively, removal of maxillary first premolars could be considered (Figure 7.25), although this may generate excessive space in the upper arch. A further alternative would be to use headgear applied to bands on the UR6 and UL7 to distalize these teeth, creating the space required for the canines. Whilst this would require more co-operation, it may provide a better occlusal outcome.

Extraction of the maxillary canines has the advantage of shortening the treatment time with fixed appliances. With this option, treatment would primarily involve tooth alignment and closure of residual space. The upper first premolars would substitute as the canine teeth. The disadvantage of this strategy is that it sacrifices the upper canines, which have long, robust roots and are resistant to decay; and a cornerstone of the dynamic occlusion.

Could the canines be transplanted?

Transplantation could be performed, although the position of the canines may make their atraumatic removal difficult, compromising the long-term prognosis. Furthermore, transplantation will also require space creation, although occasionally the canines can be transplanted with the crowns slightly rotated to reduce space requirements.

Any orthodontic treatment would need to be planned carefully. Ideally, sufficient space would need to be created prior to transplantation with a fixed appliance. However, any tooth movement prior to transplantation should be undertaken with care because of the proximity of the ectopic canines to the roots of the maxillary incisors. The permanent canines could be removed and 'parked' in the buccal sulcus, space created safely with a fixed appliance, and the canines subsequently transplanted into position in a second surgical procedure, to overcome this problem.

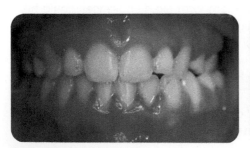 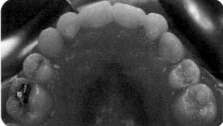 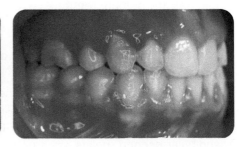

Figure 7.25

Case 7.10

This 12-year-old girl presented after referral from her general dental practitioner regarding failure of eruption of her upper canine teeth.

- Ectopic UL3, UR3 and UL5
- Crowding of both arches
- Diminutive UR2
- Mesio-buccal rotation of UL2
- Agenesis of the lower second premolars
- Retained second primary molars.

Summarize this malocclusion (Figure 7.26)

A class I incisor relationship on a skeletal class I pattern with average vertical dimensions complicated by:

What treatment plan would you suggest?

Fixed appliances on a non-extraction basis would be a suitable treatment plan. The ULE could be retained

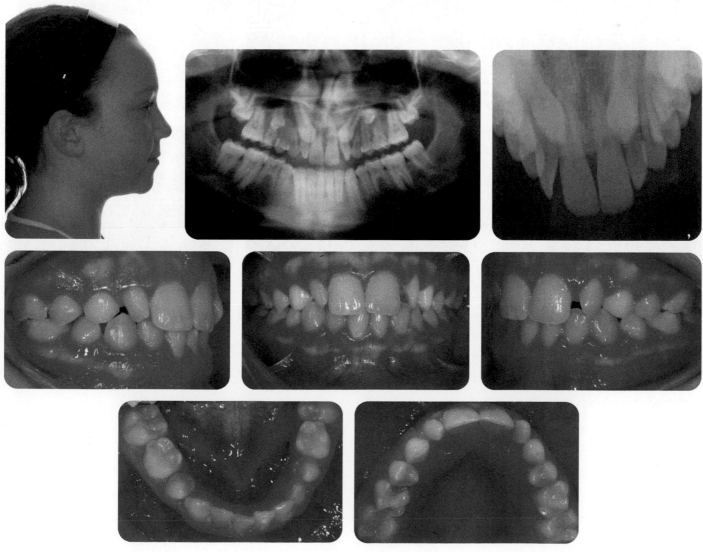

Figure 7.26

indefinitely as the UL5 is severely displaced with a poor prognosis for alignment. Placement of a lower appliance could be deferred until near the end of treatment as the majority of treatment is required in the maxillary arch. The UR2 would also benefit from restorative build-up.

Would you advocate removal of UL5?

To make this decision the risks of removal must be weighed against the risks of leaving the tooth *in situ*. Surgical risks include the risks of anaesthesia, damage to adjacent teeth and surgical morbidity. The risks of leaving the tooth *in situ* include the potential for dentigerous cystic change and resorption of adjacent teeth with intra-osseous migration. In this case, the UL5 was left *in situ* as there was no evidence of pathology and the tooth did not present an impediment to tooth movement.

What are the limitations associated with treatment?

ULE is likely to be exfoliated by the fifth decade. Maxillary primary teeth tend to have a poorer lifespan than mandibular teeth (Haselden *et al.*, 2001). This case was treated with an upper fixed appliance to bring the upper canines into occlusion and composite build-up of the UR2 (Figure 7.27).

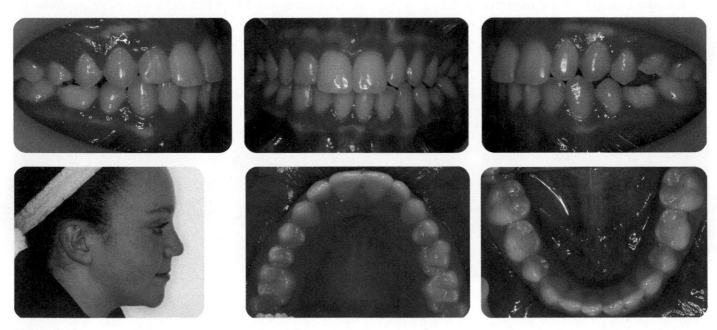

Figure 7.27

Case 7.11

This 12-year-old patient was referred by his general dental practitioner, who was concerned about the development of his dentition.

Why do you think there was concern about the development of his dentition (Figure 7.28)?

The URB and URC are retained.

At what age would you expect the UR2 and UR3 to erupt?

The maxillary lateral incisors are expected to erupt between the ages of 7 and 8 years. The maxillary canines are expected to erupt between the ages of 10 and 12 years.

What are the possible causes of delayed tooth eruption?

- Generalized delay in dental development
- Congenital absence of teeth
- Crowding
- Delayed eruption due to obstruction by a supernumerary tooth or odontome
- Primary failure of eruption

What information could you obtain from the history to make a diagnosis?

It would be helpful to confirm from the history when the contra-lateral teeth had erupted. If these have only recently erupted, there may be a possibility of delayed eruption. A family history of hypodontia may increase the likelihood of this being the aetiological factor.

What further investigations would you carry out?

Radiographic examination would confirm the presence of the unerupted teeth and identify any factors obstructing eruption.

A panoramic radiograph was taken (Figure 7.29) and revealed the presence of a disorganized mass of tooth-like tissue lying below the crown of the UR2, preventing its eruption. How would you manage this?

Arrangements would need to be made for the extraction of the retained URB and URC, and for removal of the tissue mass. It would be advisable to request the exposure and bonding of a gold chain to both the UR2 and UR3 at the same time, to allow orthodontic traction to be applied to these teeth.

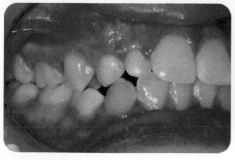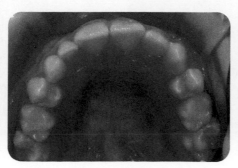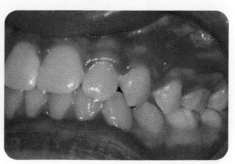

Figure 7.28

What kind of mass is suggested from its radiological appearance? How would you confirm this?

The radiograph suggests that this is a complex odontome as the dental tissue is haphazard and disorganized. This impression could be confirmed by histological examination.

Figure 7.30 shows an upper removable appliance that was used following surgical removal of the odontome, and retained deciduous teeth. Discuss the design of this appliance

Retention is provided by cribs on the upper first premolars and upper first permanent molars, and by a modified Southend clasp on the UL2 and UL1. A unilateral screw on the right of the base plate allows some additional space to be created for the unerupted UR2 and UR3 (because the retained URB and URC have a smaller combined crown width than the permanent successors). Hooks in the baseplate and a buccal arm soldered to the premolar and molar crib on the right will allow traction to be applied to the unerupted teeth.

Figure 7.31 shows the successful eruption of the UR3. The UR2 remained unerupted and there was clearly insufficient space for this tooth. How could additional space be created for the UR2?

There is insufficient space for the UR2 because the UR3 is in a ½ unit class II relationship. However, there is some space in the arch distal to this tooth and the upper centre line has deviated to the right slightly. At this stage it would be appropriate to progress to the fixed appliance stage of treatment, with a view to creating sufficient space for the lateral incisor and to start applying traction to this tooth. This space can be generated using open coil spring between the UR1 and UR3, which will help to correct the centre line and canine relationship (Figure 7.32).

At what stage of treatment would it be appropriate to start applying traction to the UR2?

Traction to the UR2 using the bonded gold chain can be started when a stainless steel archwire is in place, having created sufficient space to accommodate the tooth.

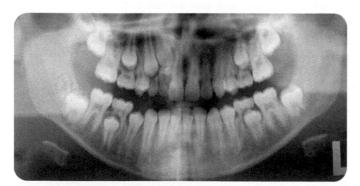

Figure 7.29

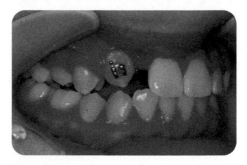

Figure 7.31

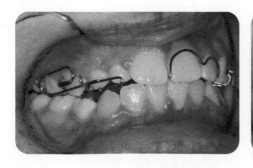

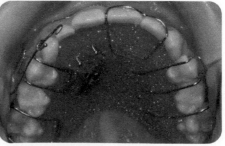

Figure 7.30

Figure 7.32 shows traction being applied to the unerupted UR2 from a rectangular stainless steel base archwire, using elastomeric string. Describe an alternative method of applying traction

Traction could be applied by the use of an auxillary archwire as a 'piggy-back'. A base stainless archwire is required to maintain arch form and provide vertical anchorage, whilst the 'piggy-back" archwire is a flexible nickel–titanium archwire that applies traction.

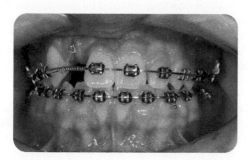

Figure 7.32

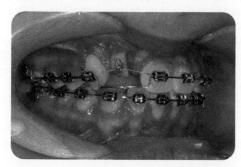

Figure 7.33

Figure 7.33 shows the 'piggy-back' mechanics being used. Why has the stainless steel archwire been 'stepped down' in the region of the partially erupted UR2?

Stepping the archwire down provides more scope to apply downward traction to the UR2 and extrude this tooth vertically.

How do you assess if an unerupted tooth is responding to traction?

To assess this, it is common practice to cut the chain to the most gingival link when applying the traction. At the following visit, if additional links of the gold chain are visible, this suggests the tooth is responding to traction and moving. If there are no signs of tooth movement after 6 months, it would be reasonable to re-radiograph the tooth. Comparison of the two radiographs allows an assessment of whether the tooth has moved.

In this case, after the partial eruption of the UR2 there appeared to be very slow subsequent movement. Over a period of time, there was an apparent change in the position of the UR2 (Figure 7.34). How would you describe what is happening?

The UR2 is not moving and the adjacent teeth appear to be intruding. This would suggest that the UR2 may be ankylosed.

What other signs would you expect to see in cases of ankylosis?

The ankylosed tooth may produce a characteristic dull tone on percussion.

How would you manage the intruded UR2?

If the UR2 were ankylosed, further traction would be inappropriate. Arrangements for removal of this tooth

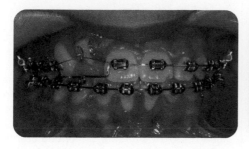
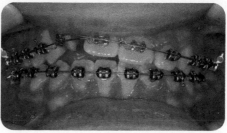

Figure 7.34

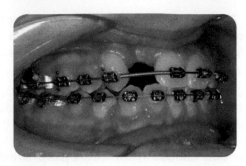

Figure 7.35

would need to be made. Realignment and levelling of the upper arch would improve the position of the UR1 (Figure 7.35).

How would you manage the resultant lateral incisor space?

In the short-term, the space could be restored with a pontic on a removable retainer. In the longer-term, an adhesive bridge or an implant-retained crown could provide definitive solutions.

References

Andreasen JO, Paulsen HU, Yu Z, Ahlquist R, Bayer T, Schwartz O (1990) A long-term study of 370 autotransplanted premolars. Part I. Surgical procedures and standardized techniques for monitoring healing. *Eur J Orthod* 12:3–13.

Ashkenazi M, Greenberg BP, Chodik G, Rakocz M (2007) Postoperative prognosis of unerupted teeth after removal of supernumerary teeth or odontomas. *Am J Orthod Dentofacial Orthop* 131:614–619.

Becker A (1995) In defense of the guidance theory of palatal canine displacement. *Angle Orthod* 65:95–98.

Becker A, Chaushu S (2003) Success rate and duration of orthodontic treatment for adult patients with palatally impacted maxillary canines. *Am J Orthod Dentofacial Orthop* 124:509–514.

Bishara SE (1992) Impacted maxillary canines: a review. *Am J Orthod Dentofac Orthop* 101:159–171.

Bondemark L, Tsiopa J (2007) Prevalence of ectopic eruption, impaction, retention and agenesis of permanent second molars. *Angle Orthod* 77:773–778.

Brin I, Becker A, Shalhav M (1986) Position of the maxillary permanent canine in relation to anomalous or missing lateral incisors: a population study. *Eur J Orthod* 8:12–16.

Chaushu S, Bongart M, Aksoy A, Ben-Bassat Y, Becker A (2009) Buccal ectopia of maxillary canines with no crowding. *Am J Orthod Dentofacial Orthop* 136:218–223.

Czochrowska EM, Stenvik A, Bjercke B, Zachrisson BU (2002) Outcome of tooth transplantation: survival and success rates 17–41 years posttreatment. *Am J Orthod Dentofacial Orthop* 121:110–119.

DiBiase DD (1969) Midline supernumeraries and eruption of the maxillary central incisor. *Dent Pract Dent Rec* 20:35–40.

Ely NJ, Sherriff M, Cobourne MT (2006) Dental transposition as a disorder of genetic origin. *Eur J Orthod* 28:145–151.

Ericson S, Bjerklin K (2001) The dental follicle in normally and ectopically erupting maxillary canines: a computed tomography study. *Angle Orthod* 71:333–342.

Ericson S, Kurol J (1987) Incisor resorption caused by maxillary cuspids. A radiographic study. *Angle Orthod* 57:332–346.

Ericson S, Kurol J (1988a) Early treatment of palatally erupting maxillary canines by extraction of the primary canines. *Eur J Orthod* 1988;10:283–295.

Ericson S, Kurol J (1988b) Resorption of maxillary lateral incisors caused by ectopic eruption of the canines. A clinical and radiographic analysis of predisposing factors. *Am J Orthod Dentofacial Orthop* 94:503–513.

Ericson S, Kurol J (2000a) Incisor root resorptions due to ectopic maxillary canines imaged by computerized tomography: a comparative study in extracted teeth. *Angle Orthod* 70:276–283.

Ericson S, Kurol PJ (2000b) Resorption of incisors after ectopic eruption of maxillary canines: a CT study. *Angle Orthod* 70:415–423.

Fleming PS, Scott P, Heidari N, Dibiase AT (2009) Influence of radiographic position of ectopic canines on the duration of orthodontic treatment. *Angle Orthod* 79:442–446.

Frazier-Bowers SA, Koehler KE, Ackerman JL, Proffit WR (2007) Primary failure of eruption: further characterization of a rare eruption disorder. *Am J Orthod Dentofacial Orthop* 131:578.e1–11.

Frazier-Bowers SA, Simmons D, Wright JT, Proffit WR, Ackerman JL (2010) Primary failure of eruption and PTH1R: the importance of a genetic diagnosis for orthodontic treatment planning. *Am J Orthod Dentofacial Orthop* 137:160.e1–7.

Grauer D, Cevidanes LS, Styner MA, et al. (2010) Accuracy and landmark error calculation using cone-beam computed tomography-generated cephalograms. *Angle Orthod* 80:286–294.

Haselden K, Hobkirk JA, Goodman JR, Jones SP, Hemmings KW (2001) Root resorption in retained deciduous canine and molar teeth without permanent successors in patients with severe hypodontia. *Int J Paediatr Dent* 11:171–178.

Hilgers ML, Scarfe WC, Scheetz JP, Farman AG (2005) Accuracy of linear temporomandibular joint measurements with cone beam computed tomography and digital cephalometric radiography. *Am J Orthod Dentofacial Orthop* 128:803–811.

Iramaneerat S, Cunningham SJ, Horrocks EN (1998) The effect of two alternative methods of canine exposure upon subsequent duration of orthodontic treatment. *Int J Paediatr Dent* 8:123–129.

Isaacson KG, Thom AR, Horner K, Whaites E (2008) *Orthodontic radiographs—guidelines for the use of radiographs in clinical orthodontics*, 3rd edn. London: British Orthodontic Society.

Iseri H, Solow B (1996) Continued eruption of maxillary incisors and first molars in girls from 9 to 25 years, studied by the implant method. *Eur J Orthod* 18:245–256.

Johal A, Cheung MY, Marcene W (2007) The impact of two different malocclusion traits on quality of life. *Br Dent J* 202:E2.

Kokich VG, Crabill KE (2006) Managing the patient with missing or malformed maxillary central incisors. *Am J Orthod Dentofacial Orthop* 129 (4 Suppl):S55–S63.

Kurol J, Bjerklin K (1982) Ectopic eruption of maxillary first permanent molars: familial tendencies. *ASDC J Dent Child* 49:35–38.

Kvint S, Lindsten R, Magnusson A, Nilsson P, Bjerklin K (2010) Autotransplantation of teeth in 215 patients. A follow-up study. *Angle Orthod* 80:446–451.

Lascala CA, Panella J, Marques MM (2004) Analysis of the accuracy of linear measurements obtained by cone beam computed tomography (CBCT-NewTom). *Dentomaxillofac Radiol* 33:291–294.

Levander E, Malmgren O, Eliasson S (1994) Evaluation of root resorption in relation to two orthodontic treatment regimes. A clinical experimental study. *Eur J Orthod* 16:223–228.

Leyland L, Batra P, Wong F, Llewelyn R (2006) A retrospective evaluation of the eruption of impacted permanent incisors after extraction of supernumerary teeth. *J Clin Pediatr Dent* 30:225–231.

Mitchell L, Bennett TG (1992) Supernumerary teeth causing delayed eruption – a retrospective study. *Br J Orthod* 19:41–46.

Othman S, Harradine N (2007) Tooth size discrepancies in an orthodontic population. *Angle Orthod* 77:668–674.

Patel S, Fanshawe T, Bister D, Cobourne MT (2011) Survival and success of maxillary canine autotransplantation: a retrospective investigation. *Eur J Orthod* 33:298–304.

Pearson MH, Robinson SN, Reed R, Birnie DJ, Zaki GA (1997) Management of palatally impacted canines: the findings of a collaborative study. *Eur J Orthod* 19:511–515.

Peck S, Peck L, Kataja M (1994) The palatally displaced canine as a dental anomaly of genetic origin. *Angle Orthod* 64:249–256.

Polder BJ, Van't Hof MA, Van der Linden FP, Kuijpers-Jagtman AM (2004) A meta-analysis of the prevalence of dental agenesis of permanent teeth. *Community Dent Oral Epidemiol* 32:217–226.

Proffit WR, Vig KW (1981) Primary failure of eruption: a possible cause of posterior open-bite. *Am J Orthod* 80:173–190.

Smale I, Artun J, Behbehani F, Doppel D, van't Hof M, Kuijpers-Jagtman AM (2005) Apical root resorption 6 months after initiation of fixed orthodontic appliance therapy. *Am J Orthod Dentofacial Orthop* 128:57–67.

Stewart DJ (1978) Dilacerate unerupted maxillary central incisors. *Br Dent J* 145:229–233.

Stewart JA, Heo G, Glover KE, Williamson PC, Lam EW, Major PW (2001) Factors that relate to treatment duration for patients with palatally impacted maxillary canines. *Am J Orthod Dentofacial Orthop* 119:216–225.

Walker L, Enciso R, Mah J (2005) Three-dimensional localization of maxillary canines with cone-beam computed tomography. *Am J Orthod Dentofacial Orthop* 128:418–423.

Wisth PJ, Norderval K, Boe OE (1976) Periodontal status of orthodontically treated impacted maxillary canines. *Angle Orthod* 46:69–76.

Woloshyn H, Artun J, Kennedy DB, Joondeph DR (1994) Pulpal and periodontal reactions to orthodontic alignment of palatally impacted canines. *Angle Orthod* 64:257–264.

8

Fixed Appliances

Introduction

Fixed orthodontic appliances form the mainstay of contemporary treatment, permitting controlled, precise and sophisticated tooth movement in three dimensions. The appliance in most common use is the pre-adjusted edgewise, or straight wire, appliance. The edgewise slot was originally developed by Edward Angle in the 20th century, improving on his earlier designs (Angle, 1928). The edgewise slot conferred significant control and precision to tooth movement, which had been lacking in previous systems.

Contemporary pre-adjusted edgewise appliances stem from later work by Laurence Andrews, who identified six characteristic occlusal features common to ideal, untreated occlusions. These include: a slight modification to the Angle class I molar relationship, correct crown angulation and inclination, absence of spacing and rotations, and a flat curve of Spee (Andrews, 1972). Subsequently, he tailored a fixed appliance system to introduce the desired degree of angulation, inclination and rotational control to produce this ideal occlusion with treatment (Andrews, 1976). The key difference, therefore, between the Andrew's pre-adjusted edgewise appliance and Angle's original edgewise system was that in the former, a prescription was placed in the bracket slot for each individual tooth, necessitating the use of specific brackets for each tooth. Previously, standard edgewise brackets were generic, with artistic archwire bends necessary to achieve appropriate three-dimensional position for each tooth. With the pre-adjusted edgewise appliance, archwire bends were theoretically unnecessary. Various modifications to the original prescription of the Andrews' system have since been introduced, with Ronald Roth altering and streamlining the bracket series and introducing a single bracket system for both extraction and non-extraction cases (Roth, 1976).

In parallel with the development of fixed appliances based on the edgewise slot, one of Angle's pupils developed an alternative fixed appliance system and treatment philosophy, furthering one of Angle's earlier appliances, the ribbon arch appliance. This appliance became known eponymously as the Begg appliance (Begg, 1956). It was based on tipping teeth initially before uprighting them later in treatment. By doing this, the heavy anchorage demands of the edgewise appliance were overcome, but the precise three-dimensional control was compromised. In an attempt to superimpose the precision of the pre-adjusted edgewise appliance on the advantages of the Begg appliance, the Tip Edge® appliance was developed. The Tip Edge® appliance also permits free tipping of teeth during the initial stages of treatment (Kesling, 1988). However, as the teeth are uprighted, the dimensions of the bracket slot reduce, imparting three-dimensional control.

More recent modifications to pre-adjusted edgewise appliances include self-ligating bracket systems and the emergence of customized systems. Self-ligating brackets have a clip or slide mechanism to engage the archwire, obviating the requirement for elastomeric or steel ties, which are time-consuming to place and believed to retard tooth movement (Harradine, 2003). Fixed appliances have also been modified to improve their appearance, with ceramic brackets available for

Clinical Cases in Orthodontics, First Edition. Martyn T. Cobourne, Padhraig S. Fleming, Andrew T. DiBiase, and Sofia Ahmad.
© 2012 Martyn T. Cobourne, Padhraig S. Fleming, Andrew T. DiBiase, and Sofia Ahmad. Published 2012 by Blackwell Publishing Ltd.

most appliance systems and a new generation of lingual orthodontic appliances gaining in popularity, particularly among adult patients. With the advancements in computer-assisted design, fully-customized labial and lingual bracket systems (Insignia® and Incognito®) are also gaining in popularity with these appliances fully-tailored to each patient. These systems raise the prospect of producing ideal results without recourse to significant archwire bending and alteration.

The mandibular canine brackets have been reversed in this case (Figure 8.1). Why has this been done?

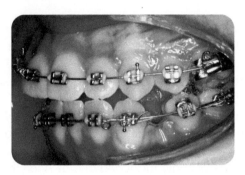

Figure 8.1

Mandibular canine brackets have prescribed mesial crown angulation. By reversing them, distal crown tipping is encouraged. This will facilitate retroclination of the lower incisors, permitting class III camouflage.

What is this auxiliary wire and why is it used? (Figure 8.2)

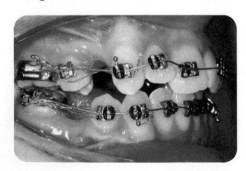

Figure 8.2

It is a laceback. Lacebacks are used to control the position of the canine crown during alignment with pre-adjusted edgewise appliances. The in-built mesial angulation in the canine bracket means that there is a tendency for the crown of this tooth to tip forwards during early alignment, particularly if this tooth is distally angulated. This can result in undesirable

proclination of the lower incisor teeth with a continuous archwire in place. Lacebacks limit this unwanted mesial tipping of the canine crown whilst allowing uprighting of the roots as the bracket prescription is expressed. However, these potential advantages have not been borne out in prospective research (Irvine *et al.*, 2004; Usmani *et al.*, 2002) and attachment of the laceback to the first molar tooth can be anchorage demanding, particularly in extraction cases with marked distal angulation of the canine teeth.

What other problems can occur during early alignment using a pre-adjusted edgewise appliance?

The mesial tip that is present in the canine bracket prescription also means that if the canine crown is upright or at a distal angulation, there will be a tendency for extrusion of the incisor teeth, which can result in an undesirable increase in the overbite during initial treatment.

The bracket on the maxillary canine has been inverted (Figure 8.3). Why has this been done?

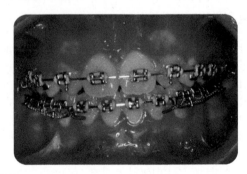

Figure 8.3

Inversion of the bracket reverses the torque prescription. The maxillary canine is occupying the lateral incisor position in this instance. Consequently, palatal root torque is desirable to simulate the lateral incisor, promoting optimal dental aesthetics and gingival position.

What type of bracket is shown in Figure 8.4?

This is a ceramic self-ligating bracket with a rhodium-plated cobalt-chromium clip.

List the main advantages and disadvantages of ceramic brackets

- **Advantages:**
  - Aesthetics

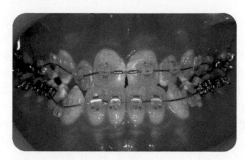

Figure 8.4

• **Disadvantages:**
  ◦ Increased friction
  ◦ Wear of opposing teeth
  ◦ Difficult removal

How can the effect of increased friction with ceramic brackets be lessened?

• Incorporation of a metal slot within the bracket
• Use of self-ligating ceramic brackets
• Space closure on round or reduced dimension stainless steel wires
• Loop space-closing mechanics

This patient has experienced root resorption, most notably on the maxillary central incisors (Figure 8.5). Why is this?

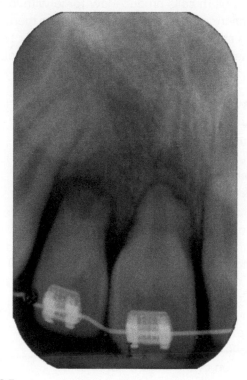

Figure 8.5

Some degree of root resorption is almost universal following orthodontic treatment; however, it has been estimated that around 5% of patients will experience more than 5 mm of root shortening during treatment (Killiany, 1999). In the long-term, teeth with severe root resorption do not appear to necessarily elicit greater mobility or discolouration (Becker and Chaushu, 2005).

Can we predict which patients are at risk from root resorption?

Whilst numerous factors have been implicated in the development of root resorption, many of these have been based on clinical observation rather than clinical trials (Levander et al., 1998; Linge and Linge, 1983; 1991; Weltman et al., 2010). Possible risk factors include:

• Heavy forces
• Continuous as opposed to intermittent forces
• Intrusive forces
• Amount of tooth movement
• Use of class II elastics
• Teeth with abnormal root morphology
• Duration of treatment
• Moving root apices into cortical bone
• A history of allergies or asthma
• Teeth with no occlusal contact.

Of these, there is only substantive evidence that heavy forces cause more root resorption (Weltman et al., 2010).

What should be done if root resorption is diagnosed during orthodontic treatment?

When severe root resorption is diagnosed, the patient should be informed and the aims of treatment modified to shorten overall duration and limit further movement of the affected teeth There is some evidence that less root resorption occurs if active forces are removed and there is a period of quiescence for 2–3 months during treatment (Levander et al., 1994).

What type of mechanics are being used in this case? (Figure 8.6)

The patient is in the end-stage of space closure and overbite reduction. To achieve this, double-delta loops have been placed in the maxillary archwire. By increasing the amount of wire vertically and horizontally, the wire is more flexible in both planes. The double-delta applies both a levelling and retractile force to the upper incisors in this case.

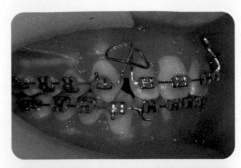

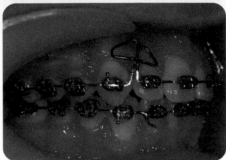

Figure 8.6

first premolars. This is being utilized to align the UR2 by redistribution of space using a compressed nickel–titanium coil spring on a round stainless steel archwire (upper panels). Once space has been created, a bracket is positioned on the lateral incisor and an auxiliary or piggy-back nickel–titanium archwire is placed beneath the main archwire to begin aligning the UR2 (middle panels). Once the UR2 has been partially aligned, the stainless steel archwire is removed and a flexible nickel–titanium archwire tied in to complete the process of alignment (lower panels).

Why are these mechanics being used?

Teeth require space to be aligned. If all the teeth are engaged on the initial aligning archwire, space will be created by uncontrolled expansion or proclination of the upper incisors. This will then require further treatment to correct, potentially extending treatment and risking root resorption. To avoid the use of uncontrolled mechanics or 'round tripping', space should be created initially to permit alignment of grossly displaced teeth. By using compressed coil on a rigid steel wire, minimal strain is placed on the anchorage units and as reciprocal anchorage is used, friction is low and arch form is maintained. An added advantage in this case is that the use of active coil spring has corrected the maxillary dental centre line. Nickel–titanium coils produce low force with long-range action, making them more efficient then stainless steel or elgiloy. To prevent adjacent teeth from rotating, they should be ligated with stainless steel ties as shown in Figure 8.7.

What type of appliance is shown in Figure 8.8?

This is the Begg light wire fixed appliance.

What are the objectives of this stage of treatment?

This is stage 1 of treatment. Rigid round stainless steel archwires are in place with circle loops placed mesial to the canine teeth and anchorage bends mesial to the first molars. Full-time light class II elastics are used in conjunction with these wires. The precise objectives of stage 1 are:

- Tooth alignment (with overcorrection of rotations)
- Overjet reduction
- Overbite reduction
- Correction of the molar relationship
- Arch co-ordination.

What are the advantages and disadvantages of looped mechanics?

Prior to the introduction of the pre-adjusted edgewise appliance, the placement of loops and bends in the archwire was a routine part of standard edgewise mechanics. The standard edgewise appliance had brackets that were identical for each tooth. Therefore, bends were placed in the archwire to achieve precise three-dimensional positioning of the teeth. With the advent of bracket prescriptions, this positioning was placed automatically in the edgewise slot and bracket base. Thus, it became possible to apply sliding mechanics to individual teeth or to groups of teeth, moving them along the archwire, simplifying treatment mechanics and improving the quality of finishing considerably.

However, loops and bends still have a place in contemporary orthodontics. The chief advantage of using loops for space closure is elimination of friction generated by sliding mechanics. The disadvantages are that the wires are often complex to bend, the force on activation tends to be high and has a short range, and the wires can cause soft tissue trauma.

What mechanics are shown in Figure 8.7?

The patient has crowding and a palatally-excluded UR2. Space has been created by extraction of the maxillary

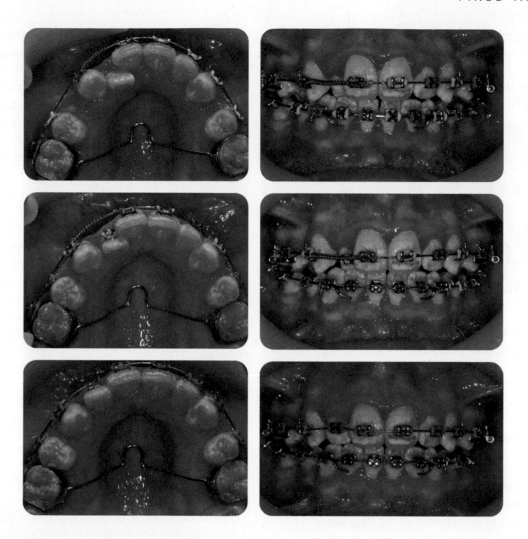

Figure 8.7

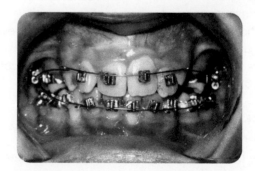

Figure 8.8

Why is this appliance no longer used?

The Begg appliance requires the placement of individual brass pins to secure the archwire into each bracket, which combined with extensive wire bending is time-consuming. It is also heavily reliant on elastic wear for successful treatment. A major disadvantage is the lack of precise control afforded by using round wires and brackets with a narrow slot.

Which bracket system has replaced the Begg appliance?

The Tip Edge® bracket is the natural successor to the Begg appliance (see Figure 4.15). This bracket incorporates a rectangular slot, but the basic design also allows for tipping. The rectangular slot allows three-dimensional control of tooth movement and appropriate torque expression as the teeth are uprighted using auxiliary springs or an additional superelastic archwire.

What are the main advantages of light wire appliances?

The main advantage of these appliances is that they can achieve overbite and overjet reduction very rapidly and early in treatment. However, this is tempered by a reliance on elastic wear, extraction-based mechanics and complex tooth uprighting during the final stages of treatment.

What type of brackets are shown in Figure 8.9?

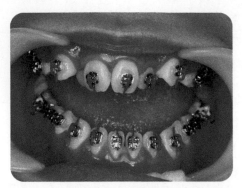

Figure 8.9

These brackets are DamonQ®, which is an example of a passive self-ligating pre-adjusted edgewise bracket. Passive self-ligating brackets are characterized by a slide that does not actively engage the wire. In other self-ligating systems, such as InOvation®, closure of the clip results in a force being imparted on the archwire. This type of self-ligation is referred to as active.

What is the purpose of the blue plastic jigs on the anterior brackets?

These allow accurate positioning of the brackets. DamonQ® brackets have a self-ligating mechanism and are not Siamese in design. They can be more difficult to position because of the lack of a vertical groove, a large antero-posterior bracket thickness and a labial face to the bracket that is not completely flat. The jig represents an attempt to address these problems.

Why have self-ligating brackets increased in popularity over the last few years?

This is primarily due to the improved quality and sophistication of the bracket systems available and the marketing that has accompanied them. Numerous systems are now available, most of which are based on a traditional twin bracket, with a clip or slide that is activated to close the slot of the bracket engaging the wire.

What are the advantages of self-ligating brackets?

Many advantages have been claimed by proponents and manufacturers of self-ligating brackets, including reduced friction, more efficient tooth movement, less discomfort, and greater, more stable expansion. Certainly there is a lot of evidence from *in vitro* studies that less friction is generated between self-ligating brackets and the archwire, particularly passively ligated brackets. However, it is very difficult to measure friction and it has proven impossible to replicate friction *in vivo*; the importance of friction on tooth movement is therefore debatable.

Do self-ligating brackets move teeth more rapidly?

There have now been several clinical studies investigating the speed of tooth movement with self-ligating bracket systems compared to conventionally ligated brackets (Fleming *et al.*, 2009b; Scott *et al.*, 2008a). To date, these studies have not found any significant advantage to using self-ligating brackets in terms of faster tooth movement. Although most have investigated just the initial alignment phase of treatment, the available evidence indicates that these brackets do not reduce overall treatment time (DiBiase *et al.*, 2011; Fleming *et al.*, 2010).

Is treatment with self-ligating brackets less painful for the patient?

In terms of subjective discomfort, one study has suggested that the initial stages of treatment with self-ligating brackets may be associated with slightly less discomfort when compared with conventional ligation (Pringle *et al.*, 2009). However, other studies have reported no difference when compared to conventionally ligated brackets (Scott *et al.*, 2008b).

Do self-ligating brackets allow for more expansion?

The use of some self-ligating brackets allows for slightly more expansion in the molar region when compared to conventional ligation, but the clinical importance of this is again open to interpretation (Fleming *et al.*, 2009a). So, at this stage, many of the claims for self-ligating brackets remain unsubstantiated.

Are there any other advantages of self-ligating brackets?

It would appear that for the experienced clinician, it can be quicker to remove and place archwires with self-ligating systems when compared with elastomeric or steel ligatures (Turnbull and Birnie, 2007).

Figure 8.10 shows the same patient as in Figure 8.9 after placement of the archwires. What type of archwires has been placed?

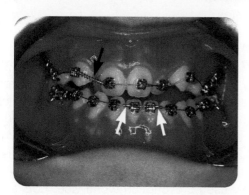

Figure 8.10

These are round 0.014-inch superelastic nickel–titanium archwires.

What are the white arrows pointing to?

These are small soft metal tubes, which are compressed onto the archwire by the orthodontist and limit unwanted sliding of the wires through the brackets. The combination of small diameter archwires and low friction means that this can be a problem with self-ligating brackets during the early stages of treatment.

What is the black arrow pointing to?

This is a section of compressed coil, which is creating space to align the UR2. An advantage of the robust, complete ligation provided by self-ligating brackets is

that space-creating mechanics such as this can be instigated much earlier in treatment and on much more flexible archwires than is advocated with conventional fixed appliances.

What are the two appliances shown in Figure 8.11 and what are they used for?

They are both forms of palatal arch and are used to reinforce anchorage in the maxillary arch. The one on the left is a trans-palatal arch and the one on the right is a palatal arch with an acrylic button in the palatal vault. They are constructed from 0.9- to 1-mm stainless steel wire soldered to bands placed on the first molars.

The trans-palatal arch, which was originally described by Robert Goshgarian, theoretically fixes the inter-molar distance and prevents mesial movement of the molars, particularly by rotation around their palatal roots. It can also be activated to correct molar rotation and produce a small amount of molar distalization and expansion. The palatal arch with an acrylic button was originally described by Hays Nance and is referred to as a Nance palatal arch. It fixes the position of the molars by using an acrylic button resting against the vault of the palatal arch for anchorage, thus preventing their mesial movement and anchorage loss.

How effective are they?

Anchorage management is a key component in effective orthodontic treatment. Maximum anchorage, where the first molars are required to maintain their position without moving mesially, is often required in the maxillary arch. This can be achieved using extra-oral traction or headgear but this form of anchorage is compliance-based. Therefore, the fixed arches shown in Figure 8.11 are available to the orthodontist for

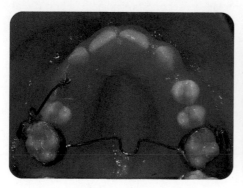
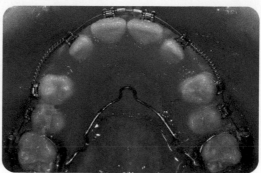

Figure 8.11

maximizing maxillary anchorage. However, there is little evidence that they are particularly effective. Indeed, in one clinical trial that compared patients with and without trans-palatal arches, no difference in terms of mesial and vertical movement of the first molars was found (Zablocki et al., 2008). However, this was a retrospective cephalometric study; it can be very difficult to clearly visualize maxillary first molars from lateral cephalograms. A more recent study using direct measurement from laser scans of models using the palatal rugae as a stable reference point, found that there was no difference between the two types of arch in terms of preventing mesial molar movement or tipping during the alignment phase of treatment (Stivaros et al., 2010).

What problems exist with these appliances?

- Neither arch provides absolute anchorage
- If there is movement of the molars, the U loop of the trans-palatal arch can become embedded in the palatal mucosa as the molars tip mesially
- The acrylic button of the Nance palatal arch can become embedded in the mucosa of the palatal vault.

List some alternatives to palatal arches?

- Headgear
- Micro-implants
- Mini-plates

Why do orthodontists use pre-adjusted bracket systems with different prescriptions?

A variety of prescriptions are available for different pre-adjusted edgewise bracket systems. The most significant differences relate to the programmed levels of tip or angulation (Table 8.1) and inclination or torque (Table 8.2). Whilst the Andrews prescription was the original, the Roth prescription is now the most commonly used prescription worldwide. Roth's modifications were based on an emphasis on dynamic occlusion with enhanced mesial tip on the maxillary canine brackets designed to promote canine guidance.

Table 8.1 Angulation values for Andrews, Roth and MBT prescriptions. Positive values represent mesial crown angulation

	Max central	Max lateral	Max canine	Max first premolar	Max second premolar	Max first molar	Max second molar
Andrews	5	9	11	2	2	5	5
Roth	5	9	13	0	0	0	0
MBT	4	8	8	0	0	0	0
	Mandibular central	Mandibular lateral	Mandibular canine	Mandibular first premolar	Mandibular second premolar	Mandibular first molar	Mandibular second molar
Andrews	2	2	5	2	2	2	2
Roth	2	2	7	−1	−1	−1	−1
MBT	0	0	3	2	2	0	0

Table 8.2 Torque values for Andrews, Roth and MBT prescriptions. Positive values signify palatal or lingual root torque

	Maximum central	Maximum lateral	Maximum canine	Maximum first premolar	Maximum second premolar	Maximum first molar	Maximum second molar
Andrews	7	3	−7	−7	−7	−9	−9
Roth	12	8	−2	−7	−7	−14	−14
MBT	17	10	0	−7	−7	−14	−14
	Mandibular Central	Mandibular Lateral	Mandibular Canine	Mandibular first premolar	Mandibular second premolar	Mandibular first molar	Mandibular second molar
Andrews	−1	−1	−11	−17	−22	−30	−30
Roth	−1	−1	−11	−17	−22	−30	−30
MBT	−6	−6	−6	−12	−17	−20	−10

The degree of buccal root torque in the maxillary molars was accentuated to avoid non-working side interferences due to hanging palatal cusps (Roth, 1976). Other popular generic prescriptions include MBT; however, some bracket systems are produced with a range of prescriptions to provide greater versatility (Damon Q®, InOvation®).

The MBT modification, which incorporates increased upper incisor torque and reduced lower incisor torque, is useful for class II malocclusions, maintaining ideal torque following removal of maxillary premolars and resisting lower incisor proclination with the use of class II inter-arch traction. Moreover, MBT brackets have smaller amounts of in-built mesial crown tip, conserving anchorage in class II malocclusions.

What stage of treatment is shown in Figure 8.12?

This is the initial stage of alignment and levelling, aiming to correct all rotations, and vertical and horizontal discrepancies. The archwires being used are round and composed of nickel–titanium, and are partially engaged. Nickel–titanium archwires exhibit high flexibility, low force, a wide range of action and shape memory, whereby they return to their original shape on deactivation. Newer, martensitic active wires are designed to exhibit 'super-elasticity', meaning they deliver a constant force over a wide range of activation. This is due to a phase shift in crystalline structure on activation from a low stiffness martensitic structure to a higher stiffness austenitic phase, represented by a plateau on the stress–strain curve. This makes them particularly suited for use in alignment when a low constant force is required. The range of activation of stainless steel wires can be increased by the incorporation of bends, or the use of multi-strand wires, where the force delivered is related to the dimensions of the individual wires within the strand.

Despite the theoretical advantages of nickel–titanium wires and their popularity, there is no evidence that they outperform multi-stranded steel wires in the initial alignment phase of treatment (Cobb *et al.*, 1998). This negative finding may be related to the large degree of individual variability in rapidity of tooth movement.

Which archwire sequence is most effective?

The requirements of archwires vary significantly, depending on the stage of treatment. In particular, strength is required throughout treatment to resist occlusal forces, although there is a greater premium on this property later in treatment. High flexibility and range are required during initial alignment to engage grossly irregular and displaced teeth. Later in treatment, greater stiffness and low range are preferable as alignment is likely to have occurred and stiffness is needed to permit overbite reduction and controlled space closure (Kusy, 1997).

The specific choice of archwire for each stage of treatment is primarily related to individual preference.

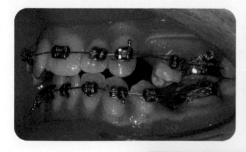
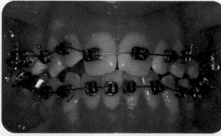
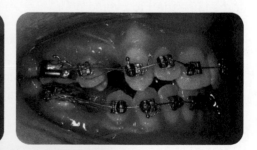
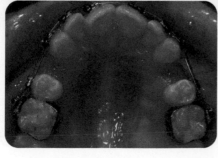
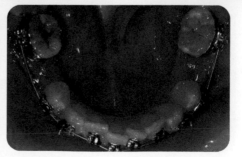

Figure 8.12

A recent randomized controlled trial has, however, compared three archwire sequences with respect to efficiency, root resorption and pain experience (Mandall et al., 2006). The wire sequences did not differ with respect to either the degree of root resorption or subjective pain experience. However, treatment with a sequence comprising 0.016-inch and 0.018 × 0.025-inch nickel–titanium, followed by 0.019 × 0.025-inch stainless steel was found to be more efficient than the use of intermediate stainless steel wires. Some practitioners, however, continue to use intermediate steel wires to promote overbite reduction before progressing to stainless steel working archwires.

What stage of orthodontic treatment is shown in Figure 8.13?

Both images show space closure. The appliances are pre-adjusted edgewise appliances and space closure is being carried out using sliding mechanics. The base working archwire is a thick rectangular stainless steel wire, which is stiff and resists deformation, maintaining arch form and permitting overbite control. Typically, a 019 × 025-inch wire will be used in a 022 × 028-inch bracket slot, as shown here, and a force is applied from hooks on the molars to hooks soldered onto the arch between the lateral incisors and canines. Stainless steel wires also present less frictional resistance than nickel–titanium or titanium–molybdenum alloy wires. Although difficult to measure clinically, friction can be an issue when using sliding mechanics and it is estimated that half the applied force is needed to overcome it.

What is the best way to apply force during space closure?

Force can be applied either using elastomeric traction in the form of power chain or an activated ligature (as shown), or activated nickel–titanium coils. Elastics undergo rapid force degradation, whilst nickel–titanium coils have the advantage of delivering a fairly consistent force over prolonged periods with a wide range of activation, although there appears to be variation between different products (Baty et al., 1994). There is some evidence that nickel–titanium coils are more effective than activated ligatures, but not power chain, although considerable individual variation exists (Dixon et al., 2002; Nightingale and Jones, 2003; Samuels et al., 1998). Care should be taken not to over-activate the coils as over-extension compromises superelastic properties (Manhartsberger and Seidenbusch, 1996). A force level of approximately 150 g has been found to be the most effective, although this too is subject to individual variation (Samuels et al., 1998).

What are the appliances shown in Figure 8.14?

These are two fixed expansion arches. On the right is a quadhelix appliance, while the one on the left is a HYRAX rapid maxillary expander. The quadhelix is constructed of 0.9–1.0-mm stainless steel or elgiloy and is soldered to bands on the maxillary first molars. The four helices increase the range and flexibility of the appliance. It can be used for expansion of the maxillary arch as well as de-rotation of the molars. The framework of the HYRAX appliance is also made of stainless steel, connecting bands on maxillary first premolars and first molars to a pre-fabricated expansion screw, which is available in various sizes, depending how much expansion is required.

How are these appliances activated and what are their effects?

The quadhelix can be activated either outside or inside the mouth. Outside the mouth, the appliance should

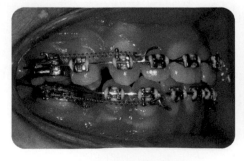
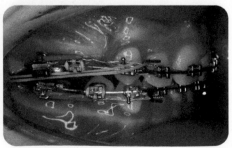

Figure 8.13

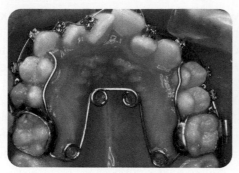
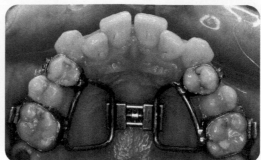

Figure 8.14

be expanded by approximately 1 cm on each side in the molar region and 1.5 cm anteriorly. Inside the mouth, triple beak pliers can be used to re-activate it at subsequent visits. This will generate over 300 g of force (Birnie and McNamara, 1980). Whilst this may have some orthopaedic effect, especially in children, the majority of the effect of a quadhelix is dento-alveolar, with teeth tipping buccally. Therefore, this appliance is contra-indicated when bodily expansion of the maxillary buccal dentition is required.

The HYRAX appliance is activated intra-orally by the patient with a key to turn the midline screw. It is used for rapid maxillary (palatal) expansion. Activation is directed at opening the mid-palatal suture, resulting in skeletal or orthopaedic expansion. The screw is activated 0.25–1.0 mm per day over a period of 2–4 weeks, producing forces up to 10 kg. A transient midline diastema usually develops as the suture opens, but closes without active intervention due to the recoil of supra-crestal fibres between the incisors. When adequate expansion has been achieved, usually when the lingual cusps of the maxillary molars are occluding on the lingual inclines of the mandibular molars, the appliance is made passive and left *in situ* for a minimum of 3 months to consolidate the expansion. Skeletal expansion can be achieved in children and adolescents due to the patency of the mid-palatal suture, although in adults the suture becomes obliterated and therefore less amendable to splitting. If skeletal expansion is required in an adult patient, the mid-palatal suture can be split surgically prior to expansion, combined with relieving cuts at the lateral maxillary buccal plates, a technique known as surgically-assisted rapid palatal expansion (SARPE).

What type of appliance is shown in Figure 8.15?

This is a customized lingual orthodontic appliance.

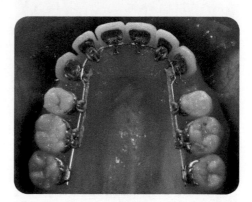

Figure 8.15

What are the advantages of this type of appliance system?

Customized appliances may limit the requirement for wire bending, simplifying orthodontic finishing. However, small adjustments are typically still necessary to produce an ideal result due to physiological variations. Lingual orthodontic appliances have significant aesthetic advantage. In addition, any decalcification arising during treatment is less likely to affect the labial surfaces.

Comment on the difference in inclination between the maxillary incisors arising during treatment (Figure 8.16)

The maxillary incisors have been torqued. Palatal root torque has been added to the UL1, UR1 and UR2. Labial root torque has been added to the UL2.

How could this be achieved?

Torque is expressed using stiff, large dimension, rectangular archwires. Supplementary torque may be added with local archwire bends, choice of prescription and local bracket alteration. Use of MBT prescription

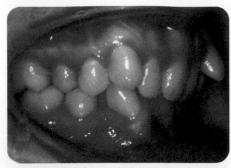

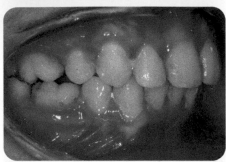

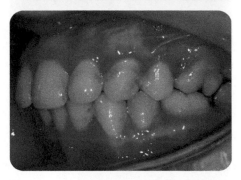

Figure 8.16

will provide additional palatal root torque to the maxillary incisors. Inversion of the UL2 attachment would reverse the torque in this tooth to impart labial root torque without altering the mesio-distal tip.

What is torque?

Torque is described as rotation without translation. It involves preferential root movement while crown position is kept stationary. Torque is usually delivered in rectangular archwires.

What factors influence torque delivery with fixed appliances?

- Archwire dimension
- Bracket dimension
- Play (or tolerance) between the wire and bracket slot. Small amounts of play permit greater torque delivery; hence, large dimension wires and correctly-sized slots are preferable
- Stiffness of bracket and wire
- Archwire and bracket materials (Gioka and Eliades, 2004). Torque delivery with flexible plastic brackets is problematic; rigid stainless steel wires permit larger amounts of torque delivery

What problems do you anticipate in placing fixed appliances in the case shown in Figure 8.17?

Bonding of the fixed appliances will be difficult. Porcelain veneers have been placed on the maxillary

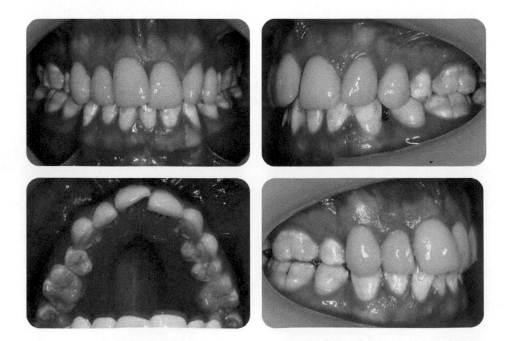

Figure 8.17

anterior teeth. There is also fluorosis affecting the lower anterior teeth.

How could this situation be managed?

Conventional appliances could be placed on the veneers using a porcelain-bonding system involving hydrofluoric acid and porcelain primer. Risks with this approach include failure of the attachments and fracture of the veneers at debond. Sandblasting of porcelain is also known to improve bond strengths, although this also risks damage to the porcelain glaze (Schmage *et al.*, 2003). Alternatives include use of lingual appliances or clear aligners.

What type of set-up is shown in Figure 8.18?

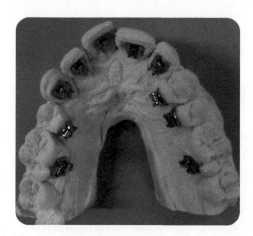

Figure 8.18

This is an example of indirect bonding of a lingual appliance. This promotes more accurate bracket positioning, although errors do still occur (Koo *et al.*, 1999). A transfer tray is fabricated to allow the position of these attachments to be replicated during appliance placement.

The panoramic radiograph in Figure 8.19 reveals an ectopically-placed UR3. Is the prognosis for orthodontic eruption good?

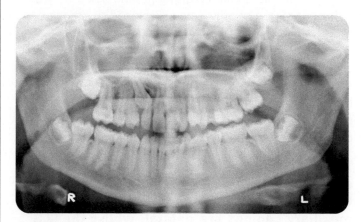

Figure 8.19

Yes. The tooth is almost vertical in orientation and is not excessively high or mesially-displaced. Furthermore, the patient is an adolescent and the tooth is palatally-placed not buccal; hence, mechanical eruption is a predictable option.

Explain the rationale for the mechanics in Figure 8.20

Piggy-back wires are shown in Figure 8.20. These are necessary to avoid unwanted reactionary effects, including intrusion, proclination and transverse changes arising during eruption of the canine. The relatively rigid base archwire, in this case 0.018-inch stainless steel, has a high elastic modulus. Therefore, unwanted reactionary forces to the vertical movement of the UR3 will be kept to a minimum.

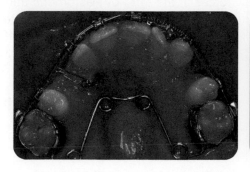 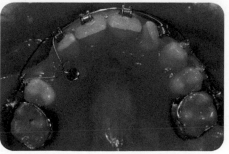

Figure 8.20

What piggy-back wires are being used in Figure 8.20?

A stainless steel auxiliary has been used in the image on the left while a nickel–titanium piggy-back has been used in the image on the right.

Nickel–titanium has a high range and flexibility with sufficient stored energy when displaced to produce tooth movement. The piggy-back has also been extended to include the UL2 to align this tooth simultaneously.

The stainless steel auxiliary is bent into a vertical loop to increase its horizontal flexibility, enhancing its range to allow a light force to be delivered that promotes vertical tooth movement.

The panoramic radiograph in Figure 8.21 shows a 14-year-old patient with three unerupted permanent canine teeth. The two maxillary canines are palatal, whilst the LL3 is in the line of the arch. Comment on the prognosis for eruption of these teeth

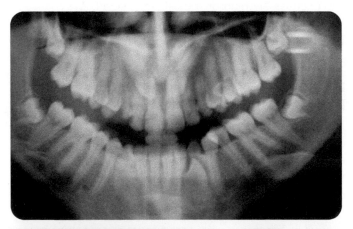

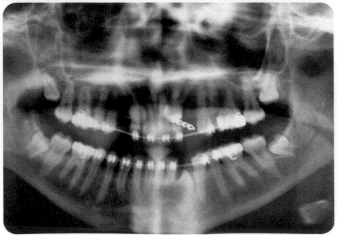

Figure 8.21

Spontaneous eruption is highly unlikely for the maxillary canines. For the LL3 there is space available in the arch but eruption of this tooth might have been expected to occur by now, given that the patient is 14 years old.

A decision was made to extract the upper primary canines, surgically expose and bond the maxillary canines, apply traction via a gold chain and accommodate them in the maxillary arch. The LLC was also extracted to encourage eruption of the LL3. Comment on the prognosis for this approach

The position of these teeth is not favourable; they are high and close to the midline. Anchorage requirements are high, both vertically and in terms of the space available from the extracted primary canines. The LL3 may erupt independently, although consideration should be given to exposing this tooth as well. Orthodontic treatment to align them will be time-consuming. There is also evidence of previous high caries levels with inter-proximal restorations in the upper labial segment.

Why do you think the panoramic radiograph in the lower panel has been taken?

This radiograph shows that fixed appliances have been placed and there has been some improvement in the position of the maxillary canines. However, the attachment on the UR3 has become detached. In addition, there has been no improvement in the position of the LL3.

How would you manage this situation?

A decision needs to be made regarding the re-exposure of the UR3, either with the placement of a new gold chain or with an open surgical exposure. The position of the UR3 was such that open exposure was carried out. In addition, arrangements were made to expose the LL3 at the same time. Eruptive forces in the form of elastomeric traction will then be applied to the 0.018-inch stainless steel archwire to erupt these teeth while providing sufficient vertical anchorage to limit reactionary effects on the dentition.

Could an alternative radiograph have been taken?

An anterior occlusal radiograph or peri-apicals could have been taken to re-assess the canines. This would have reduced exposure to ionizing radiation.

What assessments should be made during the finishing stages of orthodontics?

Both clinical and radiographic assessment should be carried out. Intra- and inter-arch occlusal features should be assessed prior to and during the finishing stage of treatment. Clinical assessment may be supplemented by radiographs to make final adjustments. In particular, a lateral cephalogram is helpful before the completion of space closure to guide final space closure and inform retention protocols. While there are well-documented limitations of panoramic radiographs (McKee *et al.*, 2002; Owens and Johal, 2008), they may be helpful to plan final refinement, particularly in respect of root angulation.

What clinical features should be assessed during finishing stages?

Inter- and intra-arch features should be assessed. Intra-arch features of particular importance include: angulation, inclination, presence of spacing, rotations, and vertical contact point discrepancies, including marginal ridge discrepancies. Inter-arch features that should be assessed are: overjet, overbite, buccal segment interdigitation, and canine and molar relationships.

What archwires would you suggest during the finishing stages?

The choice of archwire material and dimension is governed by the dictates of the residual malocclusion. Archwire choices often vary considerably between clinicians.

Archwires that could be used to address specific problems include:

- **Inadequate torque:** Large dimension rectangular wires (21 × 25-inch stainless steel, 19 × 25-inch TMA or 21 × 28-inch nickel–titanium).
- **Inadequate seating of buccal occlusion:** Flexible, light archwires (19 × 25-inch braided stainless steel; Figure 8.22) or 0.014/0.016-inch nickel–titanium.
- **First- or second-order problems:** Where brackets are not repositioned, round stainless steel archwires (0.018-inch as in Figure 8.23) or TMA archwires (Figure 8.24) may be considered as they are formable and have sufficient flexibility and range to make minor adjustments. Where brackets have been repositioned, either nickel–titanium, TMA or light stainless steel archwires may be considered.

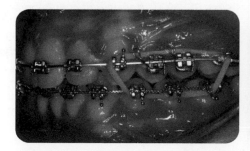

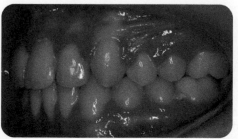

Figure 8.22

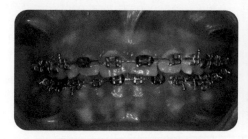

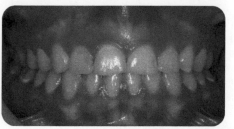

Figure 8.23

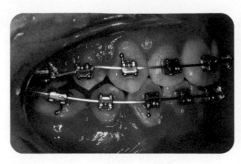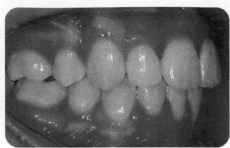

Figure 8.24

References

Andrews LF (1972) The six keys to normal occlusion. *Am J Orthod* 62:296–309.

Andrews LF (1976) The straight-wire appliance. Extraction brackets and 'classification of treatment'. *J Clin Orthod* 10:360–379.

Angle EH (1928) The latest and the best in orthodontic mechanism. *Dent Cosmos* 70:1143–1158.

Baty DL, Storie DJ, von Fraunhofer JA (1994) Synthetic elastomeric chains: a literature review. *Am J Orthod Dentofacial Orthop* 105:536–542.

Becker A, Chaushu S (2005) Long-term follow-up of severely resorbed maxillary incisors after resolution of an etiologically associated impacted canine. *Am J Orthod Dentofacial Orthop* 127:650–654; quiz 754.

Begg PR (1956) Differential force in orthodontic treatment. *Am J Orthod* 42:481–510.

Birnie DJ, McNamara TG (1980) The quadhelix appliance. *Br J Orthod* 7:115–120.

Cobb NW 3rd, Kula KS, Phillips C, Proffit WR (1998) Efficiency of multi-strand steel, superelastic Ni-Ti and ion-implanted Ni-Ti archwires for initial alignment. *Clin Orthod Res* 1:12–19.

DiBiase AT, Nasr IH, Scott P, Cobourne MT (2011) Duration of treatment and occlusal outcome using Damon3 self-ligated and conventional orthodontic bracket systems in extraction patients: A prospective randomized clinical trial. *Am J Orthod Dentofacial Orthop* 139:e111–116.

Dixon V, Read MJ, O'Brien KD, Worthington HV, Mandall NA (2002) A randomized clinical trial to compare three methods of orthodontic space closure. *J Orthod* 29:31–36.

Fleming PS, DiBiase AT, Sarri G, Lee RT (2009a) Comparison of mandibular arch changes during alignment and leveling with 2 preadjusted edgewise appliances. *Am J Orthod Dentofacial Orthop* 136:340–347.

Fleming PS, DiBiase AT, Sarri G, Lee RT (2009b) Efficiency of mandibular arch alignment with 2 preadjusted edgewise appliances. *Am J Orthod Dentofacial Orthop* 135:597–602.

Fleming PS, DiBiase AT, Lee RT (2010) Randomized controlled trial of orthodontic treatment effciency with self-ligating and conventional fixed orthodontic appliances . *Am J Orthod Dentofacial Orthop* 137:738–742.

Gioka C, Eliades T (2004) Materials-induced variation in the torque expression of preadjusted appliances. *Am J Orthod Dentofacial Orthop* 125:323–328.

Harradine NW (2003) Self-ligating brackets; where are we now? *J Orthod* 30:262–273.

Irvine R, Power S, McDonald F (2004) The effectiveness of laceback ligatures: a randomized controlled clinical trial. *J Orthod* 31:303–311; discussion 300.

Kesling PC (1988) Expanding the horizons of the edgewise arch wire slot. *Am J Orthod Dentofacial* 94:26–37.

Killiany DM (1999) Root resorption caused by orthodontic treatment: an evidence-based review of literature. *Semin Orthod* 5:128–133.

Koo BC, Chung AH, Vanarsdall RL (1999) Comparison of the accuracy of bracket placement between direct and indirect bonding techniques. *Am J Orthod Dentofacial Orthop* 116:346–351.

Kusy RP (1997) A review of contemporary archwires: their properties and characteristics. *Angle Orthod* 67:197–207.

Levander E, Malmgren O, Eliasson S (1994) Evaluation of root resorption in relation to two orthodontic treatment regimes. A clinical experimental study. *Eur J Orthod* 16:223–228.

Levander E, Malmgren O, Stenback K (1998) Apical root resorption during orthodontic treatment of patients with multiple aplasia: a study of maxillary incisors. *Eur J Orthod* 20:427–434.

Linge BO, Linge L (1983) Apical root resorption in upper anterior teeth. *Eur J Orthod* 5:173–183.

Linge L, Linge BO (1991) Patient characteristics and treatment variables associated with apical root resorption during orthodontic treatment. *Am J Orthod Dentofacial Orthop* 99:35–43.

Mandall N, Lowe C, Worthington H, *et al.* (2006) Which orthodontic archwire sequence? A randomized clinical trial. *Eur J Orthod* 28:561–566.

Manhartsberger C, Seidenbusch W (1996) Force delivery of Ni-Ti coil springs. *Am J Orthod Dentofacial Orthop* 109:8–21.

Mckee IW, Williamson PC, Lam EW, Heo G, Glover KE, Major PW (2002) The accuracy of 4 panoramic units in the projection of mesiodistal tooth angulations. *Am J Orthod Dentofacial Orthop* 121:166–175.

Nightingale C, Jones SP (2003) A clinical investigation of force delivery systems for orthodontic space closure. *J Orthod* 30:229–236.

Owens AM, Johal A (2008) Near-end of treatment panoramic radiograph in the assessment of mesiodistal root angulation. *Angle Orthod* 78:475–481.

Pringle AM, Petrie A, Cunningham SJ, McKnight M (2009) Prospective randomized clinical trial to compare pain levels associated with 2 orthodontic fixed bracket systems. *Am J Orthod Dentofacial Orthop* 136:160–167.

Roth RH (1976) Five year clinical evaluation of the Andrews straight-wire appliance. *J Clin Orthod* 10:836–850.

Samuels RH, Rudge SJ, Mair LH (1998) A clinical study of space closure with nickel-titanium closed coil springs and an elastic module. *Am J Orthod Dentofacial Orthop* 114:73–79.

Schmage P, Nergiz I, Herrmann W, Ozcan M (2003) Influence of various surgace-conditioning methods on the bond strength of metal brackets to ceramic surfaces. *Am J Orthod Dentofacial Orthop* 123:540–546.

Scott P, DiBiase AT, Sherriff M, Cobourne MT (2008a) Alignment efficiency of Damon3 self-ligating and conventional orthodontic bracket systems: a randomized clinical trial. *Am J Orthod Dentofacial Orthop* 134:470 e1–8.

Scott P, Sherriff M, Dibiase AT, Cobourne MT (2008b) Perception of discomfort during initial orthodontic tooth alignment using a self-ligating or conventional bracket system: a randomized clinical trial. *Eur J Orthod* 30:227–232.

Stivaros N, Lowe C, Dandy N, Doherty B, Mandall NA (2010) A randomized clinical trial to compare the Goshgarian and Nance palatal arch. *Eur J Orthod* 32:171–176.

Turnbull NR, Birnie DJ (2007) Treatment efficiency of conventional vs self-ligating brackets: effects of archwire size and material. *Am J Orthod Dentofacial Orthop* 131:395–399.

Usmani T, O'Brien KD, Worthington HV, *et al.* (2002) A randomized clinical trial to compare the effectiveness of canine lacebacks with reference to canine tip. *J Orthod* 29:281–286; discussion 277.

Weltman B, Vig KW, Fields HW, Shanker S, Kaizar EE (2010) Root resorption associated with orthodontic tooth movement: a systematic review. *Am J Orthod Dentofacial Orthop* 137:462–476; discussion 12A.

Zablocki HL, McNamara JA Jr, Franchi L, Baccetti T (2008) Effect of the transpalatal arch during extraction treatment. *Am J Orthod Dentofacial Orthop* 133:852–860.

9

Stability and Retention

Introduction

Whilst orthodontics is becoming ever more sophisticated and efficient, treatment should not be considered inherently stable. Relapse may be defined as a partial or complete return of the original features of the presenting malocclusion. It is one of the most difficult things to predict and manage in orthodontics, and may occur many years following treatment (Sadowsky and Sakols, 1982; Little, 1990).

It is important to understand that, in the absence of orthodontic treatment, changes in the occlusion and alignment of the teeth should be expected (Sinclair and Little, 1985; Thilander, 2009). In untreated individuals there is a tendency for crowding to increase, particularly in the lower labial segment as the lower arch becomes shorter and narrower with age. The reasons for this are not fully understood, but are thought to be related to continued growth in adulthood and a change in the soft tissue morphology and pressures with age. Other factors that have been implicated include lack of interproximal attrition, mesial drift of the dentition due to occlusal forces (Southard et al., 1990) and the eruption or impaction of third molars.

Successful orthodontic retention avoids any relapse in the post-treatment occlusion by holding teeth in their treated position through the use of fixed or removable retainers. The prescribed retention regime needs to circumvent both relapse and age-related changes, as either will be perceived as a failure of the treatment. The different regimes of wear for retainers tend to be arbitrary and loosely based on our understanding of changes and remodelling within the periodontal ligament and gingivae following treatment (Reitan, 1959; 1969). There is little evidence that one regime or type of retention is superior to another (Littlewood et al., 2006). The chosen regime should be based on shared responsibility and agreement between the patient and the orthodontist, forming part of the informed consent process.

Orthodontists should also aim, whenever possible, to avoid changes that are known to be unstable, although to achieve the aims of treatment this may not always be possible. Changes that are particularly prone to relapse include expansion of the mandibular inter-canine width, mandibular incisor proclination, arch expansion, correction of rotations and closure of a maxillary midline diastema.

As both growth-related and post-treatment relapse arise in an unpredictable manner and greater emphasis is placed on dental and facial aesthetics, an increasing premium is placed on prolonged and fixed retention in orthodontics. Retention should not be an afterthought; therefore, the proposed retention regime should be planned before embarking on a course of treatment.

Clinical Cases in Orthodontics, First Edition. Martyn T. Cobourne, Padhraig S. Fleming, Andrew T. DiBiase, and Sofia Ahmad.
© 2012 Martyn T. Cobourne, Padhraig S. Fleming, Andrew T. DiBiase, and Sofia Ahmad. Published 2012 by Blackwell Publishing Ltd.

Case 9.1

This 13-year-old female presented with a class I incisor relationship on a mild skeletal class II pattern complicated by severe tooth agenesis (Figure 9.1).

Which teeth are congenitally absent?

The UR5, UR2, UL2, UL5, LL7, LL5, LR5, LR7 and all third molars are absent.

Treatment Plan

- Upper and lower pre-adjusted edgewise appliances
- Prosthetic replacement of the UR2, UL2, LL5 and LR5
- Long-term retention: Upper and lower fixed retainers and modified Hawley-type retainers (Figure 9.2)

Why were the restorations not placed immediately?

Restorations were postponed to permit reorganization of gingival tissue, optimizing stability and allowing maturation of the gingival margins. Consequently, the emergence profile of the definitive restorations and gingival aesthetics is enhanced.

What retention regime would you suggest for this patient?

Fixed retainers were placed to maintain alignment of the maxillary central incisors and lower incisor teeth. Hawley-type retainers were used as an interim measure to replace the missing lateral incisors and mandibular second premolars. Following an initial retention phase of 3 months, definitive restorations were placed. The pontics were then removed and the removable retainer wear reduced to nights only.

Could the design of the removable retainer have been improved in any way?

Yes. Metal stops (0.7 mm) could have been added mesial and distal to the pontics. Consequently, in the event of pontic fracture, the stops would prevent migration of adjacent teeth.

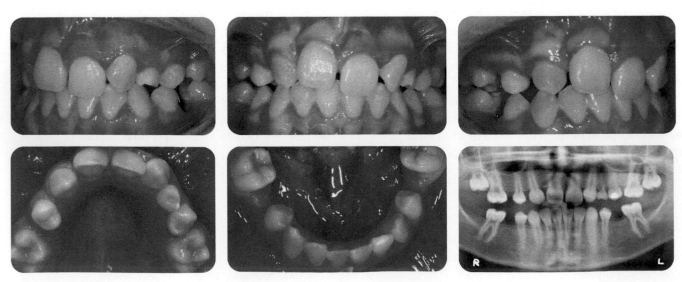

Figure 9.1

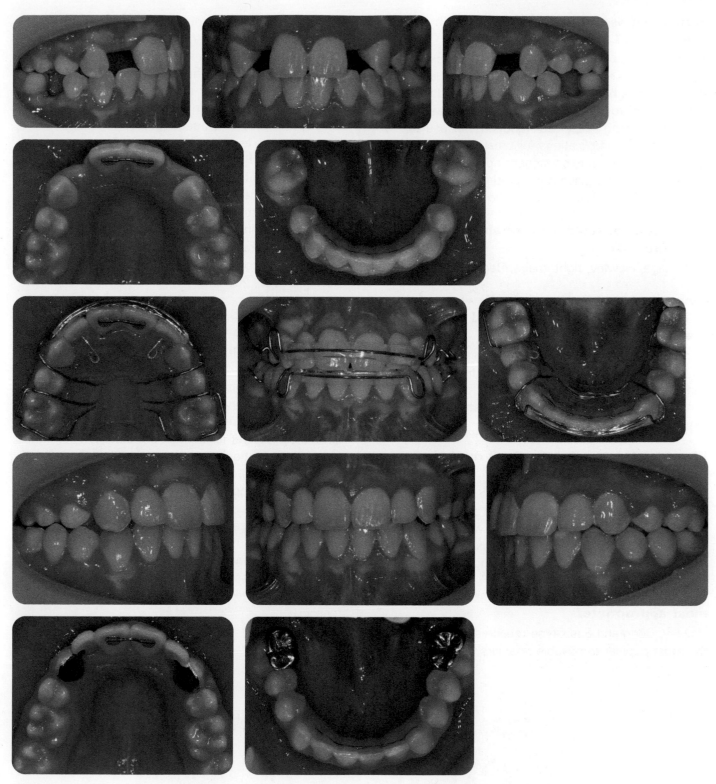

Figure 9.2

Is there an association between tooth agenesis and orthodontic relapse?

Tooth agenesis is associated with rotations and generalized spacing of teeth. Relapse potential in these cases is high because of the likelihood for recurrence of rotations and a tendency for teeth to migrate following space redistribution. Relapse can have significant implications for prosthodontic rehabilitation, which is contingent upon ideal space for bridge and implant placement, placing a premium on fixed retention following orthodontic treatment.

What types of removable retainer are shown in Figure 9.3?

Left image, Hawley; right image, Begg.

How could the design of the Hawley retainer in Figure 9.3 have been adjusted for this first premolar extraction case?

This is the standard Hawley retainer design with clasps on the first molars and a labial bow extending from canine to canine. For extraction cases, the labial bow can be extended to the first molar clasps to keep the extraction spaces closed.

Why is the design of the Begg retainer different?

The Begg retainer is designed for use with the Begg appliance, which relies upon occlusal settling after removal of the fixed appliances. The wrap-around design of the labial bow allows vertical settling and mesial space closure to take place (Figure 9.4).

Which type of removable retainer type is most appropriate?

Hawley, Begg and Essix-type retainers are amongst the most popular removable retainers. Essix-type retainers are vacuum-moulded around the teeth, transparent and relatively simple to fabricate. Perceived indications for the use of either Hawley or Begg retainers include the requirement for occlusal settling, maintenance of transverse expansion and temporary tooth replacement (pontics can be placed directly on the retainer; see Figures 4.24 and 9.2). Begg retainers are particularly useful for both mesial space closure (Figure 9.4, top two panels) and vertical settling (Figure 9.4, bottom panel). Essix retainers are cheaper to fabricate and have improved aesthetics. Results from a recent randomized controlled trial indicate that Essix retainers are generally preferable in view of patient compliance, tolerance and cost-efficacy (Hichens *et al.*, 2007; Rowland *et al.*, 2007).

Should patients wear removable retainers on a full-time or night-only basis following the removal of active appliances?

Retention protocols tend to be tailored to individual patients and to vary significantly between clinicians. However, it has been suggested that there is little difference in lower labial segment stability with either full-time or night-only wear over a 12-month period (Gill *et al.*, 2007). Therefore, night-only wear may be sufficient; this approach reduces the onus of retention wear on patients.

In the presence of tooth agenesis, however, full-time retention is necessary until edentulous spaces are restored definitively, in order to maintain the space. In these cases, patients are usually willing to wear retainers on a full-time basis for cosmetic reasons.

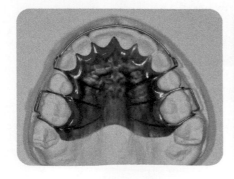 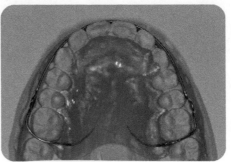

Figure 9.3

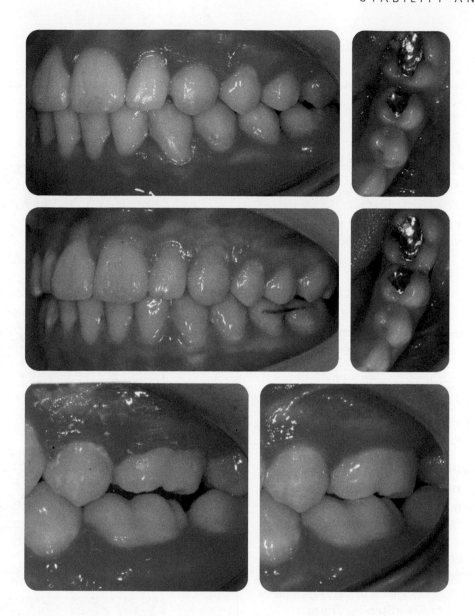

Figure 9.4

Case 9.2

This 18-year-old female was referred by her general practitioner concerned with lower incisor crowding following previous orthodontic treatment. There was no relevant medical history.

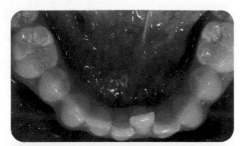

Summary

An 18-year-old female presented 3 years following dual arch fixed appliance therapy with mild crowding of the lower labial segment, lingual displacement and rotation of the LL1.

Treatment Plan

Interproximal reduction and a removable positioner to re-align the mandibular incisors (Figure 9.5).

What is a removable positioner?

Positioners are a form of 'active retainer' capable of producing tooth movements in increments of approximately 0.5 mm per appliance. Consequently, for correction of significant discrepancies a series of appliances may be necessary. This concept is incorporated into contemporary proprietary aesthetic appliances to correct malocclusions of varying degrees of severity (Invisalign™ or ClearStep™). These techniques may rely on inter-proximal reduction to generate the space to facilitate alignment. Attachments may also be necessary to produce complex tooth movements, e.g. torque and lone extrusions.

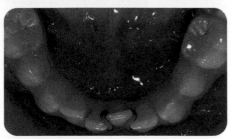

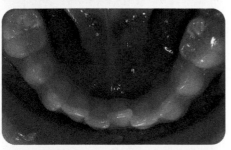

Why were separating elastics used in this case?

These elastics provide some space interproximally to allow careful and accurate interproximal reduction, creating space prior to alignment.

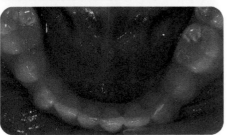

Figure 9.5

What are the advantages of removable aligners compared to fixed appliances?

- Aesthetics
- May avoid unwanted tooth movement in remote areas
- Reduced pain following initial placement of appliances (Miller et al., 2007)
- Less plaque accumulation (Miethke and Vogt, 2005)
- Improved oral health-related quality of life during the initial stages of therapy (Miller et al., 2007)

What are the limitations of removable aligners compared to fixed appliances?

- Extended treatment duration
- Reliance on compliance
- Limited tooth movement possible
- Reliant on interproximal reduction and use of auxiliaries
- Laboratory costs and dependence

How predictable is tooth movement with removable aligners?

The accuracy of tooth movement with Invisalign™ has been assessed in a prospective study (Kravitz et al., 2009). The authors concluded that Invisalign™ was capable of producing the predicted outcome with 41% accuracy. Shortcomings were noted with respect to extrusion of teeth and correction of angulation of mandibular canines. Above a threshold of 15 degrees, the accuracy of rotation for the maxillary canines fell significantly. This study confirms that further refinement may be required following an initial phase of aligner treatment.

Is there a difference in the outcome with Invisalign™ and conventional fixed appliances?

Invisalign™ appears to be less effective than conventional appliances. In a retrospective study of 96 subjects with mild malocclusions assessed using the American Board of Orthodontics Grading system, Invisalign™ scored consistently less well for control of bucco-lingual inclination, occlusal contacts, occlusal relationships and overjet (Djeu et al., 2005).

How do fixed appliances and removable aligners compare with respect to stability?

In a 3-year follow-up, patients treated with Invisalign™ experienced greater post-treatment changes than those treated with conventional fixed appliances. Changes arose in total alignment and mandibular anterior alignment in both groups. However, significant changes developed in maxillary anterior alignment in the Invisalign™ group only (Kuncio et al., 2007).

Case 9.3

This 13-year-old female was referred by her general dentist in relation to crossbite, crowding and open bite. There was no relevant medical history.

Summary

A 13-year-old female presented with a class I incisor relationship on a mild skeletal class II pattern complicated by crowding, bilateral posterior crossbites and a lateral open bite (Figure 9.6, upper panels).

Treatment Plan

- Non-extraction treatment with upper and lower pre-adjusted edgewise appliances
- Long-term retention

The initial phase of treatment was uneventful. The arches were aligned although the buccal segment inter-digitation on the right side was poor. The patient was asked to wear removable retainers on a night-only basis (Figure 9.6, second panel from top). Two years following the initial course of treatment, the patient returned complaining of irregularity of her maxillary anterior teeth. The lower anterior teeth were also crowded and the crossbite had recurred. She had failed to comply with the suggested retention regime (Figure 9.6, third panel from top). The patient requested re-treatment to realign her upper anterior teeth; this was carried out over 4 months with an upper fixed appliance. Following this second phase of treatment, an upper fixed retainer was bonded to the six upper anterior teeth (Figure 9.6, bottom panel).

What is the definition of orthodontic relapse and retention?

Relapse is the return to the original features of a malocclusion, following correction.

Retention can be defined as 'holding of teeth following orthodontic treatment in the treated position for the period of time necessary for the maintenance of the result'.

Why do changes occur following orthodontic treatment?

- **Physiological recovery:** Original features of the malocclusion reappear, e.g. rotations or spacing.
- **Growth and maturational changes:** These changes occur irrespective of orthodontic treatment.
- **Relapse:** Changes arise due to placement of teeth in unstable positions.

Therefore, retention is indicated to:
- Allow periodontal and gingival adaptation
- Limit growth-related changes
- Permit neuromuscular adaptation to the corrected tooth position
- Maintain unstable tooth positions as unstable positioning may have been required for aesthetic reasons (Blake and Bibby, 1998).

What features of this case relapsed?

- Maxillary arch expansion
- Palatal position of the UR2
- Rotational correction of incisors

How might stability have been improved?

Bonded palatal retainers could have been placed palatal to the upper anterior dentition and lingual to the mandibular incisors.

Is the result after the second treatment phase likely to be stable?

This outcome is inherently unstable as the overbite is reduced, expansion tends to be unstable and rotations (e.g. of the UR2) tend to reappear. Therefore, stability is reliant on the integrity of the upper bonded retainer and diligent wear of her Hawley retainer.

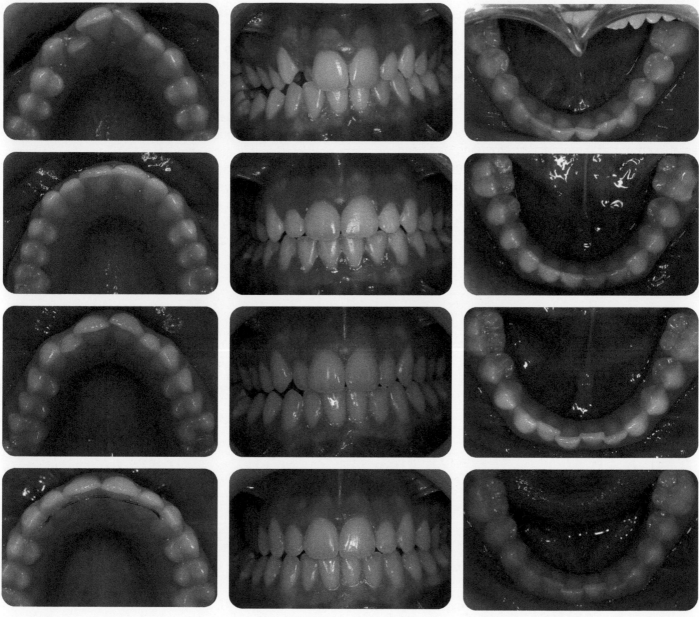

Figure 9.6

List the treatment-related factors that have an implication on prolonged stability

- Maintain inter-canine width
- Limit proclination of mandibular incisors
- Maintain arch form
- Correct rotations early during treatment
- Consider active retention of skeletal discrepancy
- Consider labial frenectomy where an abnormal frenum contributes to a diastema
- Correct edge-centroid relationship in class II division 2 cases

- Place maxillary incisors within control of the lower lip
- Optimize buccal segment inter-digitation to maintain sagittal correction

List the factors implicated in the development of late lower incisor crowding

- Tooth size and shape
- Mandibular third molars
- Mesial drift
- Lack of attrition

- Occlusal forces
- Soft tissue changes
- Late mandibular growth (Vasir and Robinson, 1991)

Is removal of the mandibular third molars indicated to relieve or prevent incisor crowding?

The prophylactic removal of third molars to prevent the establishment of lower incisor crowding has been advocated. However, research has suggested that mesial drift of the lower dentition is independent of the presence of third molars (Richardson, 1992). Consequently, removal of third molars to address incisor irregularity is not recommended clinical practice. This approach is supported by the National Institute for Health and Clinical Excellence (NICE) guidelines in the UK.

Is treatment with or without extractions more stable?

Little difference in post-treatment incisor irregularity has been demonstrated when either extraction or non-extraction treatment is performed (Luppanapornlarp and Johnston, 1993; Paquette *et al.*, 1992). To date, studies that have attempted to address this question have been retrospective in design. Consequently, there are likely to be significant pre-treatment differences, particularly in relation to crowding characteristics that may have prompted the extraction decision. The ideal study to answer this question would be a randomized controlled trial with prolonged follow-up.

Case 9.4

This 13-year-old female was referred by her general dentist in relation to an increased overjet and upper midline space. There was no relevant medical history.

Summary

A 13-year-old female presented with a class II division 1 incisor relationship on a mild skeletal class II pattern complicated by an increased overjet and maxillary median diastema (Figure 9.7).

Treatment Plan

- Modified Twin Block appliance
- Upper and lower pre-adjusted edgewise appliances
- Long-term retention (Figure 9.8)

What is a median diastema?

A median diastema is defined as a space between the central incisors. A maxillary median diastema is a common feature of the mixed dentition and is considered physiological. This diastema should close naturally with eruption of the maxillary canines. Consequently, treatment is usually not indicated until after this age. Persistent diastema may usually be corrected with fixed orthodontic appliances.

Is frenectomy indicated following closure of a median diastema?

Typically, the labial frenum, which is often low and fleshy, remodels apically following space closure. Consequently, labial frenectomy is not normally indicated following treatment. However, some practitioners advocate frenectomy (Edwards, 1977). If undertaken, a frenectomy can be carried out before (improving access) or after orthodontic space closure. It is suggested that if carried out after space closure, scar contracture of the healing tissues may consolidate space closure. Bonded palatal retainers are advised subsequent to closure of the diastema.

Is it possible to predict whether a diastema will reappear following treatment?

No association has been found between relapse and the presence of an abnormal frenum or an osseous inter-maxillary cleft (Shashua and Artun, 1999). The

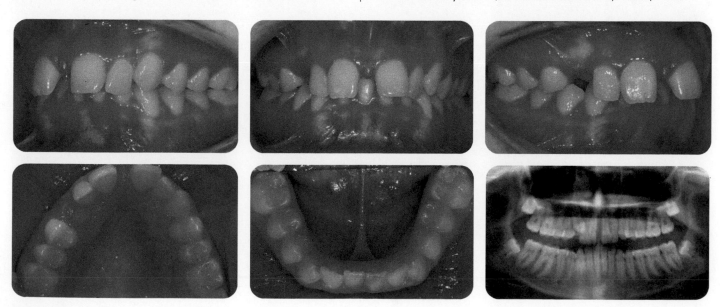

Figure 9.7

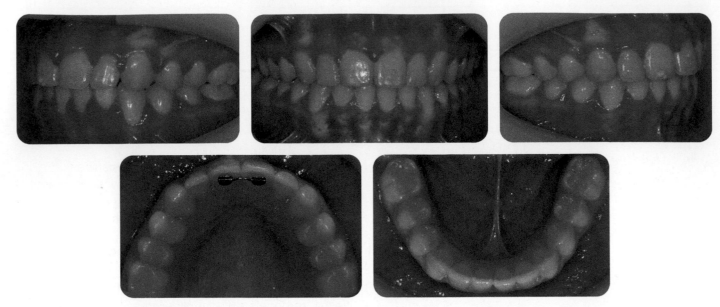

Figure 9.8

only predictors shown to increase the likelihood of relapse include pre-treatment diastema size and family history of a diastema. Therefore, fixed retainers are advisable on all patients following closure of a midline diastema.

Are there any disadvantages of the use of fixed retainers?

The increasing emphasis on fixed retention has brought the use of fixed retainers into sharper focus. In particular, bonded lingual retainers may encourage plaque accumulation with potential periodontal implications (Pandis *et al.*, 2007). Therefore, their use may not be appropriate in those with poor oral hygiene. Furthermore, failure rates with fixed retainers may be high (Booth *et al.*, 2008).

Case 9.5

This 9-year-old female had a unilateral left-sided cleft lip and palate. She was under multidisciplinary care and was referred prior to alveolar bone grafting.

Summary

A 9-year-old female presented with a class I incisor relationship on a mild skeletal class II pattern with a unilateral cleft lip complicated by a severely rotated UL1, prior to alveolar bone grafting (Figure 9.9).

Treatment Plan

- Alveolar bone graft
- Upper and lower pre-adjusted edgewise appliance
- Long-term retention

What adjunctive procedure may have been considered to retain the rotational correction of the UL1?

Circumferential supra-crestal fibrotomy (CSF) may have been considered.

What is the rationale behind this procedure?

During rotational correction of tooth position, the supra-crestal periodontal fibres can become stretched and fail to remodel as rapidly as the alveolar region. The apparent stretch of these tissues predisposes the tooth to rotational relapse and therefore by incising them, the relapse potential is reduced.

How successful is CSF?

There is little data regarding the effectiveness of this procedure. A prospective study of over 300 consecutive cases has demonstrated sustained effects

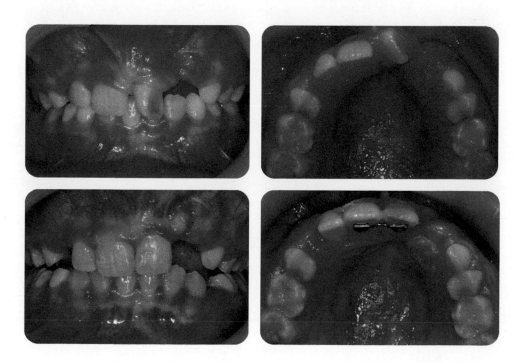

Figure 9.9

of CSF up to 14 years post-treatment, being most effective at preventing pure rotational relapse rather than labio-lingual changes; and more effective in the maxillary arch than the mandibular. However, the drop-out rate in the study was 85%; furthermore, significant relapse occurred irrespective of the intervention (Edwards, 1988).

Is CSF compatible with periodontal health?

The procedure has not been shown to have detrimental periodontal effects. No increase in periodontal sulcus depth or decrease in the labial attached gingiva has been reported 1 and 6 months following CSF (Edwards, 1988). However, periodontal parameters were not quantified in this study.

What form of removable retainer would be appropriate in this case?

A Hawley-type retainer is most appropriate. Retentive components can be placed on the first molars and central incisors. Essix retainers will not fit during the transition to the permanent dentition.

Case 9.6

This 30-year-old female underwent joint orthodontic–surgical management of her class II division I malocclusion. The surgery involved a posterior maxillary impaction and forward sliding sagittal-split osteotomy of the mandible. The pre-treatment cephalometric radiograph is shown in Figure 9.10, top left, the pre-surgical jaw position in Figure 9.10, top right, and the post-surgical jaw position in Figure 9.10, bottom left. Rigid internal fixation of the jaws was used. Two years after removal of the fixed appliances she attended for a review.

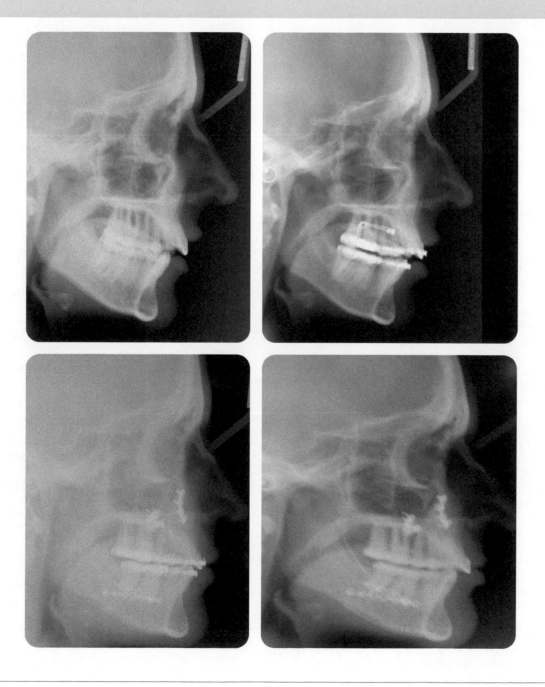

Figure 9.10

What has happened in the radiographic examination taken 2 years following removal of the fixed appliances (Figure 9.10, bottom right)?

There has been some relapse in the post-treatment occlusion. In particular, the overjet has increased.

What relapse might be expected 2 years after a posterior maxillary impaction and mandibular advancement to correct a class II division 1 malocclusion?

In around 25% of patients the maxilla and mandible would be expected to move inferiorly by 2–4 mm. Some reduction of mandibular length through remodelling of the condyles can also occur and this might have contributed to the increase in overjet seen here (Miguel et al., 1995).

Does inter-maxillary wire fixation (IMF) improve stability?

No. In fact, short-term stability over the first few weeks following surgery is poorer with this type of fixation. In particular, the mandible can move posteriorly up to 4 mm in the first 6 weeks (Miguel et al., 1995).

References

Blake M, Bibby K (1998) Retention and stability: a review of the literature. Am J Orthod Dentofacial Orthop 114:299–306.

Booth FA, Edelman JM, Proffit WR (2008) Twenty-year follow-up of patients with permanently bonded mandibular canine-to-canine retainers. Am J Orthod Dentofacial Orthop 133:70–76.

Djeu G, Shelton C, Maganzini A (2005) Outcome assessment of Invisalign and traditional orthodontic treatment compared with the American Board of Orthodontics objective grading system. Am J Orthod Dentofacial Orthop 128:292–298; discussion 298.

Edwards JG (1977) A clinical study: the diastema, the frenum, the frenectomy. Oral Health 67:51–62.

Edwards JG (1988) A long-term prospective evaluation of the circumferential supracrestal fiberotomy in alleviating orthodontic relapse. Am J Orthod Dentofacial Orthop 93:380–387.

Gill DS, Naini FB, Jones A, Tredwin CJ (2007) Part-time versus full-time retainer wear following fixed appliance therapy: a randomized prospective controlled trial. World J Orthod 8:300–306.

Hichens L, Rowland H, Williams A, et al. (2007) Cost-effectiveness and patient satisfaction: Hawley and vacuum-formed retainers. Eur J Orthod 29:372–378.

Kravitz ND, Kusnoto B, BeGole E, Obrez A, Agran B (2009) How well does Invisalign work? A prospective clinical study evaluating the efficacy of tooth movement with Invisalign. Am J Orthod Dentofacial Orthop 135:27–35.

Kuncio D, Maganzini A, Shelton C, Freeman K (2007) Invisalign and traditional orthodontic treatment postretention outcomes compared using the American Board of Orthodontics objective grading system. Angle Orthod 77:864–869.

Little RM (1990) Stability and relapse of dental arch alignment. Br J Orthod 1990;17:235–241.

Littlewood SJ, Millet DT, Doubleday B, Bearn DR, Worthington HV (2006) Retention procedures for stabilizing tooth position after treatment with orthodontic braces. Cochrane Database Syst Rev 25:CD002283.

Luppanapornlarp S, Johnston LE Jr (1993) The effects of premolar-extraction: a long-term comparison of outcomes in "clear-cut" extraction and nonextraction Class II patients. Angle Orthod 63:257–272.

Miguel JA, Turvey TA, Phillips C, Proffit WR (1995) Long-term stability of two jaw surgery for treatment of mandibular deficiency and vertical maxillary excess. Int J Adult Orthod Orthogn Surg 10:235–245.

Miethke RR, Vogt S (2005) A comparison of the periodontal health of patients during treatment with the Invisalign system and with fixed orthodontic appliances. J Orofac Orthop 66:219–229.

Miller KB, McGorray SP, Womack R, et al. (2007) A comparison of treatment impacts between Invisalign aligner and fixed appliance therapy during the first week of treatment. Am J Orthod Dentofacial Orthop 131:302 e1–9.

Pandis N, Vlahopoulos K, Madianos P, Eliades T (2007) Long-term periodontal status of patients with mandibular lingual fixed retention. Eur J Orthod 29:471–476.

Paquette DE, Beattie JR, Johnston LE Jr (1992) A long-term comparison of nonextraction and premolar extraction edgewise therapy in "borderline" Class II patients. Am J Orthod Dentofacial Orthop 102:1–14.

Reitan K (1959) Tissue rearrangement during retention of orthodontically rotated teeth. Angle Orthod 29:105–113.

Reitan K (1969) Principles of retention and avoidance of post-treatment relapse. Am J Orthod 55:776–790.

Richardson M (1992) Lower arch crowding in the young adult. Am J Orthod Dentofacial Orthop 101:132–137.

Rowland H, Hichens L, Williams A, et al. (2007) The effectiveness of Hawley and vacuum-formed retainers: a single-center randomized controlled trial. Am J Orthod Dentofacial Orthop 132:730–737.

Sadowsky C, Sakols EI (1982) Long-term assessment of orthodontic relapse. Am J Orthod 82:456–463.

Shashua D, Artun J (1999) Relapse after orthodontic correction of maxillary median diastema: a follow-up evaluation of consecutive cases. Angle Orthod 69:257–263.

Sinclair P, Little R (1985) Dentofacial maturation of untreated normals. Am J Orthod Dentofac Orthop 88:146–156.

Southard TE, Behrents RG, Tolley EA (1990) The anterior component of occlusal force part 2. Relationship with dental malalignment. *Am J Orthod Dentofac Orthop* 97:41–44.

Thilander B (2009) Dentoalveolar development in subjects with normal occlusion. A longitudinal study between the ages of 5 and 31 years. *Eur J Orthod* 31:109–120.

Vasir NS, Robinson RJ (1991) The mandibular third molar and late crowding of the mandibular incisors–a review. *Br J Orthod* 18:59–66.

10

Orthognathic Surgery

Introduction

A combined orthodontic–surgical or orthognathic approach is often indicated to address malocclusion with a significant skeletal aetiology. Collectively, these procedures have broadened the scope of orthodontic correction. It is clear that interceptive orthodontic treatment has only a minor influence on skeletal growth and in the presence of a significant skeletal discrepancy, either camouflage or orthognathic treatment is often required to obtain a class I occlusion. With the introduction of the mandibular sagittal split osteotomy and later the maxillary Le Fort 1 osteotomy, clinicians have the means to fully correct a range of skeletal discrepancies (Trauner and Obwegeser, 1957; Obwegeser, 1969). Since then, numerous other surgical techniques and variations have been described, which allow the orthodontist and surgeon to address a wide range of antero-posterior, vertical and transverse skeletal discrepancies, including asymmetry. The development and evolution of orthognathic surgery has coincided with a paradigm shift in orthodontics, away from occlusal and hard tissue-based treatment planning to soft tissue and facial treatment planning (Ackerman et al., 1999). With modern techniques, comprehensive treatment today should aim to improve not only the patient's dental aesthetics and occlusion, but also their facial aesthetics.

Indications for orthognathic surgery include cases where a significant skeletal discrepancy and orthodontic camouflage may be detrimental to facial aesthetics; where an ideal or acceptable occlusal result simply cannot be achieved with orthodontics in isolation; or where there is a desire for facial change. It is also indicated for the group of patients who present at the extremes of malocclusion, associated with a cranio-facial syndrome where the main aim of treatment is the improvement and normalization of facial appearance.

With experience, better understanding of aesthetics and more sophisticated planning, outcomes are becoming more predictable (Arnett and Gunson, 2004; 2010). There is less morbidity and inpatient stays are shorter; inter-maxillary fixation has also been largely superseded by rigid internal fixation, which permits an earlier return of masticatory function. Levels of satisfaction with orthognathic procedures are also generally very good, with significant improvement in oral health-related quality of life (Cunningham et al., 1995; 1996; 2003). Combined, these factors mean that in the last few decades, while it still remains highly specialized work that requires close collaboration between orthodontist and maxillofacial surgeon, it has become part of routine practice, allowing comprehensive treatment of skeletal problems that previously had been beyond the scope of orthodontics.

Case 10.1

This 26-year-old female was referred by her general dentist, concerned with the position of her lower jaw and the gap between her upper and lower teeth. There was no relevant medical history.

Extra-oral

Skeletal relationship

  Antero-posterior — Moderate skeletal class II

  Vertical — FMPA: Average

  Lower face height: Average

  Transverse — Facial asymmetry: Chin point to the right

Soft tissues — Lip competence: Incompetent with lower lip acting behind maxillary incisors

Naso-labial angle: Average

Upper incisor show — At rest: 3 mm

Smiling: 7 mm

Temporo-mandibular joint — Healthy with good range and co-ordination of movement

Intra-oral

Teeth present

7654321/1234567
7654321/1234567

Dental health — Good
(restorations, caries) — No restorations or active caries

Oral hygiene – periodontal Good

Lower arch — Crowding: Mild

Incisor inclination: Average

Curve of Spee: Average

Upper arch — Crowding: Mild

Incisor inclination: Proclined

Canine position: Line of the arch

Occlusion — Incisor relationship: Class II division 1

Overjet: 9 mm

Overbite: Average and complete

Molar relationship: Class II bilaterally

Canine relationship: Class II bilaterally

Centre lines: Lower to the right by 2 mm

Functional occlusion: Group function

Summary

A 26-year-old female presented with a class II division 1 malocclusion on a moderate skeletal class II pattern with average vertical dimensions complicated by an increased overjet (9 mm), mild crowding of both dental arches and a chin point displaced to the right along with the dental centre line (Figure 10.1).

Treatment Plan

- Upper and lower pre-adjusted edgewise appliances on a non-extraction basis
- Bilateral sagittal split osteotomy to advance the mandible
- Long-term retention (the final result is shown in Figures 10.2 and 10.3)

What were the main options for treatment?

There were three main treatment options in this case:

- **Alignment of the dental arches on a non-extraction basis.** This would have resulted in a residual overjet and would necessitate permanent fixed retention in both arches, as the upper incisors

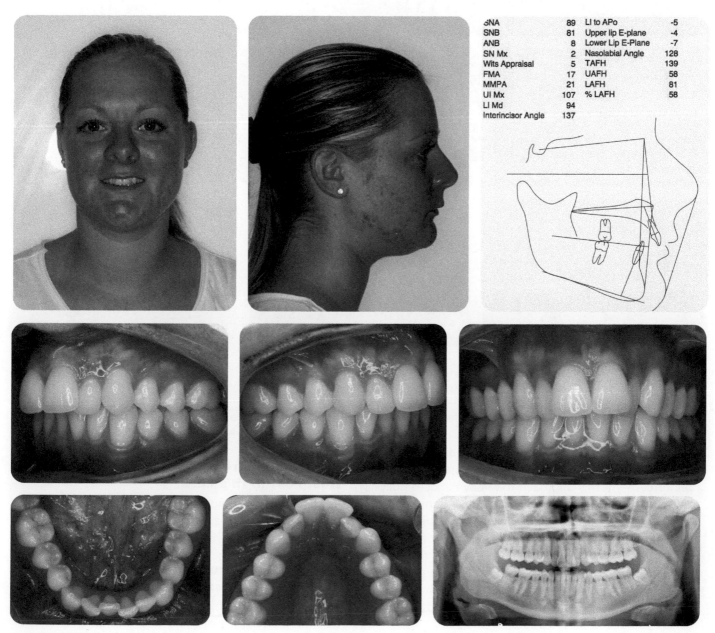

SNA	89	LI to APo	-5
SNB	81	Upper lip E-plane	-4
ANB	8	Lower Lip E-Plane	-7
SN Mx	2	Nasolabial Angle	128
Wits Appraisal	5	TAFH	139
FMA	17	UAFH	58
MMPA	21	LAFH	81
UI Mx	107	% LAFH	58
LI Md	94		
Interincisor Angle	137		

Figure 10.1

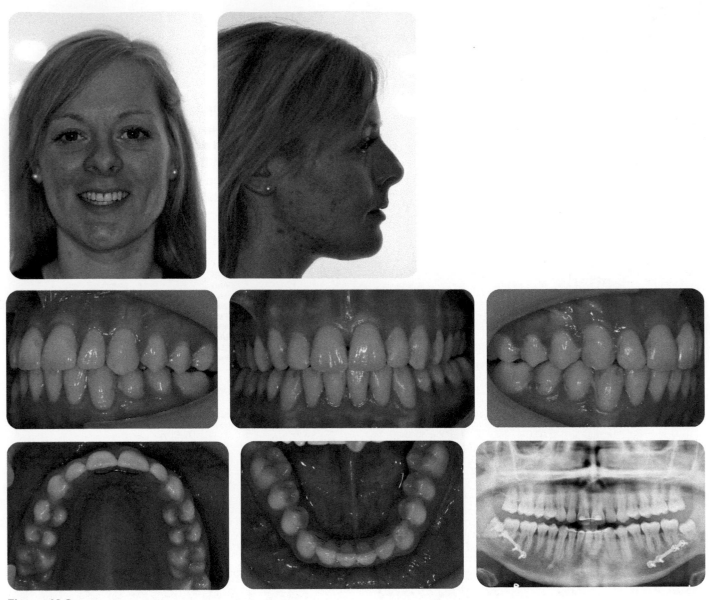

Figure 10.2

would be unsupported by the mandibular anterior segment in occlusion.

- **Orthodontic camouflage with removal of two maxillary first premolars.** With anchorage reinforcement, this approach may have successfully reduced the overjet and produced ideal arch alignment. However, occlusal improvement may have been accompanied by unfavourable soft tissue effects, including retraction and thinning of the upper lip.
- **Combined orthodontic–surgical approach.** This modality would facilitate overjet reduction by correction of the antero-posterior skeletal discrepancy with mandibular advancement surgery.

It would also be the only treatment strategy capable of correcting the mandibular chin point asymmetry.

What was the role of the orthodontic treatment in this case?

- Decompensate and co-ordinate the dental arches
- Facilitate surgical advancement of the mandible
- Finish and detail the occlusion

Why was inter-proximal reduction undertaken on the mandibular incisors?

This was undertaken to provide some space for alignment whilst maintaining their inclination and therefore facilitating mandibular advancement. The

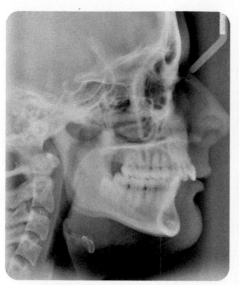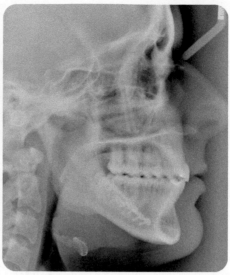

Figure 10.3

chin point and centre line discrepancy would be corrected with the mandibular surgery.

Why were mandibular premolars not extracted?

Space requirements were not high in the mandibular arch and the extraction of premolar teeth might have led to an inappropriate increase in the overjet during space closure. Too great an overjet would lead to further advancement of the mandible, which can be less stable and might also result in too prognathic an appearance post-surgery; particularly in this case, as the chin point is already quite strong.

How might the final result have differed if this patient had been treated with orthodontic camouflage?

- Clear skeletal effects are induced by surgery with increased mandibular length and anterior repositioning of pogonion (Mihalik et al., 2003).
- The dental effects would have differed significantly, with optimal inclination of the maxillary and

mandibular incisors being maintained with combined treatment. Orthodontic camouflage would have necessitated dental inclination changes to camouflage for the underlying skeletal discrepancy.
- The lower facial profile would not have been enhanced with camouflage treatment.
- The mandibular asymmetry required surgery for correction.

If orthodontic camouflage were undertaken, how much upper lip retraction would be likely to occur?

Soft tissue changes are unpredictable, being governed by soft tissue tonicity, lip competence, racial characteristics and overall fullness of the soft tissues (Ramos et al., 2005). A recent study suggests that soft tissue retraction is approximately 40% of incisor retraction (Scott Conley and Jernigan, 2006). Consequently, a 5-mm reduction in overjet may be expected to translate into 2 mm of lip retraction.

Case 10.2

This 17-year-old female was referred by her orthodontic specialist, concerned with difficulty in eating and the large gap between her front teeth.

Extra-oral

Skeletal relationship

Antero-posterior	Mild skeletal class II
Vertical:	FMPA: Increased
	Lower face height: Increased
Transverse	Mandibular asymmetry with deviation of chin point to the right side
Soft tissues	Lip competence: Incompetent
	Naso-labial angle: Normal
Upper incisor show	At rest: 1 mm
	Smiling: 6 mm
Temporo-mandibular joint	Healthy with good range and co-ordination of movement

Intra-oral

Teeth present
7 54321/1234567
7654321/1234567

Dental health (restorations, caries)	Good
Oral hygiene – periodontal	Good
Occlusion	Incisor relationship: Class II division 1
	Overjet: 5 mm
	Overbite: Reduced with an anterior open bite of 12 mm
	Molar relationship: Class I bilaterally
	Canine relationship: Class I bilaterally
	Centre lines:
	Upper centre line is correct to mid-facial plane
	Mandibular centre line is deviated 4 mm to right side
	Functional occlusion: Group function
Upper arch	Crowding: Moderate
	Incisor inclination: Proclined
	Canine position: Line of arch
Lower arch	Crowding: Mild
	Incisor inclination: Retroclined

Summary

A 17-year-old female presented with a class II division 1 malocclusion on a skeletal class II base with increased vertical dimensions and a mandibular asymmetry, further complicated by a large anterior open bite (12 mm) and crowding of both dental arches (Figure 10.4).

Treatment Plan

- Upper and lower pre-adjusted edgewise appliances on a non-extraction basis
- Bi-maxillary surgery
- Long-term retention

The final occlusion is shown in Figures 10.5 and 10.6.

What are the causes of anterior open bite?

Anterior open bites may occur for the following reasons:

- **Transitional,** as the permanent incisors are erupting.
- **Due to local factors:**
  - A prolonged digit sucking habit may impede incisor eruption and procline the maxillary incisors
  - Local pathology interfering with normal incisor eruption.
- **Skeletal open bites:** Caused by an imbalance between vertical growth of the anterior and posterior face. The Frankfort-mandibular plane angle (FMPA) and lower anterior face height are usually increased. This pattern is typically seen with a posterior mandibular rotation during growth. Skeletal open bites have a poor prognosis for orthodontic correction.
- **Soft tissue abnormalities:** Resting tongue position may contribute to anterior open bites with the tongue lying on the incisal edges of the incisor teeth, limiting vertical development. However, although this appearance may be seen in many cases, it may also occur as an adaptation to an underlying skeletal abnormality. Rarely, aberrant tongue behaviour, including endogenous tongue thrusting may contribute to anterior open bite.

How stable is the correction of open bite?

Unless an obvious habitual cause is present (e.g. digit sucking) the correction of anterior open bite is inherently unstable, irrespective of the treatment modality. In a 10-year follow-up after orthodontic correction, 35% of subjects had a vertical gap between the incisal edges of the mandibular incisors and the palatal surfaces of the maxillary incisors of 3 mm or more (Lopez-Gavito et al., 1985). However, more prolonged follow-up suggests that a slight increase in overbite may occur during the post-retention phase, up to 15 years following appliance removal (Zuroff et al., 2010). There is also evidence of greater stability of open bite correction when orthodontic treatment is undertaken with extractions (Janson et al., 2006).

Similar levels of stability have been attributed to combined orthodontic –surgical treatment, involving superior repositioning of the maxilla (Denison et al., 1989; Swinnen et al., 2001). A key predictor of open bite recurrence appears to be the presence of frank open bite pre-treatment, with 43% developing open bite in the follow-up period (Denison et al., 1989). Conversely, those with incisal contact pre-treatment demonstrated higher levels of stability.

What were the aims of pre-surgical orthodontics in this case?

- Maintain optimal inclination of the maxillary incisors to compensate for their uprighting following a posterior maxillary impaction (therefore, the orthodontist will procline these teeth prior to the surgery)
- Arch alignment
- Transverse arch co-ordination

How can maxillary incisor proclination be achieved?

- Avoidance of maxillary arch extractions
- Bracket prescription: High torque variants, e.g. MBT and increased mesial tip in the maxillary canine brackets
- Class III inter-maxillary traction
- Supplementation of maxillary incisor palatal root torque prescription with third-order archwire bends

Why was a posterior maxillary impaction employed in this case?

Posterior impaction of the maxilla allows a counter-clockwise (upward and forward) rotation of the mandible and a reduction of the anterior open bite as the lower incisors move upward.

Why was a forward mandibular osteotomy required as well (Figure 10.6)?

This was required because the degree of auto-rotation following posterior maxillary osteotomy was not

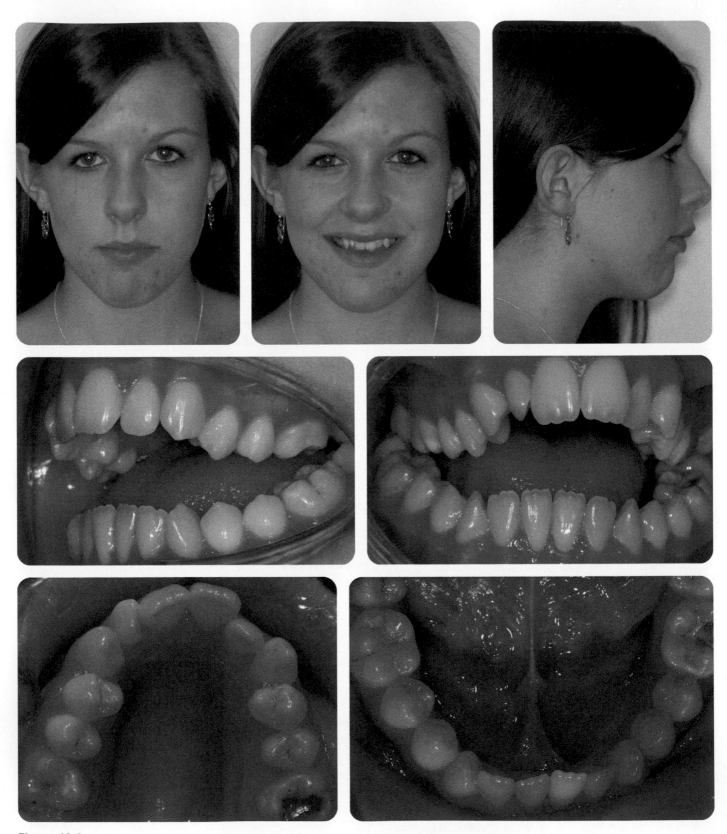

Figure 10.4

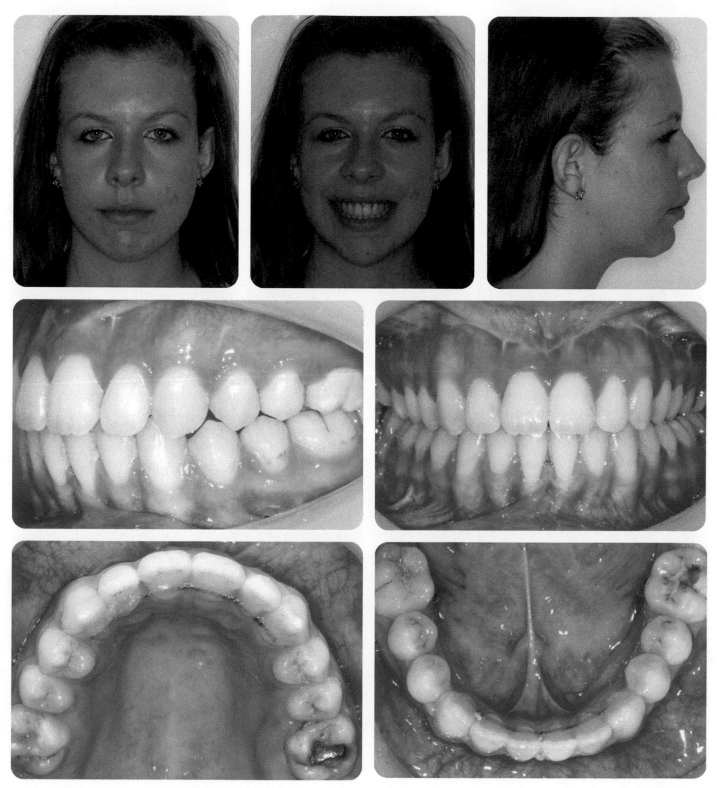

Figure 10.5

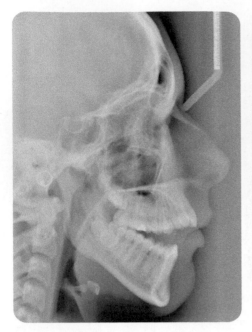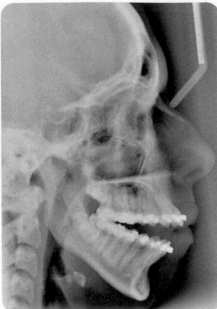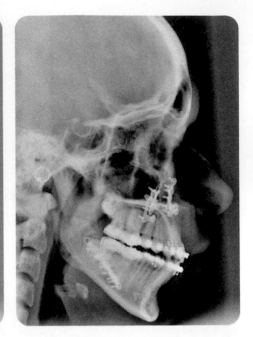

Figure 10.6

enough to produce a class I incisor relationship. The residual overjet was corrected with the mandibular osteotomy.

Could mandibular surgery in isolation (with a counter-clockwise mandibular rotation) have been used to address the anterior open bite?

Traditionally, counter-clockwise mandibular rotation in isolation to correct anterior open bites has been avoided. Pitfalls with this approach include inadvertent stretching of the pterygo-masseteric muscular sling. Following surgery, the mandibular closing muscles shorten, producing an opening mandibular rotation, which results in recurrence of the malocclusion (Iannetti *et al.*, 2007). Although recent research has demonstrated some encouraging results with this approach (Stansbury *et al.*, 2010), the degree of rotation required in this case would have been excessive and unlikely to produce prolonged stability.

Case 10.3

This 22-year-old medical student was unhappy with the appearance of her teeth and had difficulty eating certain types of food.

What are the main features of this malocclusion (Figure 10.7)?

- Class III malocclusion on a severe skeletal class III base with increased lower face height. The skeletal class III relationship has arisen because of maxillary deficiency and mandibular excess combined with increased vertical proportions.
- Class III incisor relationship with a reverse overjet, an openbite tendency, bilateral posterior crossbite and a centre line discrepancy.
- Slight gingival excess on smiling.

This patient underwent a bi-maxillary osteotomy to correct her malocclusion (Figure 10.7). What are the likely jaw movements required to achieve this?

In order to correct the open bite, the maxilla was impacted posteriorly; however, this was also accompanied by some anterior impaction to reduce gingival show and improve the aesthetics of the upper incisors. The maxilla was also moved forwards because of the underlying antero-posterior maxillary deficiency and an accompanying backward positioning sagittal split osteotomy of the mandible was carried out.

Why has the patient's profile worsened prior to surgery?

This is because orthodontic decompensation has been carried out. The upper incisors have been retroclined and the lower incisors proclined, with a resulting increase in the reverse overjet and worsening of the profile.

The appearance of the patient 12 months after removal of her fixed appliances is shown in Figure 10.8. What is the likelihood of continued stability of the surgical correction?

The surgical movements in this case are regarded as being stable over a 12-month period (little or no change in around 80% of patients). Beyond 12 months, maxillary superior movements are likely to relapse by more than 2 mm in around one-third of patients; however, these changes are not necessarily accompanied by significant changes in overjet or overbite. For bi-maxillary cases, class III correction is more stable than class II (Proffit et al., 1996; 2007).

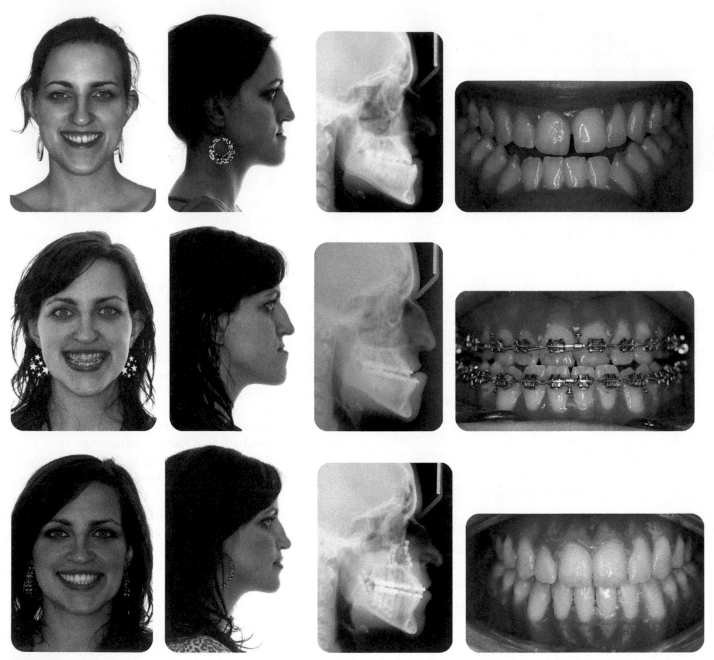

Figure 10.7

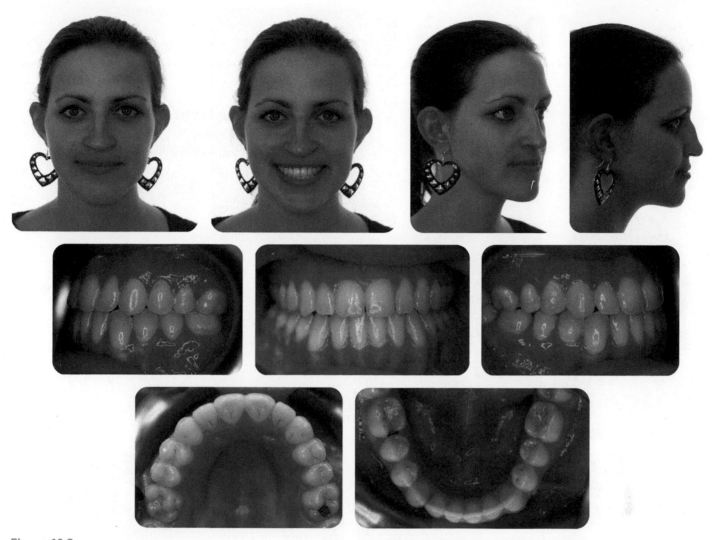

Figure 10.8

Case 10.4

This 16-year-old patient presented complaining of her small chin and the appearance of her teeth (Figure 10.9).

Describe the skeletal deformity

The patient has a skeletal class II discrepancy associated with a retrognathic mandible. She has reduced vertical proportions with a reduced FMPA and

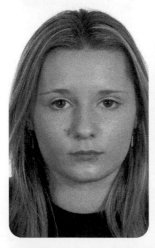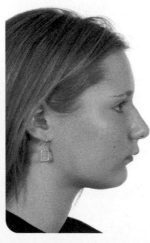

SNA	87
SNB	80
ANB	7
SN Mx	2
Wits Appraisal	3
FMA	12
MMPA	17
UI Mx	94
LI Md	102
Interincisor Angle	145
LI to APo	-2
Upper lip E-plane	0
Lower Lip E-Plane	-1
Nasolabial Angle	103
TAFH	118
UAFH	54
LAFH	63
% LAFH	54

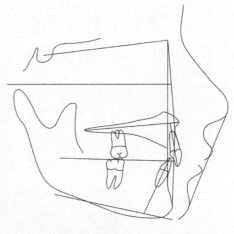

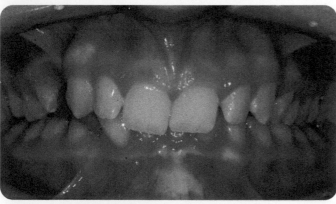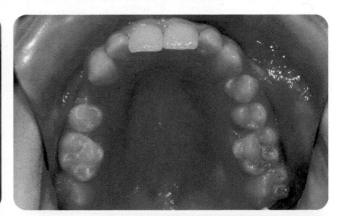

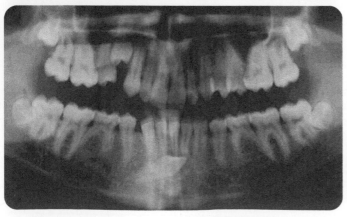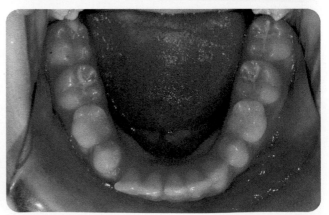

Figure 10.9

reduced lower anterior face height. There is no facial asymmetry.

Summarize the problems on intra-oral and radiographic examination

- Hypodontia: congenital absence of the LL5 and LR5, retained LLE and LRE
- Ectopic, unerupted, transmigrated LR3
- Impacted UR4
- Class II division 2 malocclusion with retroclined upper central incisors and an increased and complete (to mucosa) overbite, which is potentially traumatic

What is the Index of Orthodontic Treatment Need (IOTN) of this malocclusion?

The IOTN is 5i.

How would you assess the position of the LR3? What is the prognosis of this tooth and how could it be managed?

Clinical examination would involve visual inspection and palpation for the tooth buccally or lingually. In this case, the tooth was visible as a bulge in the buccal sulcus and could be palpated.

Radiographic assessment shows that the crown of the LR3 was lying horizontally, below the roots of the lower incisors.

The prognosis for the LR3 is poor due to the position. Orthodontic alignment would not be possible. If this were attempted, damage to the roots of the lower incisors may well occur.

What is the prognosis for the lower second primary molars? How is this assessed?

The lower second primary molars have a good prognosis. Clinically the primary teeth were firm, unrestored and showed no sign of infra-occlusion. Radiographically there was no evidence of root resorption or caries.

The UR4 is impacted. Will it be possible to align this tooth orthodontically?

The panoramic radiograph reveals that the UR4 is rotated through approximately 90 degrees. Space creation by proclination and torque of the upper labial segment should provide additional space for this tooth and, once derotated, the tooth will occupy less space in the arch. Surgical exposure and bonding of this tooth will facilitate eruption.

What are the possible treatment approaches for management of this malocclusion? Outline a possible treatment plan for each approach

- **Growth modification:** At 16 years of age, growth modification is not a realistic proposition in a female patient. A functional appliance could be considered to attempt some correction of the malocclusion through favourable tooth movement, but success is unlikely because of the lack of underlying growth and a reduced likelihood of good compliance in a 16-year-old girl.
- **Orthodontic camouflage:** Treatment would be carried out with upper and lower pre-adjusted edgewise appliances. The ectopic LR3 would be removed. In the lower arch the lower second primary molars would be retained, with a view to maintaining them as long as possible. When these teeth are lost in the future they could be replaced restoratively.

  In the upper arch, a camouflage approach would require the loss of two premolar units. In this case it would be appropriate to remove both upper first premolars, to provide adequate space for reduction of the overjet produced, which would be achieved using torque and retraction of the upper labial segment.
- **Orthodontics and orthognathic surgery:** Pre-surgical orthodontic treatment would involve removal of the ectopic LR3, and exposure and bonding of the impacted UR4. An overjet would be produced during orthodontic decompensation prior to surgical mandibular advancement.

  A decision was made to treat the patient with orthodontics and orthognathic surgery.

Describe the mechanics being used in Figure 10.10

In the upper arch, Burstone mechanics are being used to allow simultaneous correction of the torque in the upper labial segment and reduction of the overbite. In addition to a base archwire, an auxiliary arch wire with tip back bends is placed in the auxiliary tubes in the molar bands and ligated anteriorly to the base archwire with a ligature. A trans-palatal arch is in situ to prevent buccal flaring of the molars. The UR4 is brought down into the arch using elastomeric chain attached to a gold chain following previous exposure and bonding of this tooth. Powerchain is also being used to derotate

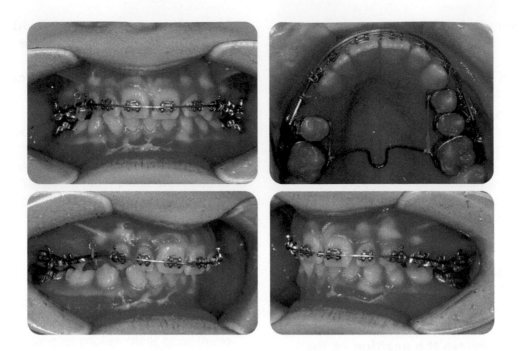

Figure 10.10

the UL4 and UR5, which have been banded and have metal cleats attached on the palatal side.

The patient is shown at the end of the pre-surgical orthodontic phase of treatment in Figure 10.11. What is the relevance of the pre-surgical overjet in this case?

The pre-surgical overjet dictates the mandibular advancement that can be achieved by the surgery. In order to check that sufficient increase in the overjet has been achieved, asking the patient to posture into a class I incisor relationship should reveal the desired change in facial profile.

Why has the overbite not been completely reduced pre-surgically?

Maintaining an increased overbite will facilitate some increase in the lower anterior face height as the mandible is advanced, which was thought desirable in this case.

What is illustrated in Figure 10.12?

Model surgery has been carried out in the laboratory. In this case the planned surgery was a mandibular advancement. The pre-surgical position has been reproduced using the articulated models on the left. On the right, the post-surgical position has been reproduced and an acrylic surgical wafer fabricated. This wafer will be used by the surgeon in theatre to

accurately position the mandible in the correct post-surgical position.

What is the rationale for model surgery?

Model surgery allows the final position of the occlusion to be checked based on the planned surgical moves. The prescription for the model surgery is planned around the clinical assessment pre-surgically. If the aims of the pre-surgical orthodontics have been achieved, the definitive surgical plan should match the original proposed plan.

The model surgery may highlight the need for additional orthodontics before the surgery to enable the proposed plan to be achieved, or more rarely may suggest the surgical plan be amended. A change in surgical plan at this stage, in order to accept the occlusion may result in a compromise in the facial aesthetics.

The model surgery also allows the laboratory to produce surgical wafers which are used in theatre to help achieve the planned surgical moves.

Why are study models mounted using a facebow record?

A facebow record is required if maxillary surgery is planned. The relationship between the Frankfort plane, maxillary base and terminal hinge axis of the mandible is recorded. Consequently, the influence of mandibular auto-rotation secondary to maxillary procedures may be gauged more accurately.

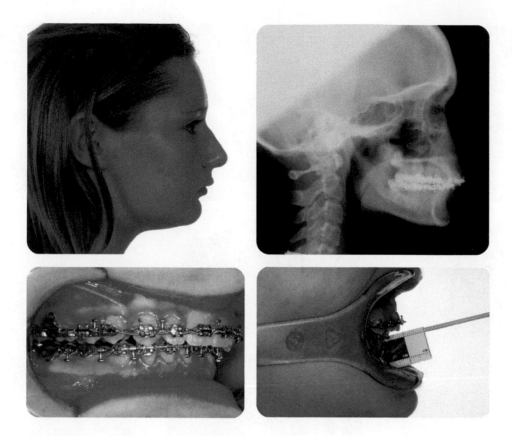

Figure 10.11

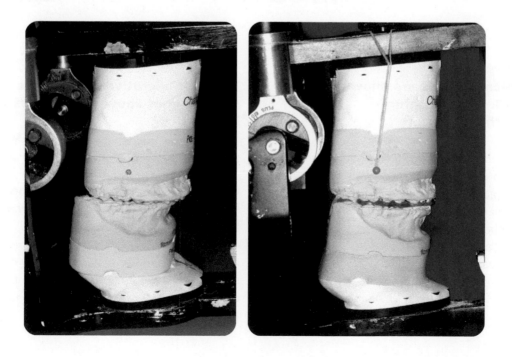

Figure 10.12

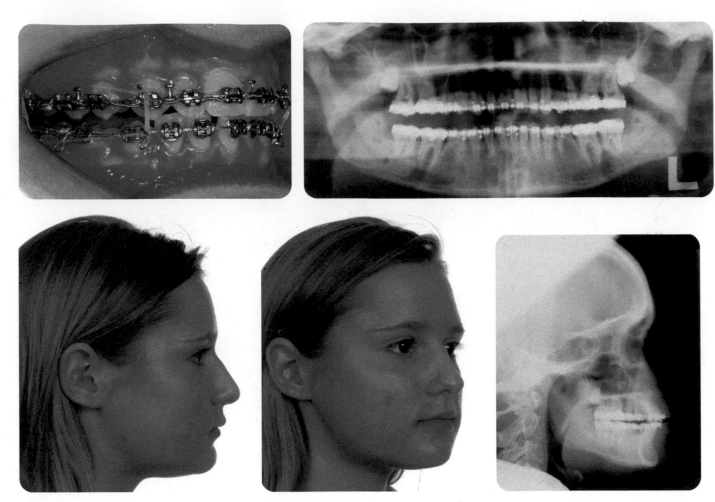

Figure 10.13

The post-surgical records are shown in Figure 10.13. What is being carried out in the upper left panel?

The lower arch was not levelled pre-surgically, by maintaining the curve of Spee, an increase in lower anterior face height can be achieved with the mandibular advancement surgery. The post-surgical mechanics involved closure of the resulting lateral open bites with the use of bilateral box elastics. In order to facilitate this post-surgical settling, the lower archwire was changed to a 19 × 25-inch braided stainless steel.

The post-operative radiographs in Figure 10.13 do not show any obvious fixation. Why is this?

In this case resorbable screws were used for the fixation, which are not visible radiographically.

On completion of treatment the dental centre lines were not coincident. Why is this (Figure 10.14)?

The treatment plan involved the loss of the LR3. In addition, both lower second primary molars were retained, which has contributed to a tooth-size discrepancy between the upper and lower dental arches.

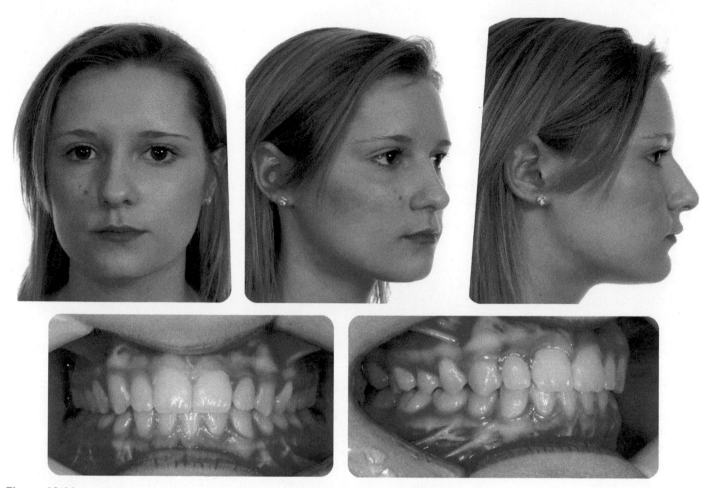

Figure 10.14

Case 10.5

This 19-year-old female was referred by her orthodontic specialist, concerned with her facial asymmetry and bite problem. There was no relevant medical history.

Extra-oral

Skeletal relationship

Antero-posterior	Mild skeletal class III
Vertical	FMPA: Increased
	Lower face height: Increased
Transverse	Mandibular asymmetry with deviation of chin point to the left side
Soft tissues	Lip competence: Competent
	Naso-labial angle: Normal
Upper incisor show	At rest: 2 mm
	Smiling: 7 mm
Temporo-mandibular joint	Healthy with good range and co-ordination of movement

Intra-oral

Teeth present

7654321/1234567
7654321/1234567

Dental health (restorations, caries)	Multiple heavily-restored and carious teeth
Oral hygiene	Poor; marginal gingivitis associated with the UR1 and UR2
Occlusion	Incisor relationship: Class III
	Overjet: 0 mm
	Overbite: Reduced and complete
	Molar relationship: Class I on left and class III on the right side
	Canine relationship: ½ unit class II on the left and class III on the bright side
	Centre lines:
	Upper centre line is correct to mid-facial plane
	Mandibular centre line is deviated 4 mm to the left side
	Functional occlusion: Group function
Upper arch	Crowding: Aligned
	Incisor inclination: Average
	Canine position: Line of arch
Lower arch	Crowding: Aligned
	Incisor inclination: Retroclined

Summary

A 19-year-old female presented with a class III malocclusion on a mild skeletal class III base with average vertical dimensions complicated by a left-sided mandibular asymmetry and unilateral posterior crossbite (Figure 10.15).

Treatment Plan

- Oral hygiene instruction and dental restorations
- Upper and lower pre-adjusted edgewise appliances on a non-extraction basis
- Asymmetric mandibular set-back surgery
- Long-term retention

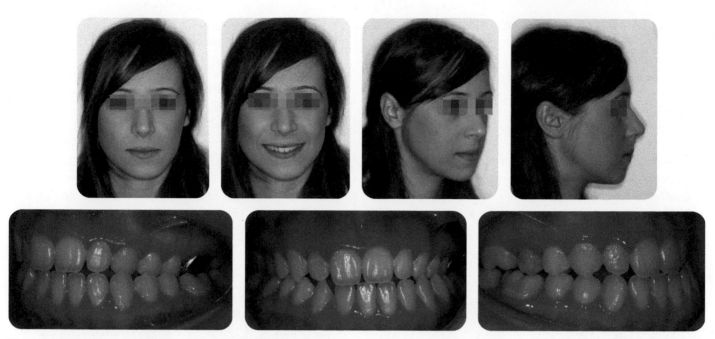

Figure 10.15

How successful is combined orthodontic–surgical treatment?

Retrospective research on the outcome of combined treatment has indicated high levels of success with excellent final occlusal outcomes (Baker *et al.*, 1999) and a mean duration of treatment of approximately 2 years (Dowling *et al.*, 1999). However, retrospective research is subject to selection bias and may fail to consider unsuccessful outcomes. Prospective research has suggested that overall treatment time may be longer than 2 years on average (O'Brien *et al.*, 2009). This study analysed the success of combined treatment in the UK and reported a non-completion rate of 28%. Younger subjects were more likely to abandon treatment. In relation to the final occlusal result, the mean PAR score was 10. This figure is slightly higher than might be expected with orthodontics in isolation, reflecting the complexity of combined care. Early success was influenced by the severity of the pre-treatment skeletal discrepancy, as larger surgical movements are more complex to achieve. However, the direction of the sagittal skeletal problem was not predictive of success or failure.

What is the hierarchy of stability for orthognathic procedures?

A scale of post-surgical stability for a range of malocclusions and jaw movements has been described, which is based upon longitudinal research carried out in the Orthodontic Department at Chapel Hill, University of North Carolina, and involves the follow-up of over 2000 patients. Most of the changes occur in relatively few subjects. Post-surgical changes of 2–4 mm are potentially clinically significant. Larger movements are beyond the scope of orthodontic correction and therefore regarded as highly clinically significant. Maxillary impaction, mandibular advancement and genioplasty are all considered highly stable. Maxillary advancement is also a stable procedure. However, single-jaw procedures involving mandibular set-back, inferior repositioning of the maxilla and maxillary expansion are less stable (Proffit *et al.*, 1996).

How is mandibular asymmetry classified?

Two main subtypes of mandibular asymmetry have been described: hemi-mandibular elongation and hemi-mandibular hyperplasia (Obwegeser and Makek, 1986). Mixed varieties also exist.

List the principle features of hemi-mandibular elongation and hyperplasia

Hemi-mandibular hyperplasia

- Three-dimensional enlargement of one side of the mandible

- Terminates exactly at the symphysis of the affected side
- Increased ramal length
- Enlarged distance between inferior dental canal and mandibular lower border
- Maxillary canting typical
- Centre lines usually coincident

Hemi-mandibular elongation

- Horizontal displacement of mandible to the unaffected side
- Mandibular rami lie at the same level bilaterally
- Maxillary canting unusual
- Contra-lateral posterior crossbite

What type of asymmetry did this patient have?

This patient had hemi-mandibular elongation. This case was typical of hemi-mandibular elongation with a mandibular midline shift, posterior crossbite on the unaffected side and absence of maxillary canting. Treatment involved asymmetric mandibular set-back only (Figure 10.16).

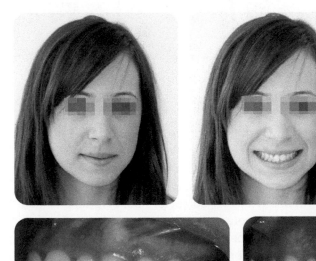
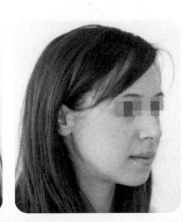
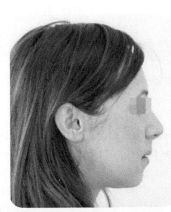
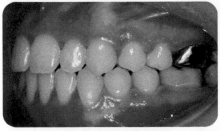
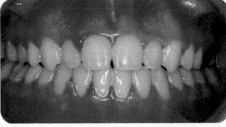
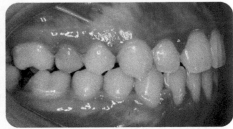
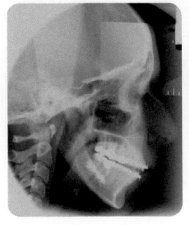
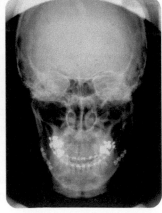
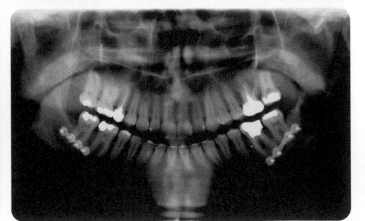

Figure 10.16

Case 10.6

This 17-year-old female was referred by her orthodontic specialist, concerned with her reverse bite and prominent chin position. There was no relevant medical history.

Extra-oral

Skeletal relationship

Antero-posterior	Moderate skeletal class III
Vertical	FMPA: Average
	Lower face height: Increased
Transverse	Facial symmetry: Chin point deviated to the left by 2 mm
Soft tissues	Lip competence: Competent
	Naso-labial angle: Normal
Upper incisor show	At rest: 3 mm
	Smiling: 8 mm
Temporo-mandibular joint	Healthy with good range and co-ordination of movement

Intra-oral

Teeth present
7 54321/1234567
7654321/1234567

Dental health (restorations, caries)	Moderate
	Restorations in UR5, UL5, UL6, LL6, LR6
Oral hygiene – periodontal	Good
Occlusion	Incisor relationship: Class III
	Overjet: −2 mm
	Overbite: Reduced and complete
	Molar relationship: Class III (although the UR6 is absent)
	Canine relationship: Class III bilaterally (greater on the right)
	Centre lines:
	Maxillary centre line is deviated 2 mm to the right side
	Mandibular centre line 2 mm to the left side
	Functional occlusion: Group function
Lower arch	Crowding: Mild
	Incisor inclination: Retroclined
Upper arch	Crowding: Mild
	Incisor inclination: Proclined
	Canine position: Line of arch

Summary

A 17-year-old female presented with a class III malocclusion on a moderate skeletal class III base with increased vertical dimensions complicated by a centre line discrepancy, early loss of the UR6 and crowding of both dental arches (Figure 10.17).

Treatment Plan
- Improve oral hygiene
- Upper and lower pre-adjusted edgewise appliances with extraction of the UL5
- Bi-maxillary surgery
- Long-term retention

When should surgery to correct a class III malocclusion be timed?

Surgical intervention to address a skeletal class III deformity should not be carried out until growth has declined to the physiological levels of adulthood. Chronological age is often used as an indicator, with surgery typically deferred until 18 years in males and at least 17 years in females. However, a recent study has suggested little long-term difference in outcomes in a comparison of females under 18 years and males under 20 years at the time of surgery with older patients (Bailey *et al.*, 2008). Consequently, cessation of growth may be more accurately predicted with superimposition of serial lateral cephalograms (Fudalej *et al.*, 2007).

Are there any early predictors available to indicate a potential need for surgery?

Combined orthodontic–surgical treatment may be indicated for the following reasons:
- Where an ideal occlusal result is not achievable with camouflage alone

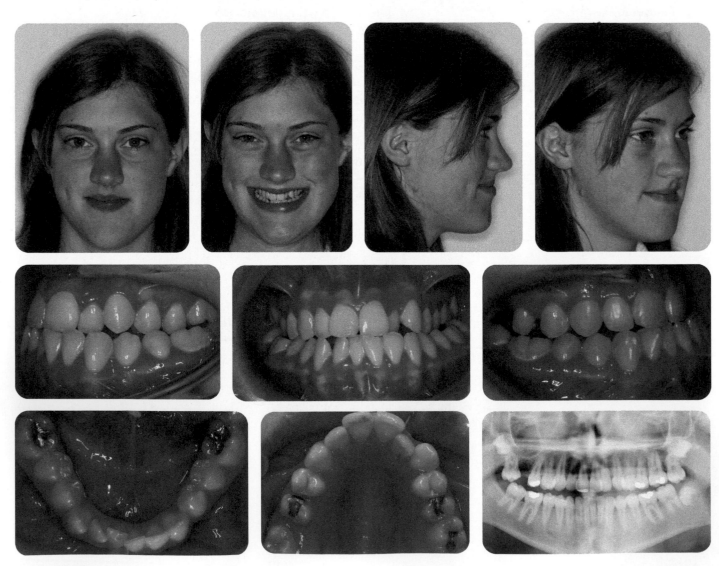

Figure 10.17

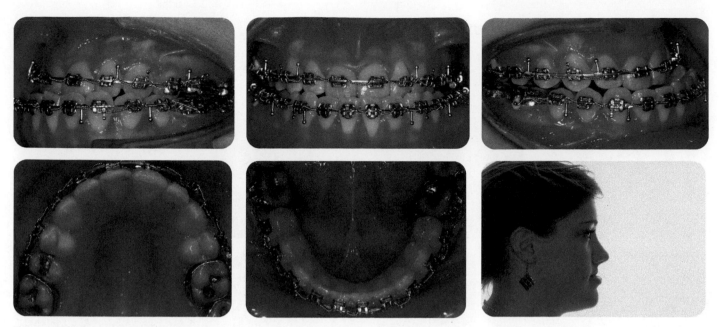

Figure 10.18

- Where facial change is required
- Where orthodontics will not produce an ideal occlusion without detrimental effects on facial aesthetics

A number of studies have assessed clinical and cephalometric predictors of the ability to camouflage for an underlying skeletal discrepancy without surgery in class III cases. Predictors include Wits, ANB, mandibular incisor inclination and Holdaway angle (Kerr *et al.*, 1992; Stellzig-Eisenhauer *et al.*, 2002). Threshold values of –4 degrees for ANB and 83 degrees for mandibular incisor inclination to the mandibular base have been suggested; with more negative values deemed more likely to necessitate surgery. Nevertheless, while these predictors are of some value, the requirement for surgery should be evaluated on an individual basis.

Comment on the rationale for extraction of the UL5 in this case

- To aid maxillary centre line correction and maxillary incisor decompensation with pre-surgical orthodontics
- This tooth is heavily-restored

What were the aims of pre-surgical orthodontics in this case (Figure 10.18)?

- Correct the maxillary centre line discrepancy
- Decompensate the mandibular incisors
- Co-ordinate the arches transversely

There was a reverse overjet of 6mm prior to surgery (Figure 10.18). Could this patient have been treated successfully with single-jaw surgery (Figures 10.19 and 10.20)?

As the amount of surgical movement required was 9mm, an acceptable occlusal outcome could have been achieved with a single-jaw procedure. However, the aetiology of the skeletal class III deformity was both mandibular prognathism and maxillary retrusion. There was also a minor mandibular asymmetry. Consequently, to optimize facial balance a bi-maxillary procedure was indicated.

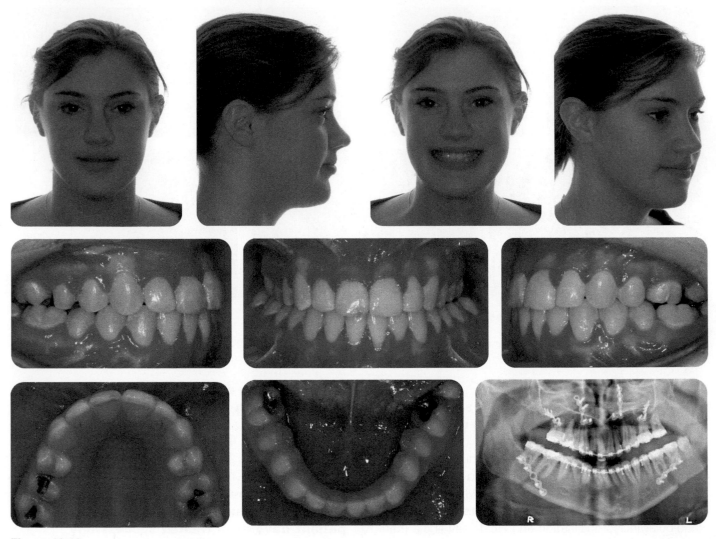

Figure 10.19

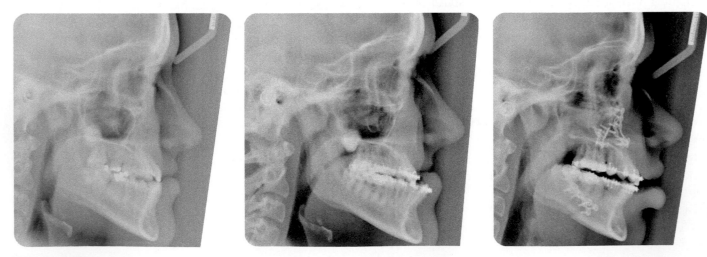

Figure 10.20

Case 10.7

This 48-year-old female was referred by her general dental practitioner, concerned with her prominent upper front teeth. There was no relevant medical history.

Extra-oral

Skeletal relationship

Antero-posterior	Moderate skeletal class II but a prominent chin button
Vertical	FMPA: Reduced
	Lower face height: Reduced
Transverse	Chin point symmetric

Soft tissues — Lip competence: Competent

Naso-labial angle: Normal

Little or no maxillary incisor show at rest or on smiling

Upper incisor show — At rest: 2 mm

Smiling: 9 mm

Temporo-mandibular joint — Healthy with good range and co-ordination of movement

Intra-oral

Teeth present

7654321/1234567
7654321/1234567

Dental health — Moderate
(restorations, caries) — Restorations in the UR5 and all molars, but sound

Acid erosion affecting the UL2, UL1; UR1, UR2

Oral hygiene – periodontal — Good

Occlusion — Incisor relationship: Class II division 1

Overjet: 8 mm

Overbite: Increased and complete

Molar relationship: ½ unit class II on the left; full unit class II on the right

Canine relationship: Class II bilaterally

Centre lines: Mandibular centre line is deviated 2 mm to the right side

Functional occlusion: Canine guidance

Lower arch — Crowding: Moderate

Incisor inclination: Average

Upper arch — Crowding: Mild

Incisor inclination: Average

Canine position: Line of arch, the LR3 distally angulated

Summary

A 48-year-old female presented with a class II division 1 malocclusion on a moderate skeletal class II pattern with reduced vertical dimensions complicated by an increased overjet, increased overbite, centre line discrepancy and a heavily restored dentition with marked acid erosion affecting the upper incisors (Figure 10.21). There was little upper incisor show, which was of concern to the patient. The pre-surgical occlusion is shown in Figure 10.22.

What technique is being used in Figure 10.23?

Surgical planning has been carried out using computer-based prediction software (in this case Quickceph®). This allows superimposition of cephalometric data derived from the lateral skull radiograph onto clinical photographs of the facial profile.

Pre-treatment data is shown in the upper left panel (the pre-treatment cephalometric radiograph has been digitized and overlaid on the pre-treatment profile photograph). In the upper right panel, the pre-surgical cephalometric radiograph has been digitized and in the middle left panel, this data has been transferred onto the pre-surgical profile photograph. Different surgical movements can then be performed. In the middle right panel, a maxillary advancement with posterior impaction has been performed in combination with forward movement, auto-rotation and reduction genioplasty of the mandible. The effect of these movements on the soft tissue profile are predicted by the computer (red outline) and these can then be simulated (or 'morphed') on the patient's profile photograph using the computer (lower left panel). The actual final surgical result is shown in the lower right panel. There is a difference between the predicted and

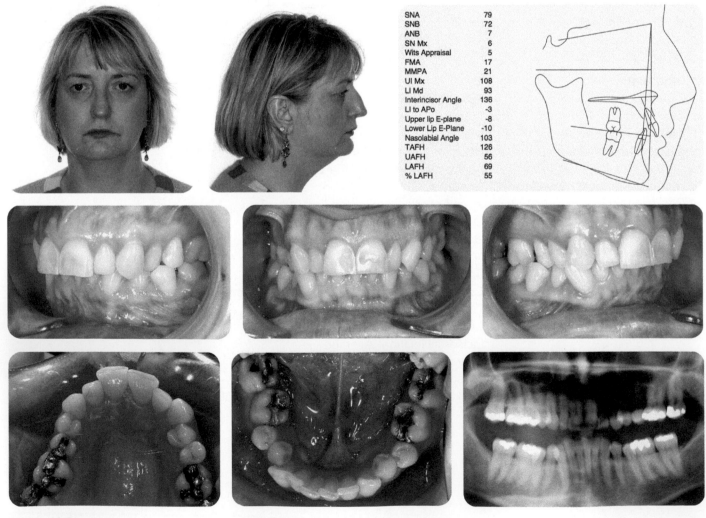

SNA	79
SNB	72
ANB	7
SN Mx	6
Wits Appraisal	5
FMA	17
MMPA	21
UI Mx	108
LI Md	93
Interincisor Angle	136
LI to APo	-3
Upper lip E-plane	-8
Lower Lip E-Plane	-10
Nasolabial Angle	103
TAFH	126
UAFH	56
LAFH	69
% LAFH	55

Figure 10.21

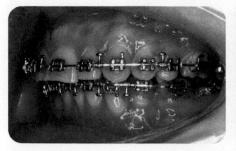
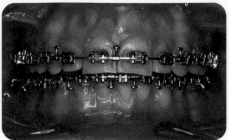
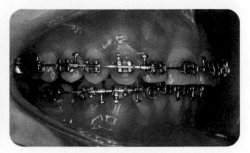

Figure 10.22

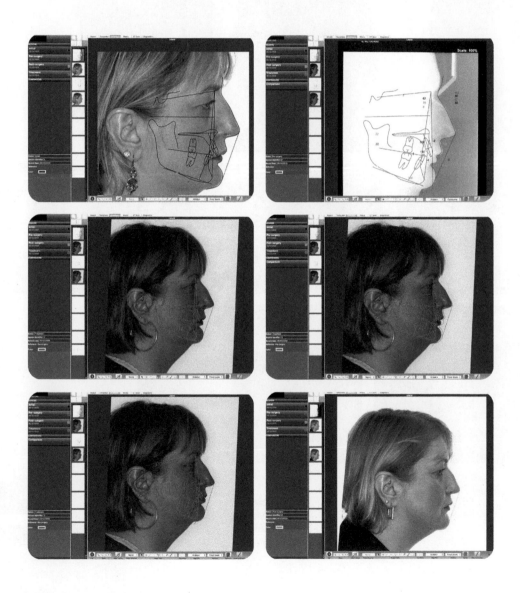

Figure 10.23

actual profiles, primarily because it was decided not to perform a genioplasty. The surgeon decided in theatre, once the maxillary and mandibular osteotomies had been carried out, that the profile was such that a genioplasty was not necessary. The final records following removal of the fixed appliances are shown in Figure 10.24.

Why do you think this surgical plan was carried out?

A maxillary advancement was undertaken to increase the amount of upper incisor show; posterior impaction was required to prevent the occurrence of an open bite following mandibular advancement. An alternative plan was mandibular advancement only and the patient

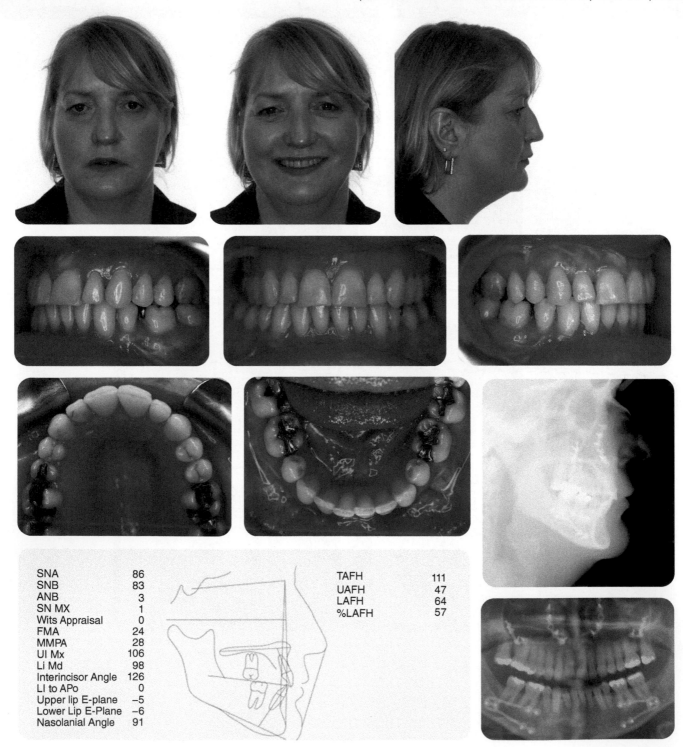

SNA	86
SNB	83
ANB	3
SN MX	1
Wits Appraisal	0
FMA	24
MMPA	28
UI Mx	106
Li Md	98
Interincisor Angle	126
LI to APo	0
Upper lip E-plane	−5
Lower Lip E-Plane	−6
Nasolanial Angle	91

TAFH	111
UAFH	47
LAFH	64
%LAFH	57

Figure 10.24

was given this option; however, she was keen to improve the upper incisor position and elected to undertake bi-maxillary surgery.

How accurate is digital prediction software?

Digital software is increasingly used as a diagnostic aid and for patient counselling. However, these techniques are not infallible, primarily because they aim to predict notoriously unpredictable changes. There is inevitably significant inter-individual variation in soft tissue response to skeletal change. In particular, soft tissue responses may vary due to ethnicity, soft tissue tonicity, lip thickness and competence. Nevertheless, reasonable levels of accuracy have been demonstrated with mean errors of less than 2 mm (Kaipatur et al., 2009; Kaipatur and Flores-Mir, 2009).

Soft tissue changes can be predicted more accurately with certain procedures and at specific anatomical locations; e.g. soft tissue changes at the chin are quite reproducible, reflecting skeletal changes in a 1:1 ratio. Less predictable changes arise at the lips, particularly the lower lip (Kaipatur and Flores-Mir, 2009). These inconsistencies mean that soft tissue prediction offers little more than a guide to expected changes and should not be relied upon completely.

In relation to individual systems, Dolphin® imaging software has demonstrated superior prediction of changes in the nasal form, chin and submandibular region. However, Dentofacial Planner Plus® outperformed Dolphin® with respect to the naso-labial angle, and upper and lower lips. However, overall there was no statistical difference between the two systems (Magro-Filho et al., 2010).

Case 10.8

This 27-year-old nurse was unhappy with the position and appearance of her teeth (Figure 10.25). She has asked for an orthodontic opinion.

From the clinical examination, how would you summarize her problem list?

- Severe class II jaw relationship
  - Increased naso-labial angle
  - Chin retrusion

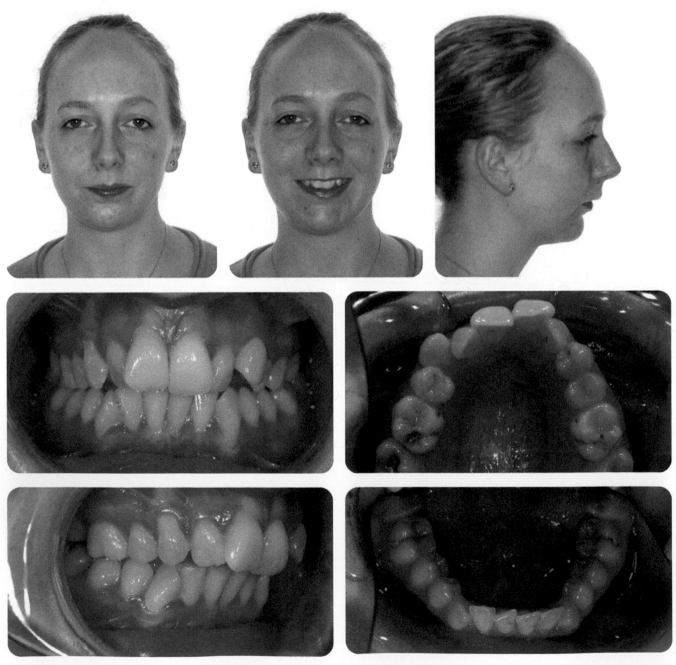

Figure 10.25

- Increased vertical proportions
- Increased overjet (actually 7 mm)
- Reduced overbite
- Moderate upper arch crowding, mild lower arch crowding
- Previous extraction of the UL3 and UR4

A decision was made to treat her malocclusion with a combination of orthodontics and surgery. Figure 10.26 shows the pre-surgical occlusion. What has the orthodontist achieved with these pre-surgical tooth movements?

- Alignment of the arches
- Some increase of the overjet
- Some reduction of the overbite
- Some expansion of the upper arch

What are the likely jaw movements required to correct this malocclusion?

- For the maxilla: Posterior impaction
- For the mandible: Advancement

Figure 10.27 shows some cephalometric predictions. What are the differences between the left and middle radiographs?

In the left radiograph, the maxilla has been impacted posteriorly and the mandible has been auto-rotated. However, the auto-rotation is not enough to correct the overjet. In the middle radiograph, the maxilla has been impacted posteriorly to the same extent as in the left radiograph, but this time, a forward mandibular sagittal split osteotomy has been introduced, which corrects the overjet and improves the chin position. In the right-hand image, the changes in the middle radiograph have been applied to the pre-surgical profile and morphed electronically to show a new predicted profile.

The final result is shown in Figure 10.28.

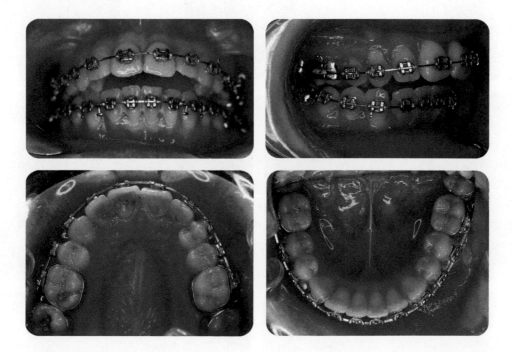

Figure 10.26

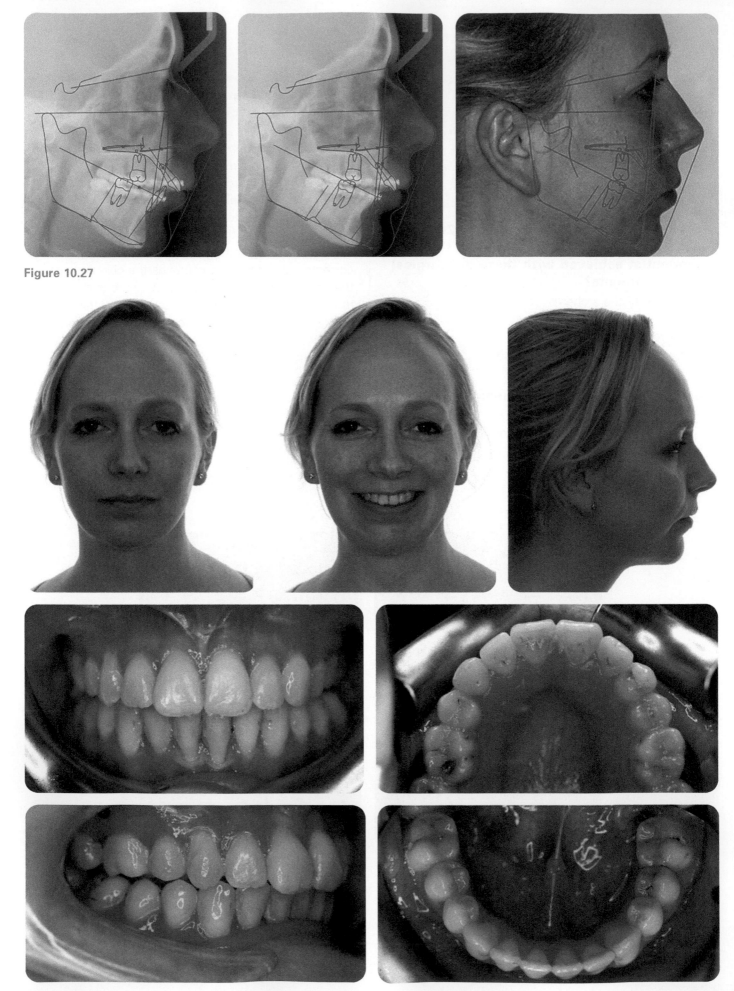

Figure 10.27

Figure 10.28

Case 10.9

This 17-year-old female was referred by her orthodontic specialist, concerned with her facial appearance and reverse bite. There was no relevant medical history.

Extra-oral

Skeletal relationship

    Antero-posterior — Mild skeletal class III

    Vertical — FMPA: Increased

        Lower face height: Increased

    Transverse — No asymmetry

Soft tissues — Lip competence: Competent

    Naso-labial angle: Normal

Upper incisor show — At rest: 3 mm

    Smiling: 8 mm

Temporo-mandibular joint — Healthy with good range and co-ordination of movement

Intra-oral

Teeth present

765 321/123 567
7654321/1234567

Dental health (restorations, caries) — Good

Oral hygiene – periodontal — Good

Occlusion — Incisor relationship: Class III

    Overjet: −2 mm

    Overbite: Reduced and complete

    Molar relationship: Class I bilaterally

    Canine relationship: Class III bilaterally

    Centre lines: Coincident with each other and mid-facial axis

    Functional occlusion: Group function

Upper arch — Crowding: Aligned

    Incisor inclination: Average

    Canine position: In line of the arch

Lower arch — Crowding: Mild

    Incisor inclination: Retroclined

Summary

An 17-year-old female presented with a class III malocclusion on a mild skeletal class III pattern with increased vertical dimensions complicated by a reversed overjet and bilateral buccal crossbites. The patient had undergone a previous course of treatment with removal of maxillary first premolars (Figure 10.29).

Treatment Plan

- Upper and lower pre-adjusted edgewise appliances on a non-extraction basis
- Maxillary advancement with differential (posterior) impaction and mandibular set-back surgery to class I
- Long-term retention (Figure 10.30)

What is the aetiology of the posterior crossbites?

This is most likely due to the sagittal discrepancy. By placing the study models into class I canine relationships, the need for expansion can be assessed.

Explain why the molar relationship is class I but the canines are class III?

This patient has had a previous course of orthodontics with loss of upper premolars bilaterally. Therefore, the class I molar relationship is misleading; the canine relationship reflects the associated malocclusion more faithfully.

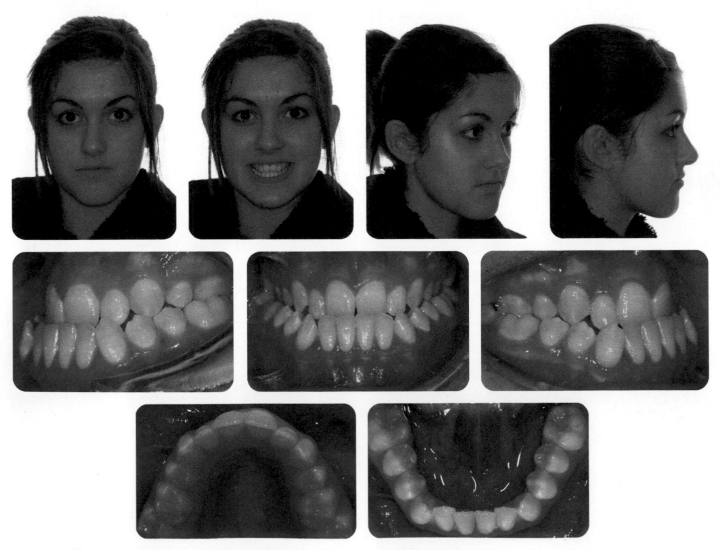

Figure 10.29

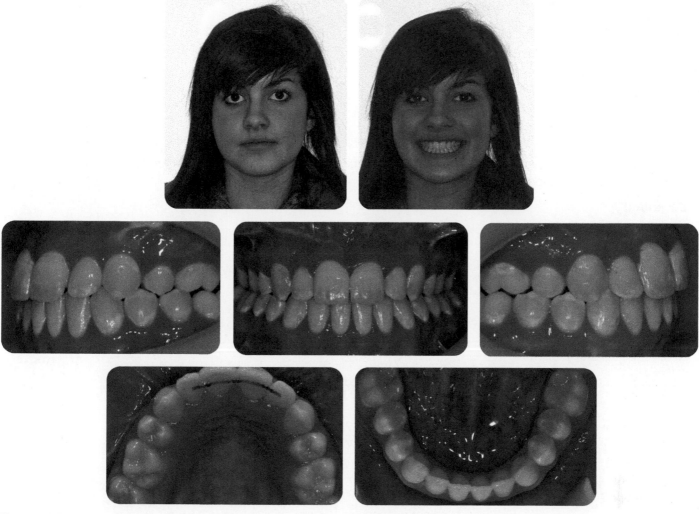

Figure 10.30

Why were maxillary first premolars removed during the first treatment phase?

First premolars were removed to provide sufficient space to allow alignment of the maxillary incisors. The previous orthodontist obviously felt the patient's malocclusion to be beyond the remit of orthodontics alone. Consequently, excessive proclination of the maxillary incisors would not be desirable, as it would camouflage the underlying skeletal discrepancy. This would limit the magnitude of surgical correction and facial change achievable.

What factors influence the stability of the surgical outcome?

- Surgical skill
- Condylar positioning
- Further growth
- Magnitude and direction of the skeletal changes
- Soft tissue and muscular effects
- Gender
- Type of fixation (Joss and Vassalli, 2008)

How likely is it that removal of surgical plates will be required?

Removal of plates is necessary in approximately 2% of cases (Fedorowicz *et al.*, 2007). Removal is typically necessitated by infection or exposure.

Case 10.10

This 16-year-old female had undergone previous unsuccessful functional appliance therapy. She was concerned about the appearance of her front teeth.

Extra-oral

Skeletal relationship

Antero-posterior	Moderate skeletal class II
Vertical	FMPA: Average
	Lower face height: Average
Transverse	No asymmetry
Soft tissues	Lip competence: Incompetent
	Naso-labial angle: Normal
Upper incisor show	At rest: 2 mm
	Smiling: 7 mm
Temporo-mandibular joint	Healthy with good range and co-ordination of movement

Intra-oral

Teeth present	7654321/1234567
	7654321/1234567
Dental health (restorations, caries)	Good
	Occlusal amalgam restorations in mandibular first molars
Oral hygiene – periodontal	Good
Occlusion	Incisor relationship: Class II division 1
	Overjet: 8 mm
	Overbite: Reduced and incomplete
	Molar relationship: Class II bilaterally
	Canine relationship: Class II bilaterally
	Centre lines: Lower to left by 1 mm
	Functional occlusion: Group function
Upper arch	Crowding: Mild
	Incisor inclination: Proclined
	Canine position: Aligned
Lower arch	Crowding: Well aligned
	Incisor inclination: Average

Summary

A 16-year-old female presented with a class II division 1 malocclusion on a moderate skeletal class II pattern with average vertical dimensions complicated by a lip trap and increased overjet (Figure 10.31).

Treatment Plan

- Upper and lower pre-adjusted edgewise appliances on a non-extraction basis
- Forward sliding sagittal split osteotomy
- Long-term retention

What was the aetiology of the increased overjet?

- Mandibular retrognathia
- Lip trap
- Proclined maxillary incisors

What were the alternatives to combined orthodontic–surgical treatment in this case? Discuss the merits of these options

- **Upper and lower pre-adjusted edgewise appliances with removal of maxillary first premolars.** This approach would have resulted in an acceptable class I incisor relationship; however, extraction of maxillary premolars would have compensated for the mandibular retrognathia rather than treating the aetiology. Their removal would result in some undesirable retraction of the upper lip with potentially detrimental effects on the facial profile.
- **Upper and lower pre-adjusted edgewise appliances on a non-extraction basis.** This plan would have involved alignment of the arches and accepting a residual overjet. Given that the arches

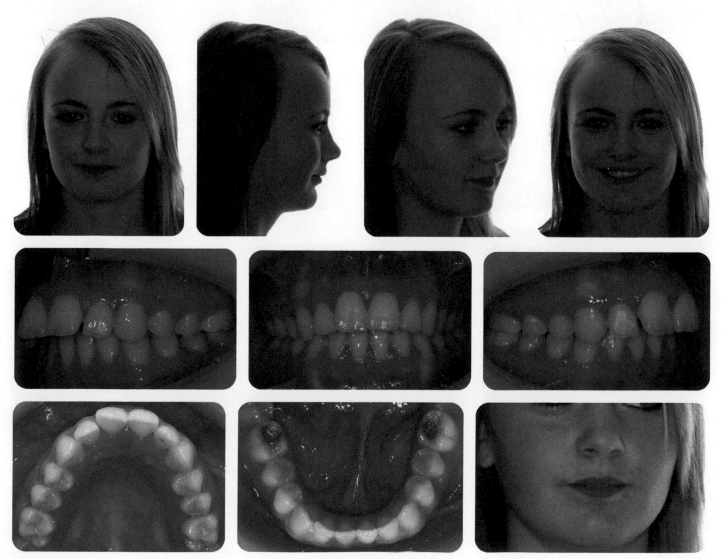

Figure 10.31

were relatively well-aligned at the outset, little would have been gained from this approach. In addition, a residual overjet is prone to relapse because the lower lip is likely to habitually sit underneath the upper incisors at rest and during function.

List the aims of pre-surgical orthodontics in this case (Figure 10.32)

- Arch alignment
- Decompensation

- Provision of surgical fixation
- Removal of occlusal interferences

This patient underwent a mandibular advancement sagittal split osteotomy (the radiographs and final result are shown in Figures 10.33 and 10.34, respectively). Comment on this choice of surgical procedure

Mandibular advancement surgery is considered a stable procedure provided advancement does not

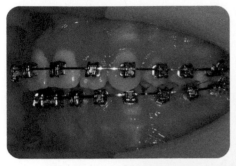
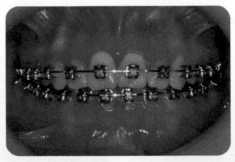
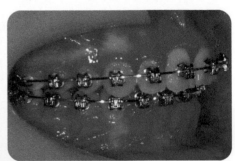
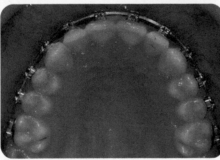
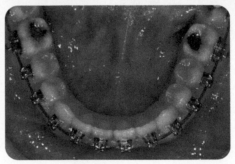

Figure 10.32

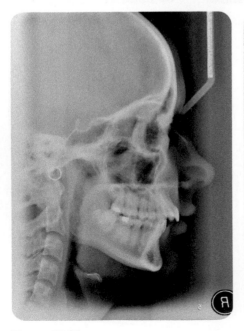
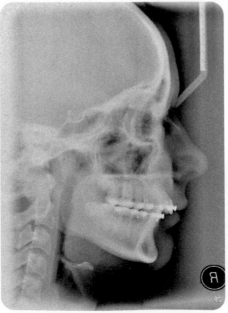
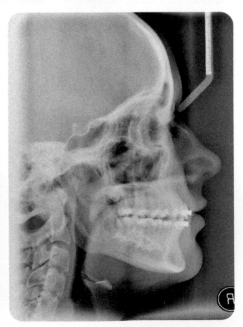

Figure 10.33

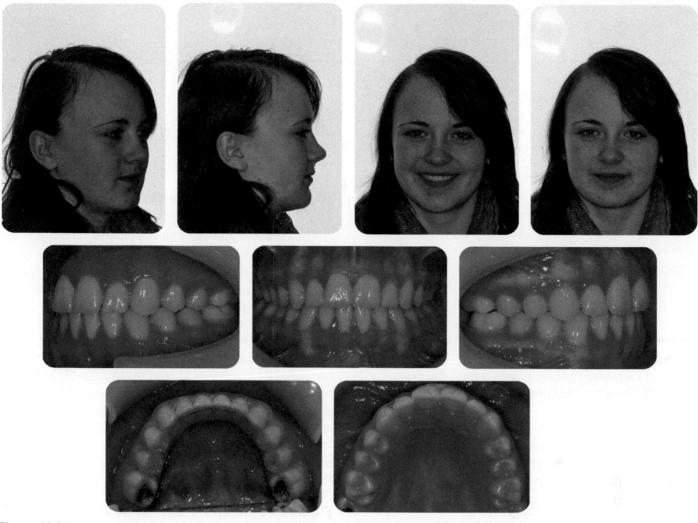

Figure 10.34

involve counter-clockwise mandibular rotation (Bailey *et al.*, 2008) or exceed 10 mm. The advent of rigid internal fixation has reduced the morbidity associated with mandibular surgery, whilst making it more predictable and stable.

How common is sensory nerve alteration following sagittal split osteotomy?

A systematic review of studies considering this question concluded that the risk of transient numbness is 63%, while permanent numbness is likely in 13% of those undergoing mandibular osteotomies (Colella *et al.*, 2007).

Case 10.11

This 16-year-old girl presented complaining about the prominence of her upper front teeth (her overjet was 12 mm) and the crowding of her lower front teeth.

Summarize her malocclusion (Figure 10.35)

A 16-year-old female presented with a class II division 1 case on a marked skeletal class II base associated with mandibular retrognathia and average vertical proportions. The overjet is increased to 12 mm and the overbite is normal but incomplete. The buccal segment relationship is class II bilaterally and the lower centre line is over to the left by 1 mm. There is severe crowding in the lower arch and mild crowding in the upper.

What does the radiographic examination reveal (Figure 10.35)?

The cephalometric radiograph demonstrates a skeletal class II pattern with marked mandibular retrognathia. The MMPA is within the normal range. The lower incisors are proclined but the upper incisors are of normal inclination. All teeth are present with the third molars unerupted. There is no caries.

Comment on the soft tissues (Figure 10.35)

The profile is retrognathic but the naso-labial angle is essentially normal. The lips are incompetent with the lower lip seemingly positioned behind the upper incisors at rest. The upper lip is quite long but there is normal upper incisor show at rest and during smiling.

What are the main problems?

- Mandibular retrognathia
- Significantly increased overjet
- Class II buccal segment relationship
- Crowding

What options are there for treatment?

This patient is too old for growth modification.

The extent of the skeletal discrepancy, the presence of crowding and the class II buccal segment relationship make orthodontic camouflage challenging. In addition, the maxillary incisor position is acceptable and retraction of these teeth is unlikely to improve the facial profile. Dento-alveolar compensation has already taken place, with the lower incisors proclined. Collectively, these findings mean that orthodontic camouflage (which would require the loss of four first premolars, anchorage reinforcement and fixed appliances) would be difficult and unlikely to produce an acceptable aesthetic result.

Mandibular advancement surgery in conjunction with fixed appliances to align, level and decompensate the malocclusion is the treatment of choice.

Figures 10.36 and 10.37 show the clinical and cephalometric appearance prior to surgery, respectively. Comment on what has taken place and what has been achieved

Pre-adjusted edgewise appliances have been used to align the teeth in conjunction with the extraction of mandibular first premolars. Alignment has been achieved, the maxillary incisor position maintained and the mandibular incisors decompensated, creating an increase in the overjet (to 15 mm). The extent of the skeletal discrepancy has also meant that a scissors bite is present on the right.

What is being carried out in Figure 10.38 and why?

This patient is undergoing distraction osteogenesis to advance the mandible. The reason for this is that the surgical advancement required to correct the overjet was too large to be carried out by a sagittal split osteotomy because movements beyond 10 mm are unstable and susceptible to relapse.

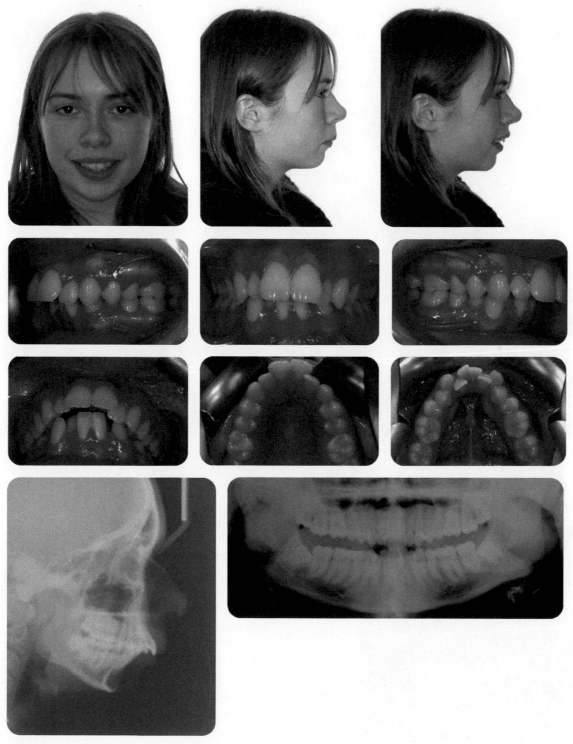

Figure 10.35

What is distraction osteogenesis of the mandible?

Distraction osteogenesis of the mandible involves a sagittal corticotomy of the body to fracture the bone into two segments. The two bone ends are then gradually moved apart mechanically during a distraction phase, which allows new bone to form in the gap. When the desired length is reached, in this case when the incisor relationship was class I, a consolidation phase follows in which the bone is allowed to continue to heal. Distraction osteogenesis has the benefit of simultaneously increasing bone length and volume,

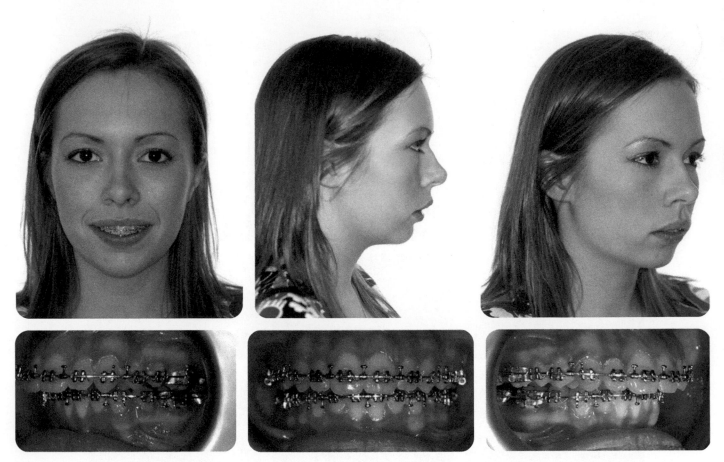

Figure 10.36

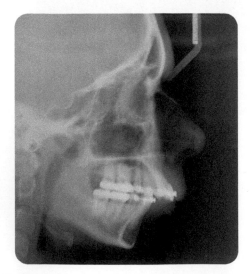

Figure 10.37

allowing lengthening of the mandibular body beyond 10 mm. A distraction rate of 1 mm per day is used and the patient activates the distractors themselves by turning a screw. If too rapid advancement takes place, fibrous tissue rather than bone is produced in the space between the two bone ends, which is undesirable.

The final occlusion is shown in Figure 10.39; why is the molar relationship class III?

The molar relationship is class III because lower first premolars were extracted prior to surgery to allow alignment of the lower incisors.

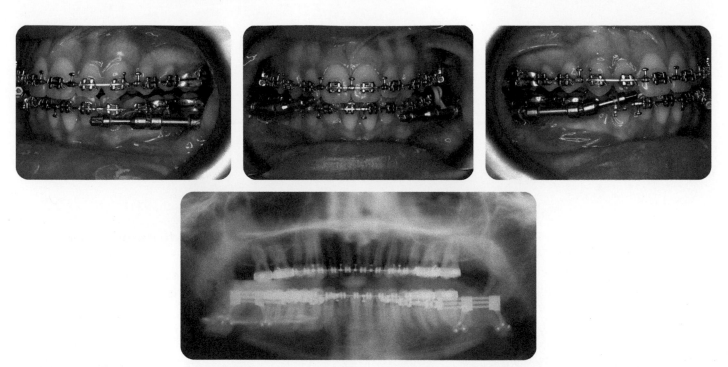

Figure 10.38

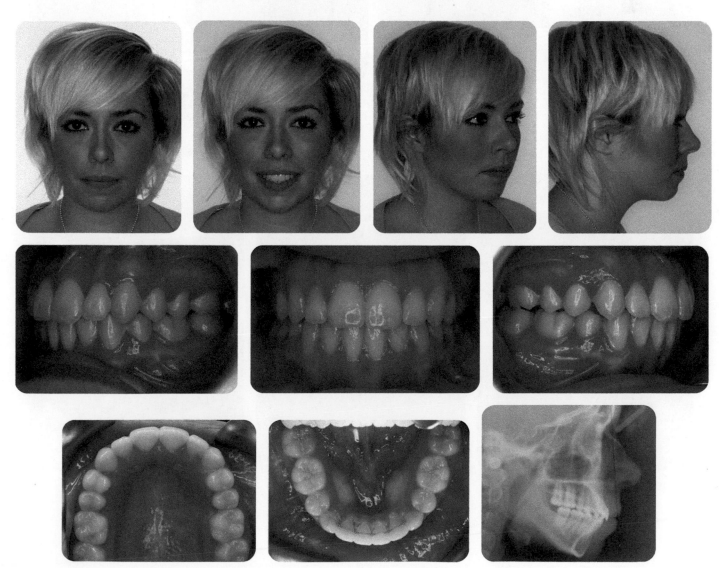

Figure 10.39

Case 10.12

This 42-year-old woman was unhappy with the appearance of her teeth. Her pre-treatment records are shown in Figure 10.40.

What are the extra-oral features of her malocclusion?

- Class II on a moderate skeletal class II base with average vertical proportions

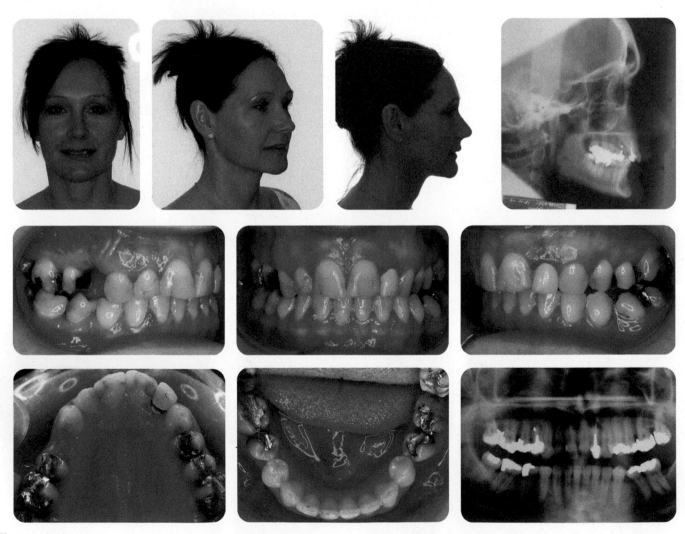

Figure 10.40

- Chin point is slightly to the patient's left
- Lip trap, with the lower lip positioned behind the upper incisors at rest
- Naso-labial angle is normal, but the presence of mandibular retrognathia and a prominent chin point has resulted in a resting lip position that is significantly behind the E-line and consequently, a poor facial profile

What are the intra-oral features?

- Class II division 1 incisor relationship with an increased overjet (8 mm)
- Overbite is within the normal range and incomplete to the palate, although the curve of Spee is increased in the lower arch
- Lower centre line is over to the left by 2 mm (½ tooth unit). The canine relationship is class I on the right and ½ unit class II on the left, which is consistent with the centre line discrepancy
- Molar relationship is class I on the right and ½ class II on the left.
- Dentition is heavily restored, with extensive amalgam restorations associated with the premolar and molar regions
- UR4 and LL7 have recently been extracted
- Oral hygiene is good
- Both arches are reasonably well aligned in the incisor regions
- Some spacing in the upper right premolar region

What information do the radiographs provide?

The cephalometric radiograph confirms the presence of a moderate class II sagittal jaw relationship and average vertical proportions. The incisors appear to be at a normal inclination and the soft tissue profile is retrusive.

The panoramic radiograph demonstrates the presence of extensive amalgam restorations (which appear to be sound, although some have overhangs), a peri-apical area associated with a root canal-treated and apicected UR4 (which has been extracted), a root-treated apicected UL2 with a post and core restoration, inter-proximal composite restorations in the upper incisor and canine regions, absent third molars and LL7. The LL5 is mesially orientated against the LL4. There has been some inter-proximal bone loss in the upper left quadrant.

What are the options for treatment?

The main options are between orthodontic camouflage or orthodontic treatment combined with orthognathic surgery.

If orthodontic camouflage is instigated with fixed appliances, what needs to be considered?

Orthodontic camouflage will require space to reduce the overjet and correct the centre line discrepancy. In this case, space would almost certainly need to be generated with orthodontic extractions.

A key decision would be whether to extract in the lower arch. The teeth are well aligned and space requirements are minimal. Extracting teeth would provide some inter-arch anchorage for overjet reduction and allow curve of Spee levelling without excessive incisor proclination. However, space closure would take a long time. The lower centre line also needs to be considered. It might be quite difficult to correct this without extracting in the lower arch.

In the upper arch, space is certainly required for overjet reduction. The UR4 has already been extracted, and extraction of the UL4 would be a reasonable choice; it is heavily restored, would provide optimal space for overjet reduction and balances loss of the UR4 nicely. Alternatively, the UL2 could be extracted (it is heavily restored and apicected), but this would have the disadvantage of requiring the UL3 to become a lateral incisor, and given that the UR2 would still be present, this asymmetry in the upper labial segment would probably not be ideal for optimal dental aesthetics.

For camouflage, extraction of the upper first premolars and non-extraction in the lower arch would probably provide the best option. In this case, some inter-proximal reduction might be needed in the lower arch to prevent excessive lower incisor proclination and help with centre line correction. In addition, some anchorage reinforcement might be necessary in the upper arch to achieve complete overjet reduction. Other problems with this strategy might be achieving complete space closure in the upper arch, particularly if the lower incisors procline.

The main disadvantage with camouflage is that it does not address the underlying skeletal discrepancy and poor profile, if anything it may worsen the profile. The lips are already quite significantly behind the E-line and further incisor retraction might not be favourable.

What are the options for surgical orthodontic treatment?

Definitive correction of this malocclusion would involve orthodontic decompensation and surgery to correct the underlying jaw discrepancy.

Given that the upper incisors have a good antero-posterior and vertical position, and that there is no vertical maxillary excess or significantly increased vertical proportions – surgery would almost certainly involve forward repositioning of the mandible. However, there is a prominent chin button and therefore, a reduction genioplasty may also be required as a supplement to the mandibular advancement surgery. Moreover, the lower centre line is to the left, along with the mid-point of the chin. Therefore, the mandibular advancement would also be planned with movement to the right to simultaneously correct the dental centre line and chin point.

A decision was made to undertake treatment with asymmetric mandibular advancement surgery and a reduction genioplasty. Figure 10.41 shows progress during archwire progression with fixed appliances. Why was the UL4 not extracted?

The UR4 was extracted because of the presence of peri-apical pathology and a previous apicectomy, which suggested a poor long-term prognosis. Minimal space was required in the upper arch and therefore, no teeth were extracted in the upper left quadrant. The upper dental centre line was coincident with the face. The UR4 could either be restored post-treatment with a bridge or implant; or space closed from behind during the orthodontic set-up. After consultation with a restorative dentist, it was decided to close space in the upper right quadrant, whilst preserving the upper centre line position. Not all of the space needed to be closed because after treatment, the heavily restored

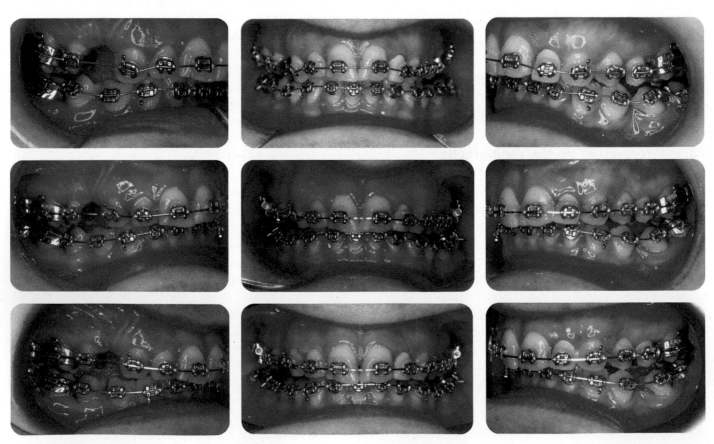

Figure 10.41

UR5 was going to have a coronal restoration and some of the excess space could be accommodated with this.

The pre-surgical records are shown in Figure 10.42. Some of the UR4 space has been closed, the centre line discrepancy has been maintained and the LL5 has been uprighted, which interestingly, generated some space in this region of the lower arch. The overjet is still increased. What other diagnostic information is required at this stage?

A set of study models should be taken to assess the transverse arch co-ordination in the final occlusal position with the overjet reduced and centre line corrected.

What has happened to the UL2?

The bracket, which had been bonded to the porcelain crown, became debonded and lost just prior to surgery! Rather than re-bond this, a decision was made to leave it until after the surgery and replace it prior to final occlusal detailing.

Why has all of the UR4 space not been closed prior to surgery?

It was felt that further space closure might result in some overjet reduction and movement of the upper centre line to the right, compromising the desired surgical movements. Therefore, final space closure was carried out following surgery.

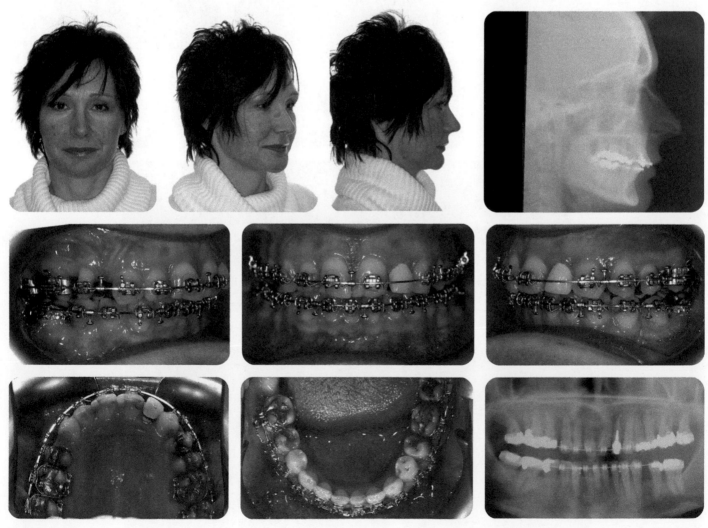

Figure 10.42

The post-treatment records are shown in Figures 10.43 and 10.44. Comment on the final result

There has been an improvement in the facial profile, although there is a slight excess of skin in the throat-chin region as a result of the mandibular advancement and reduction genioplasty. The overjet and centre line have been corrected and space closure achieved in the upper right quadrant (except for 1 mm, which will be accommodated by a coronal restoration on the UR5).

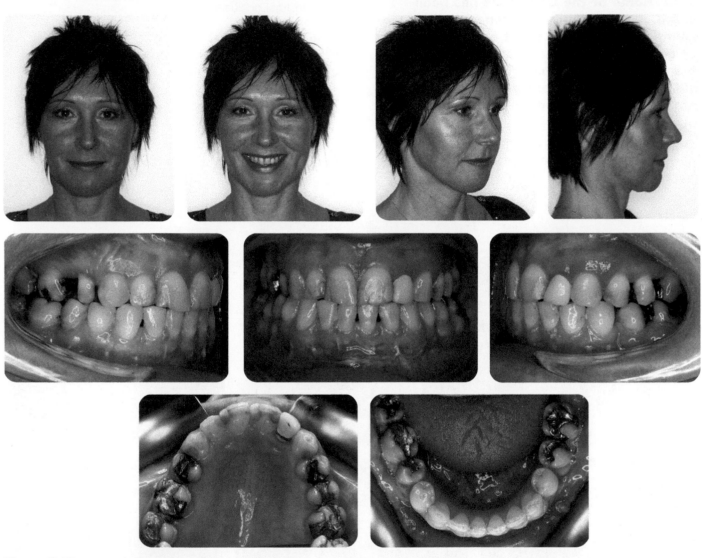

Figure 10.43

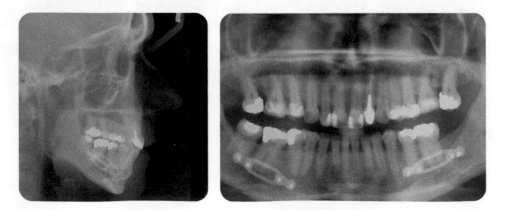

Figure 10.44

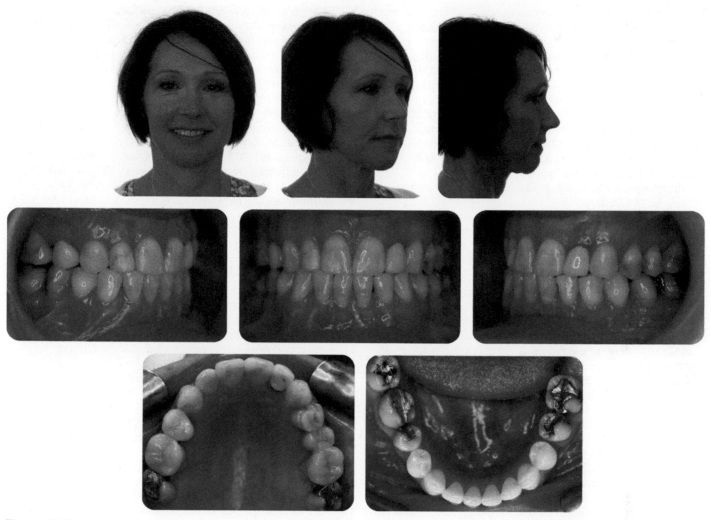

Figure 10.45

Figure 10.45 shows the occlusion 4 years post-treatment. The UR5 and UL2 have new crowns, a number of composite, composite veneer and inlay restorations have been placed and the teeth have undergone external bleaching. Removable orthodontic retainers are still being worn two nights per week.

What advice would you have regarding further maintenance of retention?

If the patient is happy, continued part-time wear of the retainers is advised on a long-term basis. Alternatively, bonded retainers could be considered, although the extensive restorative work may complicate bonding.

References

Ackerman JL, Proffit WR, Sarver DM (1999) The emerging soft tissue paradigm in orthodontic diagnosis and treatment planning. *Clin Orthod Res* 2:49–52.

Arnett GW, Gunson MJ (2004) Facial planning for orthodontists and oral surgeons. *Am J Orthod Dentofacial Orthop* 126:290–295.

Arnett GW, Gunson MJ (2010) Esthetic treatment planning for orthognathic surgery. *J Clin Orthod* 44:196–200.

Bailey LJ, Phillips C, Proffit WR (2008) Long-term outcome of surgical Class III correction as a function of age at surgery. *Am J Orthod Dentofacial Orthop* 133:365–370.

Baker NJ, David S, Barnard DW, Birnie DJ, Robinson SN (1999) Occlusal outcome in patients undergoing orthognathic surgery with internal fixation. *Br J Oral Maxillofac Surg* 37:90–93.

Colella G, Cannavale R, Vicidomini A, Lanza A (2007) Neurosensory disturbance of the inferior alveolar nerve after bilateral sagittal split osteotomy: a systematic review. *J Oral Maxillofac Surg* 65:1707–1715.

Cunningham SJ, Hunt NP, Feimann C (1995) Psychological aspects of orthognathic surgery: a review of the literature. *Int J Adult Orthodon Orthognath Surg* 10:159–172.

Cunningham SJ, Hunt NP, Feimann C (1996) Perceptions of outcome following orthognathic surgery. *Br J Oral Maxillofac Surg* 34:210–213.

Cunningham SJ, Sculpher M, Sassi F, Manca A (2003) A cost-utility analysis of patients undergoing orthognathic treatment for the management of dentofacial disharmony. *Br J Oral Maxillofac Surg* 41:32–35.

Denison TF, Kokich VG, Shapiro PA (1989) Stability of maxillary surgery in openbite versus nonopenbite malocclusions. *Angle Orthod* 59:5–10.

Dowling PA, Espeland L, Krogstad O, Stenvik A, Kelly A (1999) Duration of orthodontic treatment involving orthognathic surgery. *Int J Adult Orthodon Orthognath Surg* 14:146–152.

Fedorowicz Z, Nasser M, Newton JT, Oliver RJ (2007) Resorbable versus titanium plates for orthognathic surgery. *Cochrane Database Syst Rev* 2:CD006204.

Fudalej P, Kokich VG, Leroux B (2007) Determining the cessation of vertical growth of the craniofacial structures to facilitate placement of single-tooth implants. *Am J Orthod Dentofacial Orthop* 131:S59–67.

Iannetti G, Fadda MT, Marianetti TM, Terenzi V, Cassoni A (2007) Long-term skeletal stability after surgical correction in Class III open-bite patients: a retrospective study on 40 patients treated with mono- or bimaxillary surgery. *J Craniofac Surg* 18:350–354.

Janson G, Valarelli FP, Beltrao RT, de Freitas MR, Henriques JF (2006) Stability of anterior open-bite extraction and nonextraction treatment in the permanent dentition. *Am J Orthod Dentofacial Orthop* 129:768–774.

Joss CU, Vassalli IM (2008) Stability after bilateral sagittal split osteotomy setback surgery with rigid internal fixation: a systematic review. *J Oral Maxillofac Surg* 66:1634–1643.

Kaipatur NR, Flores-Mir C (2009) Accuracy of computer programs in predicting orthognathic surgery soft tissue response. *J Oral Maxillofac Surg* 67:751–759.

Kaipatur N, Al-Thomali Y, Flores-Mir C (2009) Accuracy of computer programs in predicting orthognathic surgery hard tissue response. *J Oral Maxillofac Surg* 67:1628–1639.

Kerr WJ, Miller S, Dawber JE (1992) Class III malocclusion: surgery or orthodontics? *Br J Orthod* 19:21–24.

Lopez-Gavito G, Wallen TR, Little RM, Joondeph DR (1985) Anterior open-bite malocclusion: a longitudinal 10-year postretention evaluation of orthodontically treated patients. *Am J Orthod* 87:175–186.

Magro-Filho O, Magro-Ernica N, Queiroz TP, Aranega AM, Garcia IR Jr (2010) Comparative study of 2 software programs for predicting profile changes in Class III patients having double-jaw orthognathic surgery. *Am J Orthod Dentofacial Orthop* 137:452 e1–5; discussion 452–453.

Mihalik CA, Proffit WR, Phillips C (2003) Long-term follow-up of Class II adults treated with orthodontic camouflage: a comparison with orthognathic surgery outcomes. *Am J Orthod Dentofacial Orthop* 123:266–278.

O'Brien K, Wright J, Conboy F, et al. (2009) Prospective, multi-center study of the effectiveness of orthodontic/orthognathic surgery care in the United Kingdom. *Am J Orthod Dentofacial Orthop* 135:709–714.

Obwegeser H (1969) Surgical correction of small or retrodisplaced maxillae. *Plast Reconstr Surg* 44:351–365.

Obwegeser HL, Makek MS (1986) Hemimandibular hyperplasia–hemimandibular elongation. *J Maxillofac Surg* 14:183–208.

Proffit WR, Turvey TA, Phillips C (1996) Orthognathic surgery: a hierarchy of stability. *Int J Adult Orthodon Orthognath Surg* 11:191–204.

Proffit WR, Turvey TA, Phillips C (2007) The hierarchy of stability and predictability in orthognathic surgery with rigid fixation: an update and extension. *Head Face Med* 3:21.

Ramos AL, Sakima MT, Pinto Ados S, Bowman SJ (2005) Upper lip changes correlated to maxillary incisor retraction–a metallic implant study. *Angle Orthod* 75:499–505.

Scott Conley R, Jernigan C (2006) Soft tissue changes after upper premolar extraction in Class II camouflage therapy. *Angle Orthod* 76:59–65.

Stansbury CD, Evans CA, Miloro M, BeGole EA, Morris DE (2010) Stability of open bite correction with sagittal split osteotomy and closing rotation of the mandible. *J Oral Maxillofac Surg* 68:149–159.

Stellzig-Eisenhauer A, Lux CJ, Schuster G (2002) Treatment decision in adult patients with Class III malocclusion: orthodontic therapy or orthognathic surgery? *Am J Orthod Dentofacial Orthop* 122:27–37; discussion 37–38.

Swinnen K, Politis C, Willems G, et al. (2001) Skeletal and dento-alveolar stability after surgical-orthodontic treatment of anterior open bite: a retrospective study. *Eur J Orthod* 23:547–557.

Trauner R, Obwegeser H (1957) The surgical correction of mandibular prognathism and retrognathia with consideration of genioplasty. *Oral Surg* 10:787–792.

Zuroff JP, Chen SH, Shapiro PA, Little RM, Joondeph DR, Huang GJ (2010) Orthodontic treatment of anterior open-bite malocclusion: stability 10 years postretention. *Am J Orthod Dentofacial Orthop* 137:302 e1–8; discussion 302–303.

11

Development of the Craniofacial Region

Embryonic Development of the Face

Figure 11.1 is a scanning electron micrograph of the face of a mouse embryo at around 10.5 days of development.

Name the structures labelled A–G

A = Fronto-nasal process
B = Medial nasal process
C = Lateral nasal process
D = Nasal pit
E = Maxillary process of the first pharyngeal arch
F = Mandibular process of the first pharyngeal arch
G = Second pharyngeal arch

Briefly describe how structures A–E contribute to formation of the developing face

Structures A–E contribute to formation of the middle third of the face. In particular, the maxillary processes (E) grow medially towards the midline, fusing with the lateral nasal processes (C) to form the naso-lacrimal duct, cheek and alar base of the nose. Further growth results in fusion with the medial nasal processes (B) in the midline to form the middle part of the nose, lip philtrum and primary palate, including the incisor teeth (Figure 11.2).

What contribution does structure F make to the face?

The mandibular process of the first pharyngeal arch will form the lower jaw or mandible, including the dentition. In addition, it will form the lower lip and muscles of mastication.

What would be the equivalent age of this embryo in relation to human development?

The equivalent is around 6 weeks.

What contribution does structure G make to the developing facial region?

Structure G is the second pharyngeal arch and will form the upper part of the hyoid bone, the styloid process, stapes of the middle ear and stylohyoid ligament. In addition, it will form muscles innervated by the facial nerve, including the muscles of facial expression.

Tooth Development

Figure 11.3 shows a developing tooth germ. Identify the labelled structures

A = Dental papilla
B = Enamel organ

What parts of the tooth will these structures give rise to?

The dental papilla is derived from neural crest cells, which form all the structures within the tooth (dentine of the crown and root, pulp, periodontal ligament) with the exception of enamel, which is derived from the epithelium of the early jaw.

Clinical Cases in Orthodontics, First Edition. Martyn T. Cobourne, Padhraig S. Fleming, Andrew T. DiBiase, and Sofia Ahmad.
© 2012 Martyn T. Cobourne, Padhraig S. Fleming, Andrew T. DiBiase, and Sofia Ahmad. Published 2012 by Blackwell Publishing Ltd.

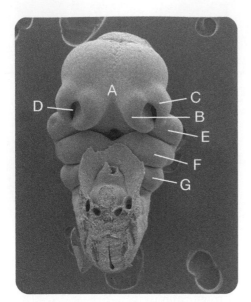

Figure 11.1

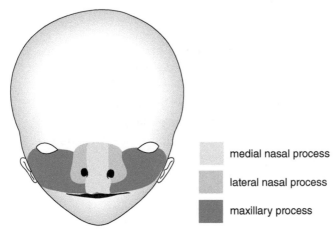

Figure 11.2

medial nasal process

lateral nasal process

maxillary process

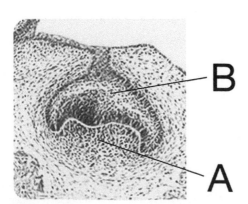

Figure 11.3

What stage of development are these tooth germs at?

They are at the cap stage.

What is the significance of this stage?

The cap stage heralds the establishment of shape within the tooth germ in the human embryo, defining a tooth germ as incisor, canine, premolar or molar.

How do the tooth germs of different tooth classes acquire their distinctive shape?

Tooth development is controlled by molecular signalling interactions between the epithelium and underlying neural crest cells within the tooth germ. The molecular instructions for shape are established early in this process, by specific domains of homeobox gene expression specifying a tooth germ as 'incisor' or 'molar'.

What are the main features identifiable on this dental panoramic radiograph (Figure 11.4)?

- Congenital absence of the UR4, UR2, UL2, LL5; this has led to associated spacing of the remaining dentition
- Retained and infra-occluded LLE
- LL4 impacted against the LLE

How would you describe the condition?

Selective tooth agenesis or hypodontia.

What is hypodontia?

Hypodontia refers to agenesis of one to six teeth, excluding the third molars; whilst oligodontia refers to agenesis of more than six teeth, excluding the third molars.

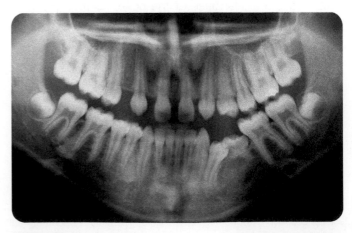

Figure 11.4

In Caucasians, what percentage of the population would be expected to have a congenitally absent maxillary lateral incisor?

Around 2%.

What is the cause of selective tooth agenesis?

Selective tooth agenesis is primarily a genetic condition, caused by gene mutation. In the majority of cases it is non-syndromic and occurs in isolation, with no other anomalies being seen in the individual.

In a minority of cases, selective tooth agenesis can be seen in association with other anomalies in a syndromic condition.

How can tooth agenesis be inherited within families?

All modes of inheritance have been described in association with tooth agenesis, including autosomal dominant and autosomal recessive Mendelian inheritance. Cases can also be sporadic, arising in families with no previous history.

Name any genes known to be mutated in cases of non-syndromic tooth agenesis

To date, relatively few human genes have been identified in cases of non-syndromic tooth agenesis. Examples include:
- *MSX1*: Encodes a transcription factor
- *PAX9*: Encodes a transcription factor
- *AXIN2*: Encodes a protein involved in stabilizing components of the Wnt signalling pathway
- *WNT10A*: Encodes a signalling protein
- *LTBP3*: Encodes a TGF-beta binding protein
- *EDA*: Encodes a signalling protein
- *EDARADD*: Encodes an intra-cellular adapter protein.

This child attended complaining of difficulty in eating. What are the main features of their dental appearance (Figure 11.5)?
- Congenital tooth absence
- Microdont, poorly-formed conical teeth
- Dental spacing

What condition is this child most likely to be affected by?

Ectodermal dysplasia, a heterogenous group of conditions characterized primarily by:

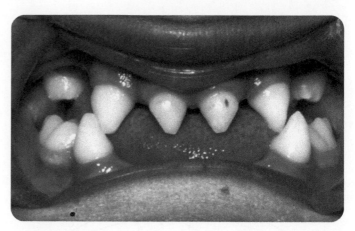

Figure 11.5

- Hypodontia (or often oligodontia) affecting both primary and permanent dentitions, with those teeth that do develop often being poorly formed
- Sparse and poorly formed hair
- Absence of sweat glands
- Nail anomalies.

How are these conditions inherited?

Sex-linked autosomal recessive inheritance is the most common form, with only males being affected. A less common autosomal recessive form also exists, affecting males and females.

Why are the teeth, hair and sweat glands all affected?

All of these organs develop in the embryo via very specific molecular interactions between their constituent epithelial and mesenchymal tissues. The disrupted molecular EDA signalling pathway in individuals affected by ectodermal dysplasia is important in the development of teeth, hair and sweat glands. Due to the common developmental mechanisms, all may be affected, giving rise to the syndrome.

Genetics

What is the mode of inheritance of the genetic disorder depicted in Figure 11.6?

This is autosomal dominant inheritance.

What are the implications of this mode of inheritance?

An affected individual possessing only one copy of a mutant allele will demonstrate the associated disorder.

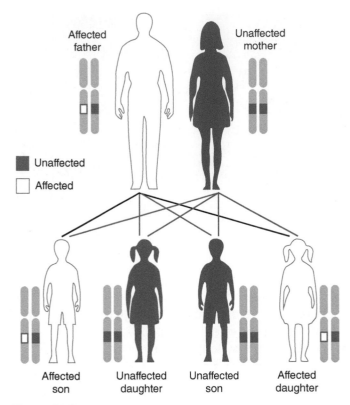

Figure 11.6

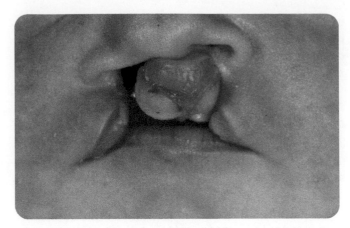

Figure 11.7

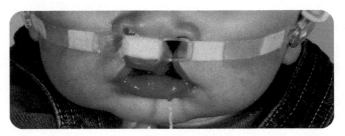

Figure 11.8

In contrast, a recessive disorder requires that an individual has two copies of a mutant allele to develop the disorder.

What are the chances of this father passing on the disorder to his offspring?

50:50.

How would the ratio of affected children change in this family if the mother was carrying one copy of the mutant allele?

Three-quarters of the offspring would have the disorder.

What is meant by the term sex-linked dominant?

Sex-linked dominant means that a single abnormal gene on the X chromosome can cause the disease. For boys, this can have serious consequences because they only have one X chromosome, meaning that they only inherit a single copy of the mutated dominant gene.

Facial Clefting

This child is 2 months old and has been born with a cleft defect that affects their face. They are otherwise quite fit and well (Figure 11.7).

What is the likely diagnosis for this condition?

This child has been born with a bilateral cleft of the lip and palate. As the child is otherwise fit and well, it is likely to be an isolated or non-syndromic form.

How common is this condition amongst Caucasian children born in the UK?

Cleft lip with or without cleft palate is seen in around 1 in 1000 live births in the UK. Males are more commonly affected than females (2:1). The non-syndromic form of this condition is responsible for around 30% of cases.

What is the normal timing of surgical repair for this defect?

The lip is usually repaired at around 3 months of age, whilst the palatal repair is usually carried out at around 9 months.

What treatment is being carried out in Figure 11.8?

The child is undergoing a period of pre-surgical orthopaedics. The appliance is worn prior to surgical repair of the lip and is designed to align the pre-maxillary segment. This alignment is aimed at facilitating the surgical repair by approximating the tissue segments and reducing the size of the tissue deficit. The effectiveness of this form of therapy has been contested, although prospective research in this area has been confined to unilateral defects.

What is the aetiological basis underlying non-syndromic cleft lip and palate? What factors can contribute to this condition?

The non-syndromic form of cleft lip and palate represents a complex multi-factorial condition. It is caused by the combined effects of gene mutation and environmental influences, exceeding a threshold of influence at a crucial stage and perturbing embryonic facial development.

A number of genes have been identified that when mutated can predispose to non-syndromic facial clefting. These encode a variety of different proteins and include members of the fibroblast growth factor (FGF) signalling pathway, transcription factors such as MSX1 and MSX2, and those encoding other molecules, including PVRL1 and IRF6. A key finding in recent years is that only a relatively small number of genes are likely to contribute to the non-syndromic form of this condition and that many of these genes are also implicated in syndromes. Environmental factors that can predispose to non-syndromic cleft lip and palate include maternal smoking or alcohol ingestion.

This child presented with a left-sided unilateral cleft lip and palate (UCLP) (Figure 11.9). List the salient features of the occlusion

- Mixed dentition
- Congenital absence of the UL2
- Class II division 2 incisor relationship
- Increased and complete overbite
- Unerupted maxillary canines
- Rotated UL1

What dental features are often seen in cases of cleft lip and palate?

- Hypodontia
- Supernumerary teeth

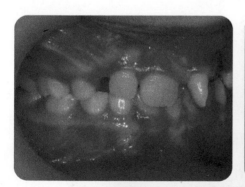 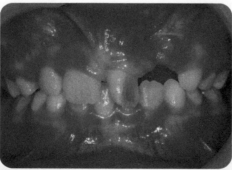 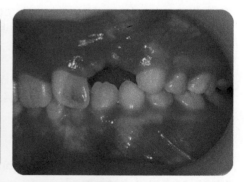

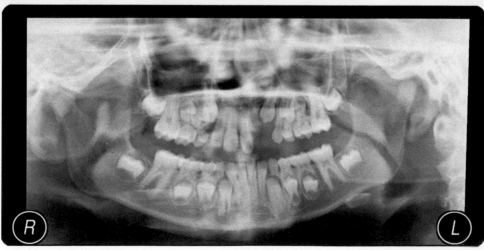

Figure 11.9

- Malformed and rotated teeth
- Ectopic eruption of maxillary first molars and canines
- Anomalies are more common in bilateral cases

Recent studies have demonstrated missing primary and permanent lateral incisors in 8% and 28% of UCLP subjects, respectively. The corresponding values in bilateral cleft lip and palate (BLCP) subjects are 17% and 60% (Lai *et al.*, 2009; Camporesi *et al.*, 2010). Congenital absence of second premolars occurs in 5% of UCLP and 9% of BCLP cases. Rotation of central incisors on the cleft side has been demonstrated in 78% of UCLP cases; this is also more common in bilateral cases. Delayed dental development on the cleft side and mesial displacement of maxillary canines are also common.

This child was born with a left-sided unilateral cleft lip and palate (Figure 11.10). At the age of 11 they underwent an alveolar bone graft. Which teeth are absent clinically in the maxillary arch?

The UL2, UL4, UL5 and UR5 are absent.

What is alveolar bone grafting?

Alveolar bone grafting is the placement of cancellous bone harvested from the axial skeleton into the maxillary alveolar defect caused by the presence of a cleft.

When is this procedure normally carried out?

Alveolar bone grafting is usually carried out around the age of 8 to 10 years, prior to eruption of the permanent canine teeth.

What is the role of the orthodontist prior to alveolar bone grafting?

The orthodontist is often required to expand the maxillary arch prior to alveolar bone grafting, usually with a fixed expander such as a tri- or quad-helix. This expansion maximizes the size of the bony defect, improves the maxillary arch form and creates access for the surgeon to place the graft during surgery.

What are the main advantages of alveolar bone grafting?

The main advantage of placing cancellous bone into the cleft defect is that it allows the permanent canine tooth to erupt. It also facilitates tooth movement in the upper labial segment, meaning space closure can be achieved if the lateral incisor is missing. If space opening is planned to replace a missing lateral incisor, grafting will enhance bone volume, facilitating implant replacement. Other advantages include the provision of good support for the pre-maxillary segment and nasal base.

This adult was referred by his general dental practitioner with concerns in relation to the tissue defect present in the roof of his mouth (Figure 11.11). He is otherwise fit and well with no relevant medical history. What is this condition?

This is isolated cleft palate, which in this case has remained unrepaired.

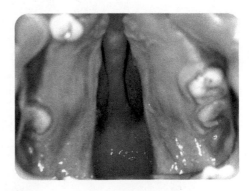

Figure 11.11

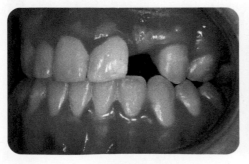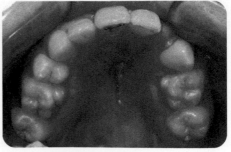

Figure 11.10

How common is this condition amongst Caucasian children born in the UK?

Cleft palate is seen in around 1 in 2000 live births in the UK. Females are more commonly affected than males (4:1). The non-syndromic form of this condition is responsible for around 50% of cases.

What other features may be seen in this patient?

The presence of an unrepaired cleft involving the primary and secondary palate in an adult will mean that there will be some difficulty with eating, particularly with food entering the nasal cavity during mastication. There may also be a significant speech defect due to the communication between nasal and oral cavities. However, facial growth is likely to have occurred relatively normally because the absence of early surgery will mean that no scar tissue will be present. It is less likely that this person will have any significant maxillary retrusion.

What are the oro-facial features seen in this neonate (Figure 11.12) and what is the likely diagnosis?

This child has a bilateral cleft of the lip and palate, and there are two large pits affecting the lower lip. This child has van der Woude syndrome.

What are the predominant features of this condition?

Van der Woude syndrome, which is the most common clefting syndrome seen in humans, is characterized primarily by lower lip pitting and cleft lip and/or cleft palate. Children with this condition also have an increased likelihood of hypodontia and may also have webbing of the soft tissues.

What is the aetiological basis of this condition?

Van der Woude syndrome is a genetic condition with autosomal dominant inheritance and variable phenotypic expression. Most cases are caused by mutation in the *IRF6* gene, which is situated on chromosome 1q32–p41.

Cleidocranial Dysplasia

This young adult is undergoing fixed appliance orthodontic treatment. What features are evident on the dental panoramic radiograph (Figure 11.13)?

There are multiple unerupted permanent teeth, multiple supernumerary permanent teeth and two retained primary maxillary canines.

A number of teeth have been exposed and chains attached to them.

What is the likely diagnosis?

Cleidocranial dysplasia.

What are the main dental features associated with this condition?

- Retained deciduous teeth
- Multiple supernumerary teeth
- Failure of eruption in the permanent dentition

How is the skeleton affected?

Cleidocranial dysplasia is characterized by defective bone formation, particularly affecting the clavicles and skull. The clavicles can be hypoplastic or absent, allowing shoulder approximation. The skull can have

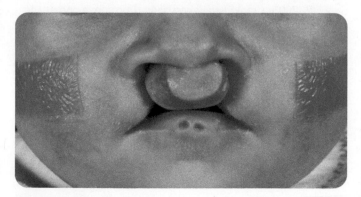

Figure 11.12

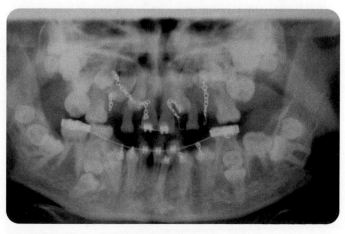

Figure 11.13

open sutures, multiple small wormian bones and delayed closure of the fontanelles. The axial skeleton can also be affected, with individuals having shortened limbs.

How do these problems manifest in the young adult?

The dental phenotype is very characteristic and often means that affected individuals have very limited permanent tooth eruption. The retained primary teeth have often deteriorated quite considerably by the mid-teenage years, with impaired aesthetics and function of the dentition. Historically, impaired eruption of the permanent dentition resulted in affected individuals undergoing widespread extractions and the provision of dentures. However, modern management attempts to accommodate as many permanent teeth in the dental arches as possible.

What is the role of the orthodontist in the management of cleidocranial dysostosis?

Accommodating the permanent dentition can be very difficult in these cases. Supernumerary teeth often have to be extracted, permanent teeth exposed and orthodontic traction applied. Although this can be successful, the whole process is often time-consuming. In addition, with limited numbers of erupted permanent teeth present within the dental arches and multiple teeth requiring traction, provision of sufficient anchorage can be problematic.

What is the Jerusalem approach to managing the developing occlusion in cases of cleidocranial dysplasia?

- At a dental age of 7–10 years (usually a chronological age of around 10–12 in these patients): All primary teeth and supernumerary teeth are extracted, closed exposure and bonding of the permanent incisor teeth is performed, and orthodontic traction is instigated, facilitated by the placement of heavy lingual and labial arches.
- At a dental age of 10–11 years (chronological age 13+): Closed exposure of the permanent teeth is carried out in the premolar and canine regions, followed by orthodontic traction to establish the permanent dentition.

Are there any alternative strategies?

The Belfast–Hamburg approach suggests extraction of all primary and supernumerary teeth, and open surgical exposure of the permanent teeth, all carried out as one procedure. This is followed by direct orthodontic traction.

The Toronto–Melbourne approach involves a staged strategy. Primary incisor teeth are extracted around 6 years of age, followed by primary canines and molars at 9–10 years. Supernumerary tooth removal and wide surgical exposure takes place separately, encouraging eruption of the permanent dentition.

References

Camporesi M, Baccetti T, Marinelli A, Defraia E, Franchi L (2010) Maxillary dental anomalies in children with cleft lip and palate: a controlled study. *Int J Paediatr Dent* 20:442–450.

Lai MC, King NM, Wong HM (2009) Abnormalities of maxillary anterior teeth in Chinese children with cleft lip and palate. *Cleft Palate Craniofac J* 46:58–64.

Further Reading

Becker A (2007) *The Orthodontic Treatment of Impacted Teeth*, 2nd edn. London: Informa Healthcare.

Cobourne MT, DiBiase AT (2010) *A Handbook of Orthodontics*. St Louis: Mosby Elsevier.

Cobourne MT (2004) The complex genetics of cleft lip and palate. *Eur J Orthod* 26:7–216.

Cobourne MT (2007) Familial human hypodontia – is it all in the genes? *Br Dent J* 203:203–208.

Jiang R, Bush JO, Lidral AC (2006) Development of the upper lip: Morphogenetic and molecular mechanisms. *Dev Dyn* 235:1152–1166.

Meikle MC (2002) *Craniofacial Development, Growth and Evolution*. Norfolk: Bateson.

Larsen WJ (1998) *Essentials of Human Embryology*. Edinburgh: Churchill Livingstone.

Rice DP (2005) Craniofacial anomalies: from development to molecular pathogenesis. *Curr Mol Med* 5:699–722.

Tucker AS, Sharpe P (2004) The cutting edge of mammalian development; how the embryo makes teeth. *Nat Rev Genet* 5:499–508.

Index

Clinical Cases in Orthodontics, First Edition. Martyn T. Cobourne, Padhraig S. Fleming, Andrew T. DiBiase, and Sofia Ahmad.
© 2012 Martyn T. Cobourne, Padhraig S. Fleming, Andrew T. DiBiase, and Sofia Ahmad. Published 2012 by Blackwell Publishing Ltd.